LABOR AND DELIVERY NURSING

A Guide to Evidence-Based Practice

About the Authors

Michelle L. Murray, PhD, RNC-OB, is an international educator, author, and expert in obstetric nursing. She has taught nursing students and nurses in the United States, Canada, and Bahrain. Dr. Murray has spent the majority of her career as a labor and delivery nurse and as an obstetric nursing educator. She was appointed by the provost at the University of New Mexico as a clinical associate professor.

Dr. Murray's company, Learning Resources International, Inc. produces clinical and educational products and seminars for labor and delivery nurses and midwives. Since 1986, more than 50,000 obstetric care providers, including nurses, physicians, and midwives, have participated in Dr. Murray's classes and seminars. Her work has been published in journals such as *Birth: Issues in Perinatal Care; The American Journal of Maternal Child Nursing (MCN)*; the *Journal of Perinatology*; the *Journal of Nursing Care Quality*; and the *Journal of Obstetric, Gynecologic, and Neonatal Nursing (JOGNN)*. Dr. Murray was also a contributor to the Association of Women's Health, Obstetric, and Neonatal Nursing (AWHONN) publication, *Nursing Management of the Second Stage of Labor*. Her best-selling books include *Antepartal and Intrapartal Fetal Monitoring* (3rd ed.) and *Essentials of Fetal Monitoring* (3rd ed.). Her books and products are available at www.fetalmonitoring.com.

Dr. Murray has been an active member and officer of the Association of Women's Health, Obstetric, and Neonatal Nursing as well as the American Nurses Association's New Mexico Nurses Association. She is an award winner in education from AWHONN (formerly the Nurses Association of the American College of Obstetricians and Gynecologists), and from the nursing honor society, Sigma Theta Tau.

Gayle M. Huelsmann, BSN, RNC-OB, C-EFM, is certified in inpatient obstetrics and holds a certificate of added qualification in electronic fetal monitoring from the National Certification Corporation in Chicago, Illinois. She has been an antepartal nurse and a labor and delivery staff nurse for 28 years. In addition, she is a maternal air transport nurse with fixed wing and rotor wing aircraft. She is also an education resource nurse at Presbyterian Hospital in Albuquerque, New Mexico. Ms. Huelsmann is the co-author of *Essentials of Fetal Monitoring* (3rd ed.) and the monograph on *Uterine Hyperstimulation: Physiologic and Pharmacologic Causes with Results from a Survey of 1000 Nurses* with Dr. Michelle Murray. Ms. Huelsmann is an award winner of the PRIDE nurse award from Presbyterian Hospital. She was nominated by her peers for her exemplary contribution to patient care.

LABOR AND DELIVERY NURSING:

A Guide to Evidence-Based Practice

MICHELLE L. MURRAY,
PhD, RNC-OB

and

GAYLE M. HUELSMANN,
BSN, RNC-OB, C-EFM

SPRINGER PUBLISHING COMPANY
New York

Springer Publishing Company, LLC
11 West 42nd Street
New York, NY 10036
www.springerpub.com

Ebook ISBN: 978-0-8261-1092-3

Acquisitions Editor: Allan Graubard
Illustrations: Ellena C. Tapia and Gary Hamrick
Production Editor: Jean Hurkin-Torres
Cover design: Steven Pisano
Composition: International Graphic Services
09 10 11 12 13 / 5 4 3 2 1

ISBN: 978-0-8261-1803-5

Library of Congress Cataloging-in-Publication Data

Murray, Michelle (Michelle L.)
    Labor and delivery nursing : a guide to evidence-based practice / by Michelle L. Murray and Gayle M. Huelsmann.
       p. ; cm.
    Includes bibliographical references and index.
    ISBN 978-0-8261-1803-5
    1. Maternity nursing. 2. Evidence-based nursing.   I. Huelsmann, Gayle.   II. Title.
    [DNLM: 1. Obstetrical Nursing—methods. 2. Delivery, Obstetric—nursing. 3. Evidence-Based Medicine. 4. Labor, Obstetric. WY 157 M983L 2009]
    RG951.M867 2009
    618.2'0231—dc22   2008047324

Printed in the United States of America by Bang Printing

DISCLAIMER

This book is not intended to replace your hospital's policies, procedures, guidelines, or protocols. It is not intended to dictate a standard of care. We recommend that the reader always consult current research and specific institutional policies before performing any clinical procedure. This book is intended for use during the process of orientation of nurses in the labor and delivery setting, and to bring experienced nurses up to date with regard to current practice and research findings. It can also be used as a reference or as a study guide by nurses preparing to take a certification examination in the field of inpatient obstetrics or labor and delivery.

This book does not include directions for equipment use or specific tests. These must be learned in the hospital setting, preferably with a mastery-based skills checklist. In addition, care should be individualized to the patient.

True/false questions appear at the end of each chapter as a complement to the learning process. Each chapter contains the information necessary to answer the questions.

The content of this book was based on the best available research at the time it was written. Some studies may appear dated and may have been the only study on the subject that was readily available at the time of this publication. Every attempt was made to provide current information that is evidence-based.

Neither the author nor the publisher shall be liable for any special, consequential, or exemplary damages resulting, in whole or in part, from the readers' use of, or reliance on, the information contained in this book. The publisher has no responsibility for the persistence or accuracy of URLs for any external or third-party Internet Web sites referred to in this publication and does not guarantee that any content on such Web sites is, or will remain, accurate or appropriate.

Knowledge comes from learning.
Wisdom comes from experience.

—Anonymous

Contents

Acknowledgments

We were helped in writing this book by many dedicated and skilled labor and delivery nurses who reviewed the manuscript and made suggestions for improvement. They are listed below in alphabetical order:

Susan Mocsny Baker, RNC
Staff Nurse
University of Massachusetts Memorial Medical Center
Worcester, Massachusetts

Darcie Beckwith, RNC, MSN
Clinical Practice Specialist
The Birthing Inn
Inova Loudoun Hospital
Leesburg, Virginia

Lynne Brengman, RN, BSN, MBA
Education Department
PeaceHealth – St. Joseph Hospital
Bellingham, Washington

Cindy Curtis, RNC, IBCLC, CCE
Staff Nurse and Director of the Lactation Center
Culpeper Regional Hospital
Family Birth Center
Culpeper, Virginia

Garla DeWall, RNC
Staff Nurse, Family Birthing Center
Presbyterian Hospital
Albuquerque, New Mexico

Becky Dunham, RNC
Staff Nurse, Labor and Delivery
Dublin Methodist Hospital
Dublin, Ohio

Donna McAfee Frye, RN, MN
Clinical Director
Women's and Children's Clinical Services
Nashville, Tennessee

Aurora Gumamit, RN, MSN, CNS
Charge Nurse, Labor and Delivery
Corona Regional Medical Center
Corona, California

Julie Holden, RN, BSN, MA
Nurse Manager
Beverly Hospital
Beverly, Massachusetts

Theresa Hyland, RNC
Yale New Haven Hospital
New Haven, Connecticut

Wanda Jeavons, RNC, MSN, PNNP
Perinatal Outreach Coordinator
Andrews Women's Hospital
Baylor All Saints Medical Center
Fort Worth, Texas

Suzanne Ketchem, MSN, RNC, CNS
Director of Women's and Children's Services
Medical Center of Aurora
Aurora, Colorado

Reta M. King, BSN, RNC
Staff Nurse, Labor and Delivery
University of New Mexico Medical Center
Albuquerque, New Mexico

Nanci Koperski, RNC, LNCC, MBA, MHSA
Legal Nurse Consultant
Omaha, Nebraska

Debra Mills, RN, BSN, MSN, CNS
Clinical Nurse Specialist, Family Birth Center
Methodist Hospital
Sacramento, California

Angela Murphy, RNC
Charge Nurse, Family Birthing Center
Presbyterian Hospital
Albuquerque, New Mexico

Nancy Powell, RNC, MSN, CNM
Clinical Educator
Shore Memorial Hospital
Somers Point, New Jersey

Michelle Rupard, MSN, RNC, FNP, LNCC
Assistant Professor, College of Nursing
The University of North Carolina at Pembroke
Laurinburg, North Carolina

Wendy Sinanan, RN
Staff Nurse, Labor and Delivery
Mt. Sinai Hospital
Toronto, Ontario, Canada

Ann Weed, RNC, MSN, CNS
Clinical Nurse Specialist
Mary Washington Hospital
Fredericksburg, Virginia

Diana Wigham, RNC, MSN
Staff Nurse, Labor and Delivery
Saint Francis Medical Center
Hartford, Connecticut

Preface

The interests of the patient are the only interests to be considered.

— *William Mayo*

The family is constant, but service systems and personnel within those systems fluctuate (Petersen, Cohen, & Parsons, 2004). Nurses are part of the service system that provides family-centered care. To be an effective care provider, nurses must develop confidence and competence. They need an open mind, an accepting attitude, hands-on skills, and a broad and deep understanding of the research related to pregnancy, labor, and birth. Ideally, they should work in a hospital that uses the latest research findings in patient care. That is rare, however (Scott-Findlay, 2007). The best care will be evidence-based. Therefore, the goal of this book is to provide you with the information to develop an evidence-based practice of labor and delivery nursing. Labor and delivery nursing requires critical thinking, constant caring, listening to your inner voice, anticipation of the needs of many, teamwork, communication, and collaboration (see Exhibit P.1).

Proper surveillance and care of the fetus and mother during labor and delivery depends on comprehensive data acquisition, attention to detail, adequate knowledge to properly understand and interpret the meaning of data, verbal and nonverbal cues, and teamwork. This book was created with these elements in mind. Figure P.1 illustrates the nursing process from admission to delivery. If possible, review the patient's prenatal record before she arrives.

Labor and delivery nurses provide patient-centered care that is "high tech" and "high touch" in settings such as a family birthing center. "High-touch" care can be thought of as "labor support," empathy, and use of touch. Labor support may play a part in shortening a woman's labor, decreasing her use of analgesia and anesthesia, labor augmentation, possibly decreasing the need for an operative vaginal delivery or a cesarean delivery, and increasing satisfaction with the birthing experience. Labor and delivery nursing or intrapartal nursing is part of the culture of obstetrics and this culture has its own myths, taboos, artifacts, and traditions.

Labor and delivery nurses are masters of anticipation, supporters of natural childbirth, and monitors of safety practices, because they are the first line of defense in preventing injury. They must understand maternal and fetal physiology, know the purpose and physiologic impact of their actions, and be able to evaluate their patients' responses to those actions. In addition, effective intrapartal nurses are fearless when advocating for their patients.

Modern obstetrics requires both high-touch and high-tech skills. Nurses need the knowledge and skills to properly use different types of machines and equipment. For example, the high-tech aspect of labor and delivery includes tests to confirm the rupture of membranes; the use of the electronic fetal monitor and its components (such as a spiral electrode); insertion of an intravenous catheter and administration of intravenous fluids, blood, or blood products; use of suction and oxygen equipment; and procedures such as amnioinfusion. This book is not intended to be a procedure or equipment manual, nor was it designed to replace hands-on bedside training. Instead, it is our hope that the information gained from reading this book will help labor and delivery nurses make wise decisions in their choices of interventions, in the creation of patient-centered plans of care, and in their communications with other members of the obstetrics team.

For those beginning their career as a labor and delivery nurse, Ray Spooner RN, BSN, an experienced labor and delivery nurse, has suggested, "Be yourself. Especially, do not feign

---

Exhibit P.1: Some characteristics of a critical thinker.

1. States the question or concern clearly
2. Creates order in complex situations
3. Diligently seeks relevant information
4. Focuses on the concern at hand
5. Persists until results are obtained in spite of difficulties
6. Is inquisitive, well-informed, open-minded, and flexible
7. Acknowledges personal biases
8. Makes prudent judgments
9. Is willing to reconsider
10. Is clear regarding the issues

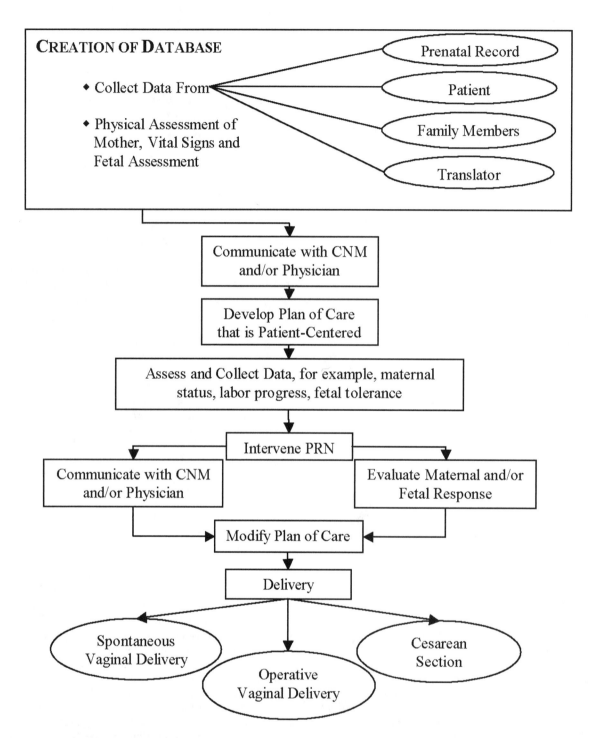

Figure P.1: The nursing process from admission until delivery. Documentation should reflect each step of this process.

knowledge. It is better to ask a stupid question than to make a stupid mistake" (Spooner, 1995).

In addition to this book, we hope nurses becoming oriented to the practice of labor and delivery nursing will read the philosophy, policies, procedures, and protocols of their facility. We encourage new nurses to ask for guidance, information, and demonstrations of procedures when they need help. We also encourage open communication with patients and other health care providers. Often the patients are the only ones who have the answers to your questions.

Benjamin Franklin once said, "The best investment is in the tools of one's own trade." Intrapartal nurses need to own equipment that aids them in their patient care (see Exhibit P.2). It is helpful to have a fetoscope in your locker, especially for those times when a patient refuses the fetal monitor or there is a power failure. As your career develops, you may find other tools that enhance your ability to meet your patient's needs.

Our combined nursing experience totals more than 50 years. The majority of our clinical time has been spent in labor and delivery settings. We hope that our experience and education

Exhibit P.2: Some "tools" of the labor and delivery nurse.

1. Stethoscope
2. Reflex hammer
3. 2 hemostats
4. Bandage scissors
5. Pen light
6. Gestational wheel
7. Measuring tape

as intrapartal nurses and educators will be transmitted to you in this book and that it will provide you with the information you need to make informed decisions and provide evidence-based care.

Michelle L. Murray, PhD, RNC-OB
Gayle M. Huelsmann, BSN, RNC-OB, C-EFM

References

Petersen, M. F., Cohen, J., & Parsons, V. (2004). Family-centered care: Do we practice what we preach? *Journal of Obstetric, Gynecologic, and Neonatal Nursing, 33*(4), 421–427.

Scott-Findlay, S. (2007). Fostering evidence-based practice. *Nursing for Women's Health, 11*(3), 250–252.

Spooner, R. (1995). Gentle reminder, *American Journal of Maternal Child/Nursing, 20,* 166.

Communication, Advocacy, and the Chain of Command

Words create our world. We want to create constructive discussions.

—Anna von Dielingen

ORGANIZATIONAL CULTURE

Health care organizations have a culture that includes norms, attitudes, values, assumptions, customs, and behaviors (Chervenak & McCullough, 2005; Lefton, 2007; Seren & Baykal, 2007). A healthy organization has a culture that is committed to honest business practices and is focused on the needs of patients, community, and society (Chervenak & McCollough, 2005). Great leaders create an environment that enables the best solutions and the best decisions (Henrikson, 2007). In a healthy organization, communication should occur among the patient, her partner, her friends and visitors, and all members of the health care team (Simkin & Ancheta, 2005).

Health care organizations may also be collaborative or competitive. In a collaborative organization, there is teamwork and team management to reach a desired goal. In a competitive organization, achievement, a sense of superiority, excellence, and possessing technology that is better than other organizations will be the goals. If the organization has a power culture, authority will be the center of attention, and tasks will be assigned by a manager.

Cynical organizations have leaders who are not supportive and who create a hostile work environment. Communication in that type of organization can be difficult or even intimidating. An unresponsive culture will have leaders with a dictatorial, top-down, threatening, and punishing style of behavior.

This type of leadership creates communication barriers. A submissive culture will be unresponsive, will have minimal expectations and communication, and will provide minimal feedback. A submissive, but responsive, culture will have people who always agree with you, who talk a lot but do not listen, who gloss over performance issues, who only provide positive feedback, and who seek harmony (Lefton, 2007). It is important that you determine the type of organization and culture within which you work.

THE CARE MODEL IN LABOR AND DELIVERY

Within the dominant health care organization culture there are subcultures. For example, the culture in postpartum care may be different from the culture in the nursery or in labor and delivery. The norms, attitudes, values, assumptions, customs, and behaviors within the subculture of labor and delivery affect the quality and quantity of communicaton (Tucker et al., 2006). Communication is also influenced by the design of the care model. The four types of intrapartal services include the nurse-managed labor model, the academic/teaching model, the nurse-to-attending physician communication-on-site model, and the nurse-to-nurse midwife communication-on-site model (Simpson, 2005). For example, if you are the primary patient care provider and the midwife or physician is not in the building, you work within a nurse-managed labor model. In that case you are responsible for recognizing problems, evaluating labor progress, providing hands-on care, and informing other team members when they are needed.

In the nurse-to-nurse midwife or physician communication-on-site model, it should be easy to communicate with the provider. However, even if the provider is in the hospital, he or she may be distracted by the needs of other patients. Since the labor nurse, midwife, and physician are part of one collaborative team, be sure to keep them up to date so that they do not miss an opportunity to make clinical decisions that promote patient safety. If you need them to come to the bedside, ask them to do so.

> **Documentation example**: Spontaneous rupture of membranes, fluid clear, nonfoul, saturated 1/3 of linen protector. Variable decelerations noted. Certified Nurse Midwife (CNM) called on postpartum unit and informed of spontaneous rupture of membranes, clear fluid, variable decelerations. Requested CNM come to bedside immediately to evaluate patient. CNM stated she was on her way.

Perhaps you work with residents in an academic/teaching model setting. In this setting, the residents will assess the cervix and fetal station and insert internal monitors such as the spiral electrode or intrauterine pressure catheter. Nurse-to-resident communication may be hindered by the resident's need to control the decision-making process. However, that does not mean you should withhold your findings or concerns. If you feel the plan of care needs to change, you must speak up.

> **Communication clinical example**: You observe late decelerations and no accelerations, and the resident orders you to administer oxytocin. You change your patient's position to her right side, place a tight-fitting face mask with oxygen at 10 liters/minute on her face, adjust the ultrasound transducer and tocotransducer, and note the continuation of late decelerations. You also note her blood pressure is normal. You say, "I'd like to wait at least 15 minutes to see if the baby's heart rate improves." The resident dons a sterile glove, rubs the fetal scalp, evokes an acceleration, and insists you administer the oxytocin immediately. You then say, "There have been no spontaneous accelerations for the last hour, variability is absent or minimal, and the late decelerations continue to persist in spite of the intrauterine resuscitation actions." You then call your team leader or charge nurse to the room using the patient call light. At that point, if the resident continues to insist on the administration of oxytocin, the charge nurse and the resident should leave the room to continue the discussion about the plan of care.

PROVIDER ROLES AND EXPECTATIONS

In order to know whom to call or with whom to share information, you need to know the roles and responsibilities of the other health care providers. Your hospital should have policies and procedures that define the maternal/child services for family practitioners, residents, obstetricians, and the anesthesia providers. For example, family practitioners may be credentialed to evaluate the condition of the mother and infant, order medications, deliver the infant when there is a cephalic presentation (or by using low forceps or a vacuum extractor), and resuscitate the infant. They may be credentialed to repair the episiotomy, but must consult with the obstetrician for certain conditions. An obstetrical consult may be required for some procedures. An obstetrician may need to be consulted for abnormal bleeding, a retained placenta, preeclampsia, prolonged labor, multiple gestation, induction of labor, polyhydramnios, before any obstetrical operation or breech delivery, for medical or surgical complications, for preterm labor and tocolysis, or for a trial of labor after a cesarean section.

Obstetricians perform duties similar to family physicians, but they also usually have privileges for midforceps and cesarean sections. Anesthesia providers evaluate the condition of the mother prior to the administration of an anesthetic agent, place and remove indwelling epidural catheters, inject medication into the epidural catheter, initiate continuous infusions administered through the epidural catheter, and remain immediately available during the induction of epidural anesthesia. They rarely know how to interpret the fetal heart rate pattern or uterine activity pattern, and you should not expect them to do so. Therefore, it is your responsibility to be sure the maternal and fetal conditions are stable prior to the administration of an anesthetic. If the mother or fetus is unstable, speak to the obstetric care provider prior to the administration of analgesia or anesthesia.

Physicians and/or certified nurse midwives may create the initial plan of care with informed consent of the patient. The nurse is responsible for coordinating care, suggesting changes in the plan of care, and knowing who else is on the team taking care of the patient. An error can be committed if the wrong plan is followed or there is a failure to complete a planned action (Institute of Medicine, 1999). Therefore, you must know the plan of care and communicate with other health care team members often during your shift to accomplish that plan of care or to change the plan of care. As the patient's condition changes, the plan of care must also change.

CHARACTERISTICS OF COMMUNICATORS

Within the subculture of labor and delivery are the people with whom you may need to communicate. They may be difficult to communicate with if they are know-it-alls, passives, dictators, "yes" people, "no" people, or gripers (see Exhibit 1.1).

NURSE–PATIENT COMMUNICATION

Patients may also take the role of know-it-all, passive, dictator, griper, or someone who always agrees with you or quickly disagrees with you. On the other hand, they may be open,

Communication, Advocacy, and the Chain of Command

Exhibit 1.1: Types of communicators.

Personality Type	Characteristics and Suggestions for Communication
Know-it-alls	Arrogant, usually have a strong opinion on every issue. When they're wrong, they get defensive. Validate their ideas. Tell them you see their point of view (if you can), then ask for their help in solving a problem.
Passives	Never offer ideas and never let you know where they stand. For example, they may perform a vaginal examination and then walk out of the room and not tell you their findings. Follow them out of the room. Establish eye contact. Ask them to tell you their findings.
Dictators	Bully and intimidate. They're constantly demanding and brutally critical. Don't try to be their friend. Just be specific in what you would like them to do and ask them if they can help you. If they refuse, ask your charge nurse or nursing supervisor to intervene or help you.
"Yes" People	Agree to cover your patient while you are on lunch break and then never see your patient. When you return from your break and see they have not charted their observations, ask them to do so. If they do not comply, notify your charge nurse or supervisor of their failure to see your patient. Document in the record the time you expected them to see your patient and their name.
"No" People	Quickly point out why something won't work and are inflexible. Avoid these people unless you have to interact with them. Keep your communications brief and clear.
Gripers	All they do is complain. See above.

honest, and genuinely interested in what you have to say. An assessment of their interaction with other family members will help you recognize their communication style and characteristics. Communication with patients, family members, and other health care providers is essential to help you prevent adverse events (JCAHO, 2000, 2004). Communication also creates relationships. Therefore, you will need to find a way to relate to your patient and her family and friends to maximize the effectiveness of your communications. By developing your emotional intelligence, you should be able to recognize your feelings and the feelings of others, and then regulate your personal feelings and expressions in response to clinical situations (Stichler, 2006).

Your first nurse–patient interaction is critical in establishing a trusting relationship with your patient and her family and friends. Introduce yourself by stating your name and licensure, and state that you will be her nurse for the next specified number of hours. When your patient speaks to you, face her, listen closely, and paraphrase what you hear. Make eye contact when it is culturally accepted, do not interrupt her, and do not multitask. It is extremely rude to look at a chart or a computer screen instead of your patient.

> **Communication example**: "Hi, Ms. Jones. I'm Michelle and I'll be your nurse today. I'm here for the next 12 hours. I understand from Gayle, your night nurse, that you are 4-cm dilated, that your plan is to have intravenous medication later in the labor, and that your husband wants to cut the cord after the birth. Is that correct? Good. It looks like you are contracting every 3 minutes and they feel strong to me. Your baby looks good. I see there are accelerations in the heart rate. Is there anything you need right now?"

Create an environment that is conducive to open communication and low stress to enhance a feeling of trust. You can enhance the environment by limiting the number of visitors, and other noise and distractions (Stichler, 2007a). Sit at eye level with your patient when you communicate. Pick your words wisely, as words might upset patients and families. For example, "failure to progress" or "noncompliant cervix" are demeaning and disparaging (Katz, 2005).

You should use open-ended questions to assess your patient's knowledge of the labor and delivery process. For example, you might say, "What questions do you have about what is going to happen today?" Some patients believe they have no questions because they have been watching birthing programs on television. They will tell you they know everything they need to know about their "epidermal." In spite of their misconceptions, it is important for you to discover their knowledge deficits and provide information during teachable moments. For example, prior to rupture of the membranes, you might want to mention that the sac around the baby has no nerves. One patient was terrified because she heard the nurse say, "The doctor will be rupturing your brains." Another patient reported she had condominiums "down there." She really had condylomata (warts). Try not to laugh. Discover the source of your patient's anxiety and fear. Perhaps her sister, cousin, or mother had a traumatic birth experience and she fears the same thing will happen to her. You will need to reassure her that you are there for her support and safety and will be in frequently during her labor. Use humor sparingly and appropriately. Listen carefully to her complaints and concerns because you may be the first person she tells or the first person who recognizes there is a problem.

To facilitate open communication, acknowledge the partner and/or labor coach and any family members present in the room. Ask them their names and recognize their supporting roles. Be sure the primary coach and the father of the baby eat and rest if there is a long labor ahead. The father-to-be may wish to play an active role during the labor process or no role at all. Assess their needs and desires as well as your patient's needs and desires. Satisfaction with the support of their partner results in less patient stress, less depression, and less anxiety for as long as three months after delivery (McVeigh, 1997).

Support family-centered care, if that is desired, by keeping the baby in the birthing room after delivery. Support skin-to-skin contact between the mother and her baby. If she chooses to breastfeed, you should support breastfeeding within the first hour of the baby's life (Phillips, 2003). Communicate with the patient to learn her expectations for labor and birth.

If there is a written birth plan, read it and acknowledge its contents. Sometimes desires or plans are more like wishes which you may not be able to fulfill. You will need courage to do the right thing for your patient's safety and health, even when it seems undesired or unpopular or goes against her birth plan or wishes.

Clinical example: A nulliparous woman in labor was four feet six inches tall. At about 5-centimeters dilation, her membranes spontaneously ruptured. There was dark green, particulate meconium in the amniotic fluid. Variable decelerations appeared on the tracing. The midwife found there was a face presentation. The physician was called into the room and decided that a cesarean section was necessary. When the patient was informed, she was sad because she had planned for a vaginal delivery. The nurse said, "I'm sorry but the baby didn't read the plan." The patient said, "Neither did my sister's baby." The nurse asked for clarification. The patient told her that her sister was also petite like her and had a baby with a face presentation. In this case, there was a good outcome for both the mother and her baby.

Nurses who communicate to discover and respond to patient needs prevent injuries (Kendig, 2006). To protect patients and prevent injury, communication should be purposeful and goal oriented. For example, there may be people in the room who are watching television and talking among themselves yet the nurse perceives the laboring woman needs a quiet room because she is preeclamptic, hyperreflexive, and hypertensive. In this case, the nurse would explain the patient's needs and ask the visitors to leave or limit their conversation. The hospital's visitor policy should provide the framework for information shared with the people in the room.

The American College of Obstetricians and Gynecologists (ACOG) believes that actively involving patients in their care will increase diagnostic accuracy, patient satisfaction, and adherence to therapy, thus resulting in improved health. They recommend that health care providers (a) speak slowly and use plain, nonmedical language; (b) limit the amount of information provided; (c) repeat information; (d) use teach-back or show-me techniques; (e) create an atmosphere in which patients can ask questions; and (f) provide written materials to reinforce oral explanations (ACOG, 2005). Naturally, if the patient does not speak English, a translator should be located. Record the name of the translator or translation service in the medical record.

ADVOCACY REQUIRES COMMUNICATION

Nurses, as well as other health care providers, are patient advocates who understand patient needs and expectations. Patient advocacy requires acceptance of other people as they are; support of their choices; the ability to help them explore their feelings, options, and possible consequences of their decisions; and the ability to speak and act on their behalf. To be an effective advocate, nurses must always err on the side of patient safety. Examples of nurse advocacy would be communication with the charge nurse when there are concerns about the current plan of care, discussing the possibility of a cesarean section with a physician, and calling the pediatrician to attend a delivery for which neonatal intubation is probable.

An effective advocate is vocal. An effective advocate does not remain silent when there is a risk of patient harm. For example, if there were two pop-offs of the vacuum extractor, the nurse may say, "Doctor, the operating room is ready. Would you like me to move the patient now?" Have confidence that your communication will make a difference in the care and outcomes for your patients. You may need to confront others when you are concerned, especially when decisions are made that are clearly wrong or when another health care provider is absent or incapacitated. For example, if the physician wishes to reapply the vacuum, thus exceeding the manufacturer's recommendations, you may say, "Doctor, please stop. The operating room is ready."

Advocacy requires empathy. There will be times when the patient or family members interfere with decisions that are in the best interest of the patient. For example, a husband may refuse to let his wife have a cesarean section because he is concerned it will mutilate her body. Empathy will be your secret weapon to defuse disruptive behavior. Try to understand these concerns and inform the physician. Disruptive behavior is personal conduct, whether verbal or physical, that affects or potentially may affect patient care negatively (Lazoritz & Carlson, 2008). You must be able to acknowledge the disrupter's point of view in such a way that you validate him or her, yet do the right thing for your patient.

Advocacy requires vigilance, and vigilance is the essence of caring. For example, if you note that the fetal heart rate pattern has evolved from a normal pattern to one with decelerations and a decrease in baseline variability with no accelerations, potentially hazardous acidemia can develop in as little as one hour (Parker & Ikeda, 2007). Your vigilance to note the change over the last 60 minutes should trigger your actions to increase fetal oxygenation and notify the physician or midwife of the changes in the fetal heart rate pattern. If the fetus needs oxygen and you do not act, the pattern may change into one with deeper decelerations or even bradycardia. Therefore, do not think, "Oh that's just a little deceleration" or "I'm reassured because I still have some variability." You should be thinking, "Wow, the fetus needs oxygen. I need to act now."

Advocacy requires the ability to make decisions that are patient centered. Decisions about patient care should be based on your knowledge of your patient's risk factors, current assessments, changes in the maternal or fetal condition following interventions, and input from the patient and her family and friends. You must be able to face problems head on and not delay decisions until it is too late. Do you know the current plan of care? If not, ask the midwife or physician, for example, "What is the plan of care for Mrs. Iminlabor?" Once you know the plan, decide if you accept the plan. Is it in the best interest of your patient and her unborn baby? If there is no clear plan of care, or if you cannot accept it, discuss your concerns with the charge nurse and midwife or physician. The plan of care must be patient centered and must prevent harm. If you believe a decision is needed to deliver by cesarean section or to expedite delivery with forceps or a vacuum extractor (an operative vaginal delivery), share your belief with the charge nurse or your supervisor first. If you do not have a charge nurse or supervisor, speak directly with the physician or midwife. It is far better to be proactive and to help the midwife or physician make a patient-centered decision now than to wait for him or her to arrive at the bedside later and make a decision at the last moment when the fetus is decompensating.

Staff nurse to charge nurse communication example: "I called you into the room because I have been seeing variable decelerations that are getting deeper and longer but the baby is still at 0 station with caput and molding. We have been pushing for 2 hours. She gained 50 pounds during this pregnancy and she is 5 feet tall. I'm concerned the baby is just not going to fit. Can you discuss the plan with the physician? He wants me to start an oxytocin infusion and I don't think that will help. I think she needs a cesarean section."

Advocacy requires support of a reasonable plan of care, anticipation of potential problems, and knowledge of what is normal and abnormal. You should know what the fetal heart rate was on admission. Is the current fetal heart rate baseline rising or falling? A rising baseline may be a fetal catecholamine (stress) response to hypoxia. Falling baselines are usually a fetal decompensation response. Both are abnormal. A generic nursing plan of care may include nursing diagnoses. Examples of nursing diagnoses are: anxiety; altered body temperature; ineffective breathing pattern; decreased cardiac output; ineffective coping; fatigue; fear; fluid volume deficit or excess; hyperstimulation; hyperthermia; high risk for infection; high

Exhibit 1.2: Elements of a generic nursing plan of care.		
1.	Problem:	Alteration in self-perception related to anxiety.
	Outcome:	Patient will understand procedures and processes and adapt without undue additional anxiety.
2.	Problem:	Alteration in comfort related to progress in labor and delivery.
	Outcome:	Patient will become comfortable.
3.	Problem:	Potential for infection related to rupture of membranes.
	Outcome:	Patient will be free of infection.
4.	Problem:	Alteration in maternal and/or fetal perfusion and oxygen delivery related to contractions and labor process.
	Outcome:	Patient will progress through labor and delivery without complications.
5.	Problem:	Alteration in self-perception related to expanded role.
	Outcome:	Patient will experience time to bond with her infant after delivery.
6.	Problem:	Potential for hemorrhage following delivery related to altered hemodynamics.
	Outcome:	Patient will recover without unusual blood loss.

risk for injury; knowledge deficit; impaired mobility; non-reassuring fetal heart rate pattern; altered nutrition; pain; post-trauma response; powerlessness; self-care deficit; impaired social interaction; urinary elimination, altered patterns; and, altered tissue integrity. Your hospital may have a list of nursing diagnoses. Nursing diagnoses have also been called the problem or potential problems (see Exhibit 1.2).

Advocacy requires a nurse to recognize, verbalize, and mobilize. In some cases, you have to mobilize the operating room crew to expedite delivery before fetal decompensation, neurologic injury, or death. However, this is a rare event. Examples of acute events where the fetus quickly decompensates, include a ruptured vasa previa when an amniotomy is performed, a uterine rupture, or an amniotic fluid embolism. In those cases, it will be crystal clear that delivery needs to be expedited. Good communication occurs when you inform the charge nurse of your actions. When cesarean sections are not performed on your labor and delivery unit, you will need to inform the operating room crew through your house supervisor that you need help to mobilize the operating room crew if the pattern continues or worsens. Ask the physician to come to the bedside. If there is fetal tachycardia, especially with decelerations or minimal or absent variability and no accelerations, the fetus is in jeopardy. Initiate intrauterine resuscitation measures. Communicate to mobilize resources. If you have no charge nurse, ask another nurse to prepare the operating room and mobilize the crew while you call the physician to come to the bedside. Call the anesthesia provider and the neonatal team so that they are on their way to the hospital. You will need to be proactive and request the presence of the obstetrician at the bedside any time you see tachycardia, bradycardia, or decelerations that last more than 30 seconds, especially if they are becoming deeper and longer.

NURSE-TO-NURSE REPORT

When you receive the report, you must know if the amniotic fluid was clear and now has meconium in it. You must know the time of the last acceleration. It should have occurred within the last 90 minutes, even if narcotics were administered. You must know how to interpret the tracing, and over time you will become more comfortable with its physiologic meaning.

You are the conduit through which information flows to the midwife and/or physician. It has been said that the nurse is the "eyes and ears" of the midwife and physician. You are the one who keeps the charge nurse informed of changes. You have the power to make a difference. Therefore, it is your duty to advocate for the physician's presence at the bedside when the parents have requested it. You have a duty to update him or her at reasonable intervals so that they stay abreast of the maternal and fetal condition throughout the labor process. The change of shift report should be comprehensive (see Exhibit 1.3). By the end of the report you should know events that happened during the last shift, changes in the mother's or baby's status, and the interdisciplinary plan of care. You will need to decide if the current plan of care is safe and reasonable for your patient. If not, request a change in the plan of care after you report your findings and share your concerns.

> **Communication example requesting a change in the plan of care**: "Dr. Imallears, may I speak with you a moment about the current plan of care. I just learned in report that your patient, Jane Doe, now has a fever. Her temperature is 100.8 degrees. In addition, her pulse is 116 beats per minute. She's been dilated 5 centimeters for the last 3 hours. There's caput at 0 station. There are variable decelerations that are getting deeper. I just discontinued the Pitocin infusion that was at 30 mU/minute. Would you please come and evaluate her and let me know if you'd like to make any changes in the current plan of care.

If a medication is due at the time of change of shift, for example 7 p.m. or 1900, the departing nurse should administer that drug and inform the arriving nurse that the medication was given. It is also important to report the patient's intake and output, and her dietary restrictions.

Exhibit 1.3: Elements of a complete nurse-to-nurse report.

1. Patient's name and name of her partner or guardian, patient's age, gravida, parity, due date or weeks of gestation, number of fetuses, and reason for admission or diagnoses, height and current weight.

2. Provider's name, location, and telephone number.

3. Allergies, including allergy to latex, and Group B streptococcus status.

4. History of transfusion reactions or prenatal laboratory results that might affect care during labor or birth.

5. Current medications and past medications if they affect or potentially affect her current condition or care, for example, antidepressants after her last delivery.

6. Maternal habits, for example, alcohol, tobacco, or street drug use.

7. Prenatal/obstetric and medical history.

8. Last vital signs and any abnormal findings.

9. Physical assessment of abnormal findings.

10. Fetal normal baseline rate (based on past nonstress tests and/or the admission report).

11. Current fetal baseline rate and other features of the fetal heart rate pattern.

12. Current uterine activity.

13. Last cervical examination, fetal station, status of membranes, including color, amount, and odor of amniotic fluid.

14. A review of progress, for example, abnormally slow dilatation or arrest of descent.

15. Last dose of medications, including prostaglandins, oxytocin, antibiotics, narcotics, insulin, antihypertensives, etc.

16. Current pain level and ability to cope with the labor, and patient desires for pain management.

NURSE–PROVIDER COMMUNICATION

Physical or psychological needs that promote patient well-being should be communicated to midwives and physicians (Henrikson, 2006). Nurses should also communicate to clarify orders, discuss therapeutic plans, report changes in the patient's condition, share questions the patient or her family members have, and report abnormal or significant findings.

Strong nurse-physician relationships affect both nurse and patient satisfaction. If nurses and physicians have equal power

---

Exhibit 1.4: Certified nurse midwife management without a requirement for a physician consultation.

1. Gestational diabetes (diet controlled).

2. Fetus that is 36 or more weeks of gestation.

3. Internal and external fetal monitoring, including insertion of a fetal spiral electrode and intrauterine pressure catheter.

4. Meconium with reassuring fetal heart rate pattern.

5. Group B streptococcus prophylaxis according to protocol.

6. Urinary tract infection diagnosis and treatment.

7. Initiation of anesthesia request when a normal spontaneous vaginal delivery is expected.

8. Amnioinfusion.

9. Episiotomy.

10. First- and second-degree laceration repair.

Exhibit 1.5: Example of certified nurse midwife intrapartal management that may require a physician consultation (consult your hospital's requirements).

1. Multiparous woman (with more than 5 pregnancies).

2. Severe anemia (hemoglobin less than 9 mg/dL).

3. Estimated fetal weight greater than 4,500 grams.

4. Postterm pregnancy (gestation of 42 weeks or more).

5. Pregnancy less than 36 weeks gestation.

6. Induction of labor.

7. Oxytocin-induced augmentation of labor.

8. Maternal fever.

9. Preeclampsia.

10. Thick and/or particulate meconium-stained amniotic fluid.

11. Regional anesthesia in the presence of dystocia.

12. Arrest of labor.

13. Second stage greater than 2 hours (without an epidural) or greater than 3 hours (with an epidural).

14. Nonreassuring fetal heart rate pattern.

15. Suspected chorioamnionitis.

---

within their respective practice areas and they collaborate to provide patient care, staff nurses will continue to work at that hospital. In fact, increased communication between nurses and physicians reduces bad outcomes (McClure & Hinshaw, 2002). Communication and relating to others requires a sense of social competency (Stichler, 2007b). Social competence includes the ability to assess the emotions of others and relate to them in a manner that diffuses anger and conflict, provides encouragement, or inspires them. Social management is part of emotional intelligence or being intelligent in our relationships (Goleman, 2002).

If you work with certified nurse midwives, you should work to develop a positive relationship with them. It will help if you know that they probably are limited in what they can do without the consultation of the back-up obstetrician (see Exhibits 1.4, 1.5, and 1.6).

Nurses must notify the midwife or physician when an order should not be followed. The American Medical Association (AMA) supports communication between a nurse and a physician when the nurse finds an order to be in error or contrary to customary medical or nursing practice. The AMA has opined that "the physician has an ethical obligation to hear the nurse's concern and explain those orders to the nurse involved. The ethical physician should neither expect nor insist that nurses follow orders contrary to standards of good medical and nursing practice" (AMA, 1997).

If you encounter a clinical situation in which you believe a physician's opinion, attention, or care is needed, discuss this with the midwife. If the midwife refuses to communicate with her consulting physician and you still feel a physician's care is needed for your patient, share your concern with the midwife in the presence of the charge nurse or supervisor. The charge nurse or supervisor possess the authority and responsibility to act in the best interests of the patient. If the charge nurse also finds that a physician is needed, it is his or her responsibility to discuss the need for a physician evaluation with the midwife. After that conversation, if the midwife fails to call the physician to the bedside, the charge nurse or supervisor has the responsibility to make that call.

To improve your communication abilities, develop your emotional intelligence. Do not let others push your buttons. In the event you work with a "know-it-all" who hangs up on you after you make a reasonable request for your patient, do not chart "Provider hung up on me." Instead, notify your charge nurse of the situation and your patient's needs. Ask the charge nurse to make the next call. This action is invoking the chain of command or chain of communication. That is the right thing to do. Alternatively, if you do not have a charge nurse, ask another nurse to listen on another line (if possible) and call the "know-it-all" again. In the second call, let him or

---

> **Exhibit 1.6: Example of midwife and physician intrapartal collaborative management (consult your hospital's requirements).**
>
> 1. Insulin-dependent diabetic or not well-controlled gestational diabetic without suspected fetal macrosomia.
>
> 2. Known intrauterine growth restriction (IUGR).
>
> 3. Nonreassuring fetal heart rate (FHR) patterns not resolving with in utero resuscitation. Interventions such as:
>   A. position change
>   B. correction of hypotension (e.g., administration of Ephedrine slow IV push)
>   C. discontinuation of oxytocin
>   D. hyperoxia (using a tight-fitting face mask at 10 liters/minute)
>   E. stop pushing or push with every other contraction
>   F. tocolysis (e.g., IV bolus or Brethine (terbutaline) 0.25 mg SQ or slow IV push)
>
> 4. Preeclampsia with "mild" laboratory abnormalities.
>
> 5. Excessive bleeding during labor.
>
> 6. Fetal malpresentation.
>
> 7. Greater than 30-minute, third stage (delivery to placenta time).
>
> 8. Less than 1-cm change in station during pushing in the second stage.
>
> 9. Vaginal birth after cesarean section (VBAC).
>
> 10. Excessive uterine tenderness or rigidity.
>
> 11. Suppression of preterm contractions.
>
> 12. Sickle-cell anemia or disease.

tive behavior. Throwing things such as instruments or lap sponges in your direction is disruptive behavior. No person with whom you work should ever hurt you. Abuse and battery must not be tolerated — and must always be reported. If you feel you are the victim of disruptive behavior in the workplace, speak with your nurse manager and discuss the incident. Disruptive behavior cannot and must not be tolerated and silence on your part is not an option. Speak to the "disrupter" privately with your supervisor present. In the meeting, state the disruptive behavior by explaining what you found to be disruptive. Keep your statement brief, factual, and descriptive. Also share how you felt when the disruptive behavior occurred. When confronted, the disrupter may argue or yell or dispute what you say. If this happens politely thank the disrupter for his or her time and leave. Write an occurrence or problem/resolution report and include his or her response. Continue to act professionally, even if the disrupter is rude to you. If the behavior continues, follow the same plan: meet, discuss, report. The report provides an opportunity for the disrupter to change his or her behavior (Lazoritz & Carlson, 2008).

Communication is necessary to gather and to share information and to mobilize help. Use a translator service if you feel you are not communicating effectively with your patient. Communicate and collaborate with the primary health care provider to ensure there is an appropriate plan of care and evaluation of the patient's condition prior to beginning a procedure such as cervical ripening or induction. For example, you might say to the midwife or obstetrician, "I'm really worried about the baby. Can you please come in and evaluate the tracing for me?" If you do not get the response you desire, it may be because you did not communicate your degree of concern. Try again and say, "I guess I didn't communicate well. I'm very concerned about the baby and I'd like you to come to the bedside now to evaluate the tracing." If you still do not get the response you desire, use your chain of command process.

Obstetricians are used to four basic types of telephone calls (see Exhibit 1.7).

If you are trying to decide whether to call the physician or midwife, just make the call. The time of day should not stop you from sharing important patient information. Call when the patient needs a medication, is not tolerant of labor, or is

her know that your colleague is listening in. Your colleague should say, "hello." Then ask the provider again for what your patient needs. If he or she hangs up or refuses to come in, activate the chain of command and record who you notified in the chain.

DISRUPTIVE BEHAVIOR IS INAPPROPRIATE BEHAVIOR

Disruptive behavior includes intimidation, violence, inappropriate language or comments, sexual harassment, and/or inappropriate responses to patient needs or staff requests. Hanging up midsentence or refusing to come in are examples of disruptive behavior. If someone verbally threatens you, that is disrup-

> **Exhibit 1.7: Telephone calls from a nurse to a physican or midwife.**
>
> 1. Patient has arrived.
>
> 2. Status update and request for new orders.
>
> 3. New, significant findings and a need to come to the unit to assess the patient.
>
> 4. There is an emergency and we're taking the patient to the operating room for a cesarean section.

ready to push, or any time there is concern for the fetus. Call for orders, to clarify orders, or to change orders.

When there are new and/or significant findings, it is especially important that you report information in a timely manner (meaning within a few minutes of knowing the information) to the midwife or physician. For example, if your patient complains of constant pain in the suprapubic area and her bladder is empty, think about the fit of the fetal head in the pelvis. Is it pressing down above her pubic bone? Ask the midwife or physician to come to the bedside and evaluate this unusual pain. If you are given an order, be sure you accept that it is safe to follow that order. If you are concerned about a risk of harm, discuss it with the person who wrote the order. It is your responsibility to question orders that may harm the patient and you must not follow harmful orders.

SBARR

The letters S, B, A, R, and R represent the words *situation*, *background*, *assessment*, *recommendation*, and *response*. The situation is the patient's current condition and your major concern. The background includes the pertinent facts from the patient's history. The assessment is what you think the problem is. The recommendation is what you recommend the provider do. The response is what he or she said or did when you made your recommendation (Cherouny, Federico, Haraden, Leavitt Gullo, & Resar, 2005; Guise & Lowe, 2006; Nunes & McFerran, 2005).

To help midwives and physicians make good decisions, they need you to provide them with relevant facts, abnormal findings or laboratory results, and any other information that paints a complete picture in their minds. For example, if there is fetal tachycardia, you will also want to inform them of the maternal pulse and temperature. Both are elevated when there is chorioamnionitis. If there is vaginal bleeding, they will need to know about contractions and details related to pain, such as the location of the pain, whether it is constant or intermittent, sharp or dull, how the patient is responding to the pain, and the fetal status. If you need a physician or midwife at the bedside, you might say "I need you to come to the hospital now" or "The patient (fetus or mother) needs you to come to the bedside now." When the midwife and/or physician respond to your request without delay, they promote a safe, reliable organization that is patient-centered.

Documentation example: Jane Doe, CNM, called at 2330. Informed her of patient's BP 156/92, facial and hand edema, and hyperreflexia with unrelenting headache and abdominal pain, but no vaginal bleeding, with contractions every 1 to 2 minutes. Patient reported no history of preeclampsia. Recommended CNM come to bedside immediately. CNM informed this nurse she was on her way.

COMMUNICATION DURING EMERGENCIES

The Association of Women's Health, Obstetric and Neonatal Nurses (AWHONN, 2004), supports nursing action that may be contrary to a physician's order when fetal well-being is in question and the external fetal monitor tracing is not reassuring or is unreadable. They have taken the position that a registered nurse may apply a fetal spiral electrode (FSE) through intact membranes for the purpose of obtaining additional assessment data and treatment provided the nurse has had appropriate education and has met competence requirements in accordance with institutional policy and state or provincial nurse practice legislation. Throughout your career in nursing, you may be confronted with a decision to not follow a standing order because it may harm the patient.

Nurses communicate when they believe the plan of care needs to change. Nurses also identify care issues that need ethical, legal, or risk intervention. In either case, communication with the supervisor is required to advocate for a change in the plan of care. If communication with a provider intimidates you, talk to your charge nurse or a more experienced nurse and ask for help. Once you have communicated the patient's information and needs, you should document in the medical record the time you communicated, whom you spoke to, what you said, what the person said, and any actions taken by you, your supervisor, or the provider.

Documentation example: Subtle late decelerations, fetal heart rate pattern sinusoidal-like. Dr. Seinwave called at home. Informed of baseline 130 to 140 bpm, recurrent subtle late decelerations, contractions every 2 minutes lasting 50 seconds, moderate to palpation. Telephone order for Pitocin received and read back to physician. This nurse refused order and requested physician come to bedside now to evaluate patient and tracing.

Documentation example: Repetitive variable decelerations with baseline 140 bpm, minimal variability. Dr. Listo called to bedside. This nurse reviewed tracing with physician. Cesarean section ordered.

Nurses recognize, verbalize, and mobilize. "In emergencies, when prompt action is necessary and the physician is not immediately available, a nurse may be justified in acting contrary to the physician's standing orders for the safety of the patient" (AMA, 1997). Staffing should be based on the acuity of patients and standardized protocols should be followed for emergencies (Fariello & Paul, 2005). Therefore, if you recognize a problem, notify other nurses, and tell them what you want them to do. A pilot once said, "In a storm, just keep the wings level. Tough it out. Fall apart after you land."

CHAIN OF COMMAND

Each hospital should have a chain of command policy, procedure, or protocol. You may need to activate your chain of command to resolve conflicts over patient management plans (Mahley & Beerman, 1998). The chain of command is a process that is used when the nurse feels that ethical or practice standards are not being maintained or there are unresolved conflicts or clinical issues that affect patient well-being. Prior to invoking the chain of command, every effort should be made to clearly and fully communicate with the midwife, resident, or physician directly involved in the patient's care. If the communication fails, the chain of command policy must be followed.

Unresolved conflicts often involve a disagreement in patient care, such as the need to apply oxygen or a spiral electrode. The chain of command or chain of communication is invoked as the patient's safety net. Your role as a patient advocate creates an ethical duty to prevent harm, and requires courage to acknowledge the disagreement and seek its resolution. You might say to the midwife or physician (away from the patient's bedside), "We have an unresolved disagreement here. I've asked the charge nurse to help us resolve this issue." You can also say, "I'm activating our chain of command policy." The charge nurse may decide to assume care of your patient or assign another nurse to care for your patient. The charge nurse can be asked to speak with the midwife and may need to speak with the next highest level in the chain, that is, the midwife's back-up physician or the attending physician. If the provider is the Chief of Obstetrics, involve your nursing chain of command, for example, the charge nurse and nurse manager. If the Chief of Obstetrics is also the Chief of the Medical Staff, involve your charge nurse or supervisor, who may need to involve the Vice Chief of the Medical Staff to resolve the conflict.

Documentation of the chain of command should include the observations and events that created a need to use the chain of command, specific facts, and the time of events and communications.

Documentation example: Dr. Noetaul ordered oxytocin. Physician was informed at nurses' station at 1205 that patient was contracting every 2 minutes x 50 to 70 seconds, and was moderate to palpation. Order to administer oxytocin was questioned. Charge nurse Sally Smith was informed of communication with physician. Nurse Smith spoke with physician who insisted on oxytocin administration. Chief of OB was called by charge nurse at 1210.

The nurse's responsibility is to advocate for the patient's safety. It is imperative that the nurse continue to communicate with the charge nurse or supervisor until the conflict is resolved. The nurse must act to prevent injury.

Patients really want a nurse who cares for them as if they were a family member. They want a nurse who is responsive to their needs, including their physical, emotional, and spiritual needs. They want a nurse who is willing to do extra things and who follows through on promises (Trossman, 2007). Sometimes our communications are ineffective in moving toward a patient-centered goal. For example, what would you do if the physician asked you to do something in front of the patient that you felt was not best for the patient or her baby?

If you receive a verbal order at the bedside, but are concerned that following the order may harm the patient, do not follow the order. When the provider leaves the room, repeat the order. For example, an order you should question is "Begin oxytocin per protocol on this patient" but you know the patient has a baby in a transverse lie. When the provider leaves the room, follow him or her. In the hallway ask if he or she wanted oxytocin to be administered to this patient who has a transverse lie. If the answer is yes, do not follow the order. Instead, speak to your charge nurse or supervisor and inform him or her of the order, the provider's response, and your concerns. The charge nurse or supervisor has the responsibility and authority to speak with the provider so that the order is changed. Your responsibility is to continue to care for your patient.

In your career, there will be times when you need to initiate the chain of command and involve your charge nurse or house supervisor — or even the Chief of Obstetrics. If you have a clinical nurse specialist, he or she often works with the Patient Care Manager as a dyad and may also be able to help you obtain the care you need for your patient. In some cases, the Director of Maternity Services or Maternal Child Services, the Assistant Vice President for Women and Children's Services, or the Executive Vice President for Patient Care Services will be called. When the chief nursing officer is called, the entire nursing chain of command will be involved.

You can develop your own list of names and phone numbers of people in your chain of command. It is a good idea for the hospital to give you a copy of the chain of command policy. It is your responsibility to find it if you do not receive it. From time to time you may want to return to the policy for guidance or to refresh your memory. In general, there are two "chains" of command that compose the overall "chain of command," the nursing chain of command and the medical chain of command (see Figures 1.1 and 1.2).

Activate the chain of command or chain of communication whenever there are unresolved issues related to patient care or if you have concerns related to a provider. If resolution of the conflict or issue is not achieved at any step up the chain of command, continue up the chain until a mutual resolution is met. Perhaps once in your entire career, you may follow the chain all the way to the top (Chief Nursing Officer and Hospital Medical Director).

If discussions with the midwife or physician do not result in appropriate care, the nurse is responsible to ensure timely and appropriate actions (Simpson & Chez, 2001). Advocacy for the patient may require you to invoke your hospital's chain of command.

A retrospective review of 90 risk manager files from 1995 to 2001 revealed that adverse outcomes are directly related to procedures and people (White, Pichert, Bledsoe, Irwin, & Entman, 2005). Half of those files were related to labor and delivery, the rest were related to gynecologic surgery (38%) and ambulatory care (12%). Communication failures were associated with 31% of the adverse events. For example, there

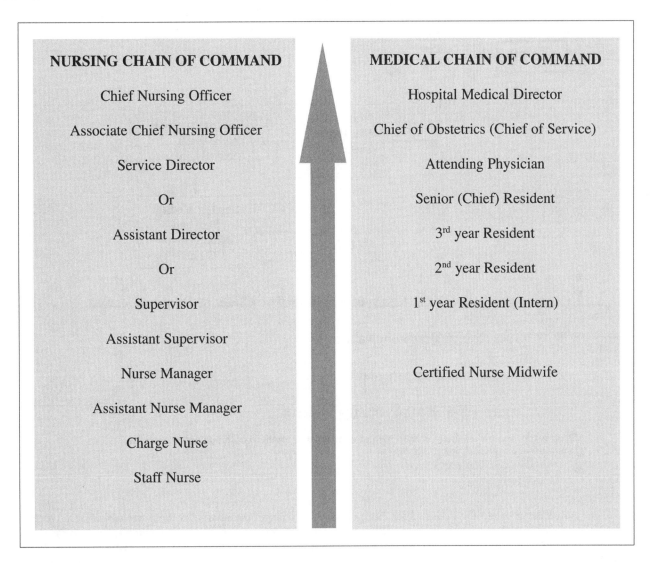

Figure 1.1: Sample chain of command with the staff nurse as the first link in the chain.

were disruptions in the flow of critical information from one caregiver to another, or there were communications that upset the patient or her family.

Example of the need for the chain of command: Dina was 29 years old, a gravida 4, having her second baby at 40 weeks of gestation. She arrived in labor and delivery with bloody show and a thick, closed cervix with a high, vertex fetal station. The unit was a nurse-managed labor unit and there was no charge nurse on duty. Dina was contracting and dilated to 5 centimeters within 6 hours of admission. However, she remained at 5 centimeters for the next 3 hours. The fetal heart rate pattern demonstrated a loss of accelerations and baseline vari-

ability decreased. Oxygen was applied at 10 liters per minute using a nonrebreather mask. The attending family physician wanted oxytocin to be administered. The nurse started the oxytocin infusion. Within 30 minutes there were late decelerations. The nurse showed the tracing to the family practice physician who asked that she continue the oxytocin infusion. The nurse continued the infusion but informed the physician she would be calling the obstetrician for a second opinion. The obstetrician arrived and the oxytocin was discontinued. Both physicians remained on the unit. Within another 3 hours, Dina had progressed to an anterior lip but the fetal heart rate fell to a bradycardic level below 90 beats per minute. There were also late decelerations and prolonged decel-

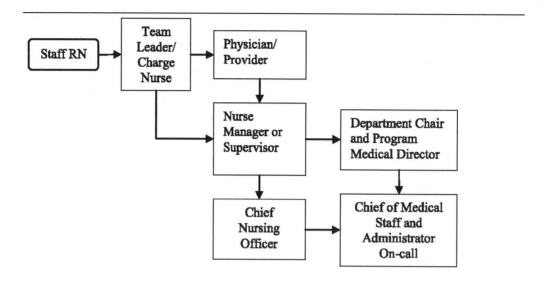

Reasons to Activate the Chain of Command or Chain of Communication

1. Issues requiring communication.

2. Issues surrounding patient care.

3. Concerns related to physican/provider.

Figure 1.2: Another example of the chain of command or chain of communication with the staff nurse as the first link in the chain.

erations. The nurse never called the house supervisor or her unit supervisor. One hour later and after use of the vacuum extractor, the baby's head was delivered. There was a shoulder dystocia. The Zavanelli maneuver and a cesarean section were performed. The Apgar scores were 0 at 1 minute and 3 at 5 and 10 minutes. The newborn weighed 4,345 grams and suffered from severe perinatal asphyxia.

Dystocia is derived from the Greek word for "abnormal" or "difficult" and the Greek word *tokos* for "labor" or "delivery." A difficult delivery of the shoulders was encountered. In fact, all maneuvers failed to deliver the baby. The nursing chain of command should have been activated when Dina's baby was bradycardic but remote from delivery. The plan of care needed to change to a cesarean section, however, the nurse remained silent. Failure of the nurse to discuss a change in the plan of care, including a cesarean section, and to activate the nursing chain of command were considered by the plaintiff's nurse expert to be substandard nursing care. The case settled prior to the trial.

This example illustrates the nurse's need to advocate for the patient and use the chain of command when the midwife or physician is unresponsive to reasonable concerns about the patient's condition or is making inappropriate patient care decisions. Any order or plan that is not consistent with standard medical practice should be questioned by the nurse.

The plan of care should be more than "monitor" or "expect vaginal delivery." It should provide a road map toward a safe outcome. Sometimes the plan of care is in conflict with the patient's needs. To resolve clinical issues related to patient care conflicts, your hospital should have a "Resolution of Clinical Issues" or "Resolution of Conflict" procedure. This procedure should define the channels of communication and decision making that you should follow when there are questions or concerns regarding medical or nursing care. Knowing your patient should be the basis for clinical decisions and judgments and individualized care.

When orders deviate from the plan of care or customary or safe practices, discuss the situation and your concerns with the midwife and/or physician(s) responsible for the patient. If the issue needing clarification is not resolved, the chain of command should be initiated and your charge nurse or immediate supervisor must be notified. The charge nurse or supervisor will discuss the concern with the midwife or physician. If the issue remains unresolved, other individuals in the "chain of command" will become involved so that the conflict can be resolved. Avoid documentation that reflects a disagreement between yourself and others. Instead, document your assessments, plans, actions, evaluations, and communications.

Example of documentation that reflects disagreement between a nurse and a physician: "Dr. Disreguarde aware of FHR throughout second stage of labor. Dr. desires no interventions at this time. Nurse manager in room. Dr. orders pushing to continue. Dr. informed of meconium and nonreassuring FHR pattern. Dr. still refuses to order any interventions at this time. Dr. asked if NICU should be called. Dr. said they are not needed. Dr. reminded of particulate meconium. Dr. said there is no meconium."

Example of appropriate documentation: Frequent discussions with Dr. Disreguarde during second stage about FHR pattern, including meconium and nonreassuring pattern at this time. No new orders. Nurse manager in the room at this time. NICU called by nurse manager to attend delivery.

The first narrative note demonstrates the lack of collaboration and teamwork. The second note demonstrates how well the chain of command worked to secure personnel for delivery.

FATIGUE AND FAULTY COMMUNICATION

Successful decision makers and communicators are well rested, not driven by pressures, and aware of their biases. To eliminate bias, you must recognize and acknowledge what the bias is and be willing to change (Cudé & Winfrey, 2007). Being well rested may be a difficult goal, but it is an important goal that prevents errors and patient injuries. Research shows that error rates increase when nurses work more than 12 hours a day, or more than 40 hours a week (Rogers, Hwang, Scott, Aiken, & Dinges, 2004). Unfortunately, nurses often work more than 40 hours per week. Some nurses work more than six days in a row and many rotate shifts (Trinkoff, Geiger-Brown, Brady, Lipscomb, & Muntaner, 2006). If you do the same, you increase your risk of becoming overtired, chronically stressed, or injured — and you therefore increase the risk of injuring a patient. For example, sleep-deprived military gunners hit their targets but shot at the wrong target (Kushida, 2005). An error-prone environment is one that has inadequate staff to get the job done, rude coworkers or supervisors, insufficient resources, ever-changing technology, too little training, excessive paperwork, and communication failures (Welker-Hood,

2006). If you work in an error-prone environment, share your concerns with nursing management.

Clinical reasoning, good problem solving, sound judgment, and effective clinical decision making require clear thinking, knowledge, and experience (Croskerry, 2003, 2005, 2006). Experience will help you develop your clinical reasoning. Good clinical reasoning means inductive, fast, and intuitive recognition of a problem. Some people call this "having a gut feeling." However, it is based on knowledge and experience, not just a feeling. For example, when a pregnant woman presents with decreased fetal movement, frequent mild contractions, a nonreassuring fetal heart rate pattern, a closed cervix, and blood in her shoes (known by skilled nurses as "the positive shoe sign"), an experienced nurse will think there is a placental abruption. The obstetrician will be called and the patient will be prepared for surgery.

Other decisions are a result of a slower, rational, deductive, rule-based, analytical process. This process takes more time, but is valuable because it results in fewer errors (Croskerry, 2006). Errors in our decisions increase when we are uncertain, hurried, pressured, or have biases (Croskerry, 2003). Therefore, if you are new to the practice of labor and delivery nursing and/or you feel something is amiss, or you feel hurried but lack the confidence, knowledge, or motivation to make a decision or to call the midwife or physician, it is best to admit you need help and confer with a more experienced nurse or your charge nurse. By constantly expanding your experiences and knowledge base, you should become a better decision maker and communicator, and you will increase your ability to see the broad range of possibilities in any given clinical situation.

CONCLUSIONS

Communication is necessary to provide the best care for patients and to prevent errors and injury (Cherouny, Federico, Haraden, Leavitt Gullo & Resar, 2005). However, mistakes do occur, especially when there is poor communication, poor documentation, a lack of planning, a lack of action, and a lack of appropriate decisions. Ideally you will work in a healthy culture where communication is open and collaborative, and health care providers know their role and work to provide patient-centered care. But if concerns exist or issues related to care arise, you should consult members of your chain of command. You are a vital part of the health care team, the patient's advocate, and the person responsible for patient well-being.

REVIEW QUESTIONS

True/False: Decide if the following statements are true or false.

1. It is best to avoid words like "noncompliant" or "failure" when communicating with patients or their families, because these words can be hurtful or demeaning.
2. A cynical health care organization is not supportive or is hostile, which impedes communication.

3. Experience is not an important factor that influences decisions.
4. Family-centered care requires care providers to make choices for the mother about the labor and birth process.
5. A reason to communicate with a midwife or physician is when the patient has a physical or psychological need.
6. Patients can provide valuable information to increase the ability of physicians to diagnose their condition.
7. A collaborative culture promotes communication with and among the patient, her significant other or family, and members of the health care team.

8. A nonreassuring fetal heart rate pattern that does not resolve after in utero resuscitation interventions should be reported to the midwife or physician.
9. The last R in SBARR stands for the patient's response to your interventions.
10. Patients want a nurse who follows the physician's orders even when they have the potential to harm the patient.

References

American College of Obstetricians and Gynecologists. (2005). Partnering with patients to improve patient safety. Committee opinion number 320. *Obstetrics & Gynecology, 106*(5), 1123–1125.

American Medical Association. (1997). *Code of medical ethics: Current opinions and annotations.* Chicago: Author.

Association of Women's Health, Obstetric and Neonatal Nurses. (2004). *Amniotomy and placement of internal fetal spiral electrode through intact membranes.* Washington, DC: Author.

Cherouny, P. H., Federico, F. A., Haraden, C., Leavitt Gullo, S. & Resar, R. (2005). *Idealized design of perinatal care.* IHI Innovation Series white paper. Cambridge, MA: Institute for Healthcare Improvement.

Chervenak, F. A., & McCullough, L. B. (2005). The diagnosis and management of progressive dysfunction of health care organizations. *Obstetrics & Gynecology, 105*(4), 882–887.

Croskerry, P. (2003). Cognitive forcing strategies in clinical decision-making. *Annals of Emergency Medicine, 41*(1), 110–120.

Croskerry, P. (2005). The theory and practice of clinical decision-making. *Canadian Journal of Anesthesia, 52*, R1. Retrieved June 2, 2006. Available: http://www.cja-jca.org/cgi/content/full/52/suppl_1/R1

Croskerry, P. (2006). Critical thinking and decision-making: Avoid the perils of thin-slicing. *Annals of Emergency Medicine, 48*, 720–722.

Cudé, G., & Winfrey, K. (2007). The hidden barrier. Gender bias: Fact or fiction? *Nursing for Women's Health, 11*(3), 255–265.

Fariello, J. Y., & Paul, E. (2005). Patient safety issues in a tertiary care hospital's labor and delivery unit. *AWHONN Lifelines, 9*(4), 321–323.

Goleman, S., Boyatzis, R., & McKee, A. (2002). *Primal leadership: Realizing the power of emotional intelligence.* Boston: Harvard Business School Publishing.

Guise, J. M., & Lowe, N. K. (2006). Do you speak SBAR? *Journal of Obstetric, Gynecologic, and Neonatal Nursing, 35*(3), 313–314.

Henrikson, M. (2006). Great leaders are made, not born. *AWHONN Lifelines, 10*, 335–338.

Henrikson, M. (2007). Great leaders are made, not born. *AWHONN Lifelines, 10*(6), 510–515.

Institute of Medicine (IOM). (1999). *To err is human: Building a safer health system.* Washington, DC: National Academies Press.

Joint Commission on Accreditation of Healthcare Organizations (JCAHO). (2000). *Operative and post-operative complications: Lessons for the future (Sentinel Event Alert No. 12).* Oak Brook, IL: Author.

Joint Commission on Accreditation of Healthcare Organizations (JCAHO). (2004). *Preventing infant death during delivery (Sentinel Event Alert No. 30).* Oak Brook, IL: Author.

Katz, A. (2005). Think before you speak. *AWHONN Lifelines, 9*(2), 105–106.

Kendig, S. (2006). Primary care safety. *AWHONN Lifelines, 10*(6), 502–509.

Kushida, C. A. (2005). *Sleep deprivation: Clinical issues, pharmacology, and sleep loss effects.* New York: Marcel Dekker.

Lazoritz, S., & Carlson, P. J. (2008). Don't tolerate disruptive physician behavior: Bad behavior harms both staff and patients. Reporting it benefits everyone. *American Nurse Today, 3*(3), 20–22.

Lefton, C. (2007). Does your workplace culture need CPR? *American Nurse Today*, 32–35.

Mahley, S. & Beerman, J. (1998). Following the chain of command in an obstetric setting: A nurse's responsibility. *Journal of Legal Nurse Consulting, 9*(1), 7–13.

McClure, M. L., & Hinshaw, A. S. (Eds.). (2002). Magnet hospitals revisited: Attraction and retention of professional nurses. Washington, DC: American Nurses Association.

McVeigh, C. (1997). Motherhood experiences from the perspective of first-time mothers. *Clinical Nursing Research, 6*(4), 335–348.

Nunes, J., & McFerran, S. (2005). Perinatal patient safety project. *Permanente Journal, 9*(2). Retrieved February 26, 2006. Available: http://xnet.kp.org/permanentejournal/spring05/perinatal.html

Parer, J. T., & Ikeda, T. (2007). A framework for standarized management of intrapartum fetal heart rate patterns. *American Journal of Obstetrics and Gynecology, 197*(1), 26.e1–26.e6.

Phillips, C. (2003). *Family-centered maternity care.* Sudbury, MA: Jones and Bartlett.

Rogers, A. E., Hwang, W., Scott, L., Aiken, L., & Dinges, D. (2004). The working hours of hospital staff nurses and patient safety. *Health Affairs, 23*(4), 202–212.

Seren, S., & Baykal, U. (2007). Relationships between change and organizational culture in hospitals. *Journal of Nursing Scholarship, 39*(2), 191–197.

Simkin, P., & Ancheta, R. (2005). *The labor progress handbook* (2nd ed.). Oxford, England: Blackwell Publishing.

Simpson, K. R. (2005). The context and clinical evidence for common nursing practices during labor. *MCN, 30*(6), 356–363.

Simpson, K. R., & Chez, B. F. (2001). Professional and legal issues. In K. R. Simpson and P. A. Creehan (Eds.), *AWHONN's perinatal nursing* (2nd ed., pp. 21–52). Philadelphia: Lippincott.

Stichler, J. F. (2006). Emotional intelligence. A critical leadership quality for the nurse executive. *AWHONN Lifelines, 10*(5), 422–425.

Stichler, J. F. (2007a). Is your hospital hospitable? How physical environment influences patient safety. *Nursing for Women's Health, 11*(5), 506–511.

Stichler, J. F. (2007b). Social intelligence: An essential trait of effective leaders. *Nursing for Women's Health, 11*(2), 189–193.

Trinkoff, A., Geiger-Brown, J., Brady, B., Lipscomb, J. U., & Muntaner, C. (2006). How long and how much are nurses now working? *American Journal of Nursing, 106*(4), 60–72.

Trossman, S. (2007). Issues up close: The science behind caring. *American Nurse Today, 2*(12), 40–41.

Tucker, S., Klotzbach, L., Olsen, G., Voss, J., Huus, B., & Olsen, R. (2006). Lessons learned in translating research evidence on early intervention programs into clinical care. *MCN: American Journal of Maternal Child Nursing, 31*(5), 325–331.

von Dielingen, A. (2008). Energizing the work environment: Appreciative inquiry. *Nursing News & Views, 3*(1), 14.

Welker-Hood, K. (2006). Does workplace stress lead to accident or error? *American Journal of Nursing, 106*(9), 104.

White, A. A., Pichert, J. W., Bledsoe, S. H., Irwin, C., & Entman, S. S. (2005). Cause and effect analysis of closed claims in obstetrics and gynecology. *Obstetrics & Gynecology, 195*(5, Part 1), 1031–1038.

2

Patient Assessment

If I have ever made any valuable discoveries, it has been owing more to patient attention, than to any other talent.

—Sir Isaac Newton

PURPOSE OF ASSESSMENT

The admission assessment identifies patient needs, helps the obstetric provider determine a correct diagnosis, and ensures that appropriate care is provided. The time needed to complete the collection of admission assessment data and the depth of data collected should be based on the patient's condition. For example, if the woman is talkative, smiling, and not in pain, a full head-to-toe assessment should be completed. If she is moaning and grunting and telling you the baby is coming, the assessment may include a vaginal examination and a call to the midwife while you set up for delivery.

If you receive a telephone call alerting you that a patient will be coming in, you should begin data collection by reviewing her prenatal record. Further data can be collected after she arrives, as time permits, through physical, psychological, and social screenings. The time to complete and document the assessment may depend on hospital protocol. A plan of care is then developed based on the medical diagnoses, nursing diagnoses, and expressed needs. This plan of care must be continually evaluated and revised to reflect the changing needs of the patient.

PRENATAL CARE

Prenatal care is important because the woman's health can affect her baby's health (American College of Obstetricians and Gynecologists, 2005a). Prenatal care is a preventive health service that can improve outcomes for women and their infants. Some women who receive prenatal care reject medical recommendations, continue to use illegal drugs, or engage in behaviors that can harm their fetus (Maloni, Cheng, Liebl, & Maier, 1996).

In the United States 1.5 to 2% of women do not receive prenatal care. Poverty creates a barrier for these women and prevents them from seeking prenatal care. More than 15% of women live below the poverty level. Sixty percent (60%) of impoverished families have a female head of the household, with children less than 18 years of age (Luke, 1998). Due to poverty, as many as one in four pregnant women will not receive prenatal care, even when it is available. Women who received no prenatal care were most likely to be Black or Hispanic, unmarried, young, less educated, foreign born, multiparous, and urban dwelling. The largest group was young Black women with low education and high behavioral risks such as smoking and alcohol use. Birth outcomes for the "no prenatal care" group were two to four times worse than for the total population. The preterm birth rate was 9.6% for the total population and 26.9% for the "no prenatal care" group (Taylor, Alexander, & Hepworth, 2005).

In addition to poverty, a lack of health literacy may prevent some women from seeking prenatal care. Health literacy includes the skills and competencies that people develop to seek out, understand, evaluate, and use health information and concepts to make informed choices, reduce health risks, and increase the quality of life. Limited health literacy may therefore be a barrier to obtaining adequate prenatal care (Wood, Kettinger, & Lessick, 2007).

Prenatal health care serves to detect and monitor health problems and, when health problems are detected, appropriate interventions can be implemented to protect the health of the fetus. For example, during the second trimester women may have serum screening for alpha-fetoprotein (AFP), human chorionic gonadotropin, unconjugated estriol, and inhibin-A (Wax, 2007). Such screening can help to detect the risk of Down syndrome. Maternal serum AFP (MSAFP) is a screening test for open neural tube defects and abnormal values associated with ventral wall defects, recent fetal demise, imminent miscarriage, preterm labor, risk of intrauterine growth restriction, and hypertension. Low MSAFP levels are associated with Down syndrome.

Women may also have ultrasounds to determine fetal anatomy or fetal size. For example, the ultrasound may reveal cleft lip and/or palate, which are more frequent in women who smoke during pregnancy (Shi, Wehby, & Murray, 2008). Antenatal test results will assist care providers in determining maternal risks and problems so that diseases can be recognized and treated to decrease maternal and infant mortality (Maloni, Cheng, Liebl, & Maier, 1996). In addition, an action plan can be determined to reduce the impact of these diseases and risk factors to improve maternal and infant outcomes.

"Risk" is a word that describes the chance that loss or harm will occur (Cragin & Kennedy, 2006). For example, a history of preterm birth is a risk that increases the likelihood of another preterm birth. In fact, there may be a gene related to preterm labor and birth (Ward, Argyle, Meade, & Nelson, 2005). Women are often classified as low-risk or high-risk patients.

WHAT IS HIGH RISK?

A high-risk patient has risk factors that increase the risk of injury for herself or her infant. She may have more than one risk factor. Some common risk factors are smoking, alcohol use, hypertension, diabetes, and infections such as human immunodeficiency virus (HIV).

If a woman seeks prenatal care in her first trimester, risks will be determined at that time. In addition, teaching and counseling to promote health to decrease the impact of risk factors may occur. Some women do not realize they are pregnant during the first trimester, which delays the assessment of risk factors. Women who realize they are pregnant after the first trimester may include those younger than 20 years of age, women with an unplanned pregnancy, and women who are simply not aware they are pregnant (Braveman, Marchi, Egerter, Pearl, & Neuhaus, 2000). When women "deny" they are pregnant, it is highly unlikely that they will seek prenatal care, and the lack of prenatal care increases risk.

Being labeled as a high-risk patient may increase a woman's stress and uncertainty. Such a women may feel fear, anxiety, guilt, grief, alienation, and aloneness. Her connectedness to her unborn child may be threatened. She may use her spiritual beliefs and practices to help her cope with the complications of her pregnancy. Prayer is one example of a coping mechanism used by women who have a high-risk pregnancy (Price, Lake, Breen, Carson, Quinn, & O'Connor, 2007).

RISK INFLUENCES THE PLAN OF CARE

The intrapartal nursing goal is "to ensure a safe passage for both mother and baby, to minimize risks, and to promote a healthy outcome and positive experience" (Martin, 2002, p. 129). The preparations for a safe delivery begin as soon as the pregnant woman arrives in your birthing center. To accomplish this safety goal it is important to appreciate the relationship between the mother's physical and psychological condition, her preparedness for labor and birth, and her ability to cope with pain. This includes her passenger (fetus), the passageway (pelvis), and the powers (contractions).

If the prenatal records are available and there is time to read them, identify risk factors that may affect labor and birth, such as obesity, a nongynecoid pelvis or suspected fetal macrosomia. All risk factors must be considered when the intrapartal plan of care is developed with the patient, the nurses, the midwife, and/or the physician(s). A woman's feeling that the labor and birth experience was satisfactory depends on a match between her expectations and her perception of the care that was provided (Schug, 2001).

The patient's prenatal history may have an impact on her labor or her baby's health. Her history, including habits and personal characteristics, should trigger thoughts about her current status (see Exhibit 2.1). For example, if she had urinary tract infections during the pregnancy, there is an increased risk that her child will have mental retardation and developmental delay (McDermott, Callaghan, Szwejbka, Mann, & Daguise, 2000). If she has gestational diabetes, there is an increased risk of fetal macrosomia, which may delay descent.

AGE AND CESAREAN SECTION RISK

Women who are younger than 20 years of age have an increased risk of preterm birth and perinatal death. They have a greater risk of dehydration, poor nutrition, insufficient weight gain or obesity, and lack of social support. They also have an increased risk of anemia and preeclampsia compared with older women (Usta, Zoorab, Abu-Musa, Naassan, & Nassar, 2008).

Age is related to the risk of a cesarean section (Alkazaleh, Seaward, Ryan, Malik, & Farine, 2001). For example, women less than 20 years of age had a 15.7% cesarean rate (Alkazaleh et al., 2001). Women between 20 and 30 years of age had a 23% cesarean section rate, and women who were 30 to 40 years of age had a 30% cesarean section rate (Perez-Delboy, Shevell, Cleary, Smok, & Simpson, 2002). In another study, women who were less than 25 years of age had an 11.6% cesarean section rate (Ecker, Chen, Cohen, Riley, & Lieberman, 2001). Women of advanced maternal age, defined as 35 years of age or older, have an increased risk for a cesarean section, especially if they are nulliparous. In addition, they have an increased risk of stillbirths (Heffner, Elkin, & Fretts, 2003; Miller, 2005). The reason for the increased number of stillbirths is unknown.

Exhibit 2.1: History, habits, and characteristics may affect pregnancy and labor outcomes.

Abortion (elective)	Did an instrument puncture her uterus? If so, she has an increased risk of uterine rupture.
Age	The older she is, the greater her risk of cesarean section.
Allergies	Which medications or substances is she allergic to? Latex?
Bleeding	Is placenta previa or abruption possible?
Blood type	Rh negative? Immunoglobulin given? When? History of miscarriage without immunoglobulin? Risk of fetal hemolysis from isoimmunization.
Caffeine use	Increased risk of miscarriage.
Cigarette smoking	Number of cigarettes per day is related to fetal growth and fetal and placental health.
Diabetes screen	Also known as the 1-hour glucola screen(ing) test.
Glucose tolerance test	If the diabetes screen was abnormal, it will be followed with a 3-hour glucose tolerance test.
Group B streptococcus	If the vaginal/rectal GBS culture is positive, she will need antibiotics during labor.
Height	Short women have more cesarean sections.
Weight	High prepregnancy BMI? Obesity is related to macrosomia, more cesarean sections due to cephalopelvic disproportion and failure to progress, and shoulder dystocia, especially if this is her first baby (Young & Woodmansee, 2002). Weight gain of 33 or more pounds? She will have an increased risk of a cesarean section or shoulder dystocia if she continues labor and has a vaginal delivery.
Membranes ruptured	Risk of infection.
Nausea/vomiting	Liver capsule distention, preeclampsia?
Prepregnancy weight	Overweight (BMI 25.0 to 29.9 kg/m^2) and obese (BMI 30 or more) women have an increased risk of stillbirth (Stephansson, Dickman, Johansson, & Cnattingius, 2001).
Prior birth(s)	Note the date, type of delivery, and weight of her babies. Ask her if this baby seems larger or smaller than her last baby. If there is a different father, the anticipated weight may change (due to different genetics). The time between the last cesarean section and the current date is related to her risk of uterine rupture if she decides to have a trial of labor after cesarean (TOLAC).
Urinary tract infection or pyelonephritis	Risk of permanent neonatal brain damage related to pyelonephritis and the fetal inflammatory response syndrome (McDermott, Callaghan, Szwejbka, Mann, & Daguise, 2000).

Women who were 40 or more years of age and who were treated for infertility had a 71.4% cesarean section rate versus a 41.3% rate for women 40 years of age and older who did not have infertility treatment (Sheiner, Shoham-Vardi, Hershkovitz, Katz, & Mazor, 2001). Some of these women will have become pregnant as a result of assisted reproductive technology (ART), which increases their ability to deliver later in life (Suplee, Dawley, & Bloch, 2007). They have an increased risk of having a child with a chromosomal abnormality and it is important to review the prenatal record for the results of any testing, such as chorionic villus sampling, ultrasounds for fetal anatomy, and blood work such as maternal serum alpha fetoprotein. Ecker and colleagues (2001) also reported a cesarean section rate of 41.3% in women who were 40 years of age or older, regardless of infertility treatment.

In addition to pregnancy-associated risks, women of advanced maternal age may have medical conditions that increase risk, such as cardiovascular disease, cancer, diabetes, hypertension, or chronic diseases such as lupus. This may affect the care provided. A holistic approach will be needed to provide for her physical, emotional, and social needs (Suplee et al., 2007).

Induction increases the risk of a cesarean section in any age group (Gülmezoglu, Crowther, & Middleton, 2006; Heffner,

Elkin, & Fretts, 2003). However, older women have more cesarean sections regardless of whether labor is spontaneous or induced. They have a higher incidence of prolonged labors, failure to progress, and fetal distress (Ecker et al., 2001; Greenberg, Cheng, Sullivan, Norton, Hopkins, & Caughay, 2007).

Clinical example: The patient is a 42-year-old nulliparous woman with a history of infertility treatment and gestational diabetes at 38 weeks of gestation. She is 5 feet 2 inches tall and weighs 185 pounds, a gain of 45 pounds. She is being admitted at 0700 (7:00 a.m.) for an induction of labor. She has a birth plan and has attended childbirth classes with her significant other. She desires as little intervention as possible. The nurse confirmed the contents of the birth plan and acknowledged she would do all she could to support the plan. Prior to starting the intravenous line, the nurse confirmed the woman understood the medical plan of care for intravenous piggyback (IVPB) oxytocin. She also examined the cervix and found it to be 1-cm dilated, 50% effaced with a −3 station. Contractions were irregular and 6 to 10 minutes apart lasting 30 to 40 seconds and mild. The fetus had a normal heart rate pattern with accelerations and no decelerations. Ten hours later, the patient was 5-cm dilated, the baby was at a −2 to −3 station, and there were variable decelerations and meconium in the amniotic fluid. The oxytocin was infusing at 14 mU/minute for the past 2 hours and contractions were every 2 to 3 minutes for the past 5 hours. The nurse discontinued the oxytocin infusion and called the attending physician, who came to the bedside and determined the fetus would not fit, the fetal heart rate pattern was abnormal, and a cesarean section was needed. Because the nurse recognized at the time of admission that there was a heightened risk of a cesarean section due to the patient's age, height, weight gain, and fetal size, she had already prepared the paperwork she would need prior to a cesarean.

ALCOHOL AND OTHER SUBSTANCE ABUSE

Tennessee and Ohio, women who abused alcohol or street drugs, smoked cigarettes, or who were Black had a higher incidence of periodontal disease. Bad breath, smoking, and the use of alcohol are some of the factors related to periodontal disease. Periodontal disease may be related to preterm birth (Beazley et al., 2001; Vergnes & Sixou, 2007). If you note missing teeth or bleeding gums, document your findings. Review her prenatal record for a history of alcohol and/or substance abuse. If you suspect your patient is drunk, ask her what she has been drinking. If she is slurring her words and having difficulty walking, record your observations in the nursing notes. Notify the midwife or physician of your observations. He or she may order a toxicology screen.

ALLERGIES

If the patient has allergies, apply an allergy identification band. If your hospital has a protocol, place a label on her chart with

Exhibit 2.2: Weight status based on body mass index (BMI).

WEIGHT STATUS	BMI	RECOMMENDED WEIGHT GAIN DURING PREGNANCY
Underweight	< 18.5	28 to 40 lbs.
Normal	18.5 to 24.9	25 to 35 lbs.
Overweight	25 to 29.9	15 to 25 lbs.
Obese	> 30	15 lbs.

her allergies. Ask her if she has a latex allergy. There are two classifications for latex allergies, Type I, which affects breathing, and Type IV, which causes a rash or blisters. If she reports she is allergic to latex, determine and document her reaction when she is exposed to latex products. A latex allergy will cause heightened anxiety because of fear that the health care providers will forget. Be sure to mention you are aware of her allergy and remove all latex products from her room unless your hospital is already a latex-safe facility.

BODY MASS INDEX

The body mass index (BMI) is calculated using a person's weight and height to determine if he or she is underweight, overweight, obese, or morbidly obese. The person's weight in kilograms is divided by height in meters squared (kg/m^2). Pounds and inches may also be used to calculate the BMI. In that case, the BMI is 703 times the weight in pounds, divided by the height in inches squared (see Exhibits 2.2 and 2.3). The Institute of Medicine classifies a BMI of less than 19.8 as underweight or less than the 5th percentile of BMI (Groth, 2007). Therefore, the information in Exhibit 2.2 should be considered relative and not absolute. In general, obesity in pregnancy is indicated by a BMI of more than 29 (Stotland, Haas, Brawarsky, Jackson, Fuentes-Afflick, & Escobar, 2005).

A BMI of 25 or more (overweight or obese) is associated with difficult labor or dystocia. It is also associated with an increased risk of a cesarean delivery (Shy, Kimpo, Emanuel, Leisenring, & Williams, 2000; Walker, 1996). Overweight and obese women have a higher incidence of hypertension. Hypertension occurred in 14.8% of women who were overweight and 26.9% of women who were obese, but in only 3.3% of women who were underweight and 5.3% of women who were normal weight (Samuels-Kalow et al., 2007). Overweight and obese women also have a higher incidence of preeclampsia, eclampsia, and fetal macrosomia (LaCoursiere, Bloebaum, Duncan, & Varner, 2005; Samuels-Kalow et al., 2007). Macrosomia is also related to maternal diabetes, a previous macrosomic infant, prolonged gestation, excessive weight gain, a male fetus, and multiparity (Zamorski & Biggs, 2001). Sixty-five percent of women who delivered one baby weighing more than 4,500 grams later also delivered a second baby weighing more than 4,500 grams (Mahony, Foley, Daly, & O'Herlihy, 2005).

BODY MASS INDEX AND WEIGHT GAIN DURING PREGNANCY

A woman's weight before and during pregnancy affects neonatal outcomes. For example, a low prepregnancy BMI was associated with preterm delivery. Overweight women were more likely to deliver after 42 weeks of gestation (Stotland, Washington, & Caughey, 2007). Nulliparous obese women were six times more likely to have a cesarean section due to cephalopelvic disproportion (CPD) and failure to progress than nulliparous women with a BMI of less than 20 kg/m^2 (Young & Woodmansee, 2002). More than 50% of morbidly obese women developed chorioamnionitis during a trial of labor after cesarean (TOLAC) (Chauhan et al., 2001).

A high pregnancy weight gain (over 33 pounds or 15 kilograms) increases the risk of an adverse outcome (Johnson, 2000). If your patient's BMI is 30 or higher and she has gained 33 or more pounds during the pregnancy, you should report findings related to CPD. CPD is associated with early decelerations due to significant fetal head compression, the lack of fetal descent, formation of caput or molding at a high station, and an abnormal labor curve. Any of these findings should be promptly reported to the midwife or physician.

If a woman weighs 500 pounds in a bed that weighs nearly 500 pounds, and you need to move her to the operating room, it may be helpful to determine who will help you move the nearly 1,000 pounds down the hall if it becomes necessary to do so (see Figure 2.1). If the pregnant woman weighs more than 500 pounds, the physician will need to determine the plan of care, which may include an elective cesarean section in the main operating room. The main operating room may have an operating room table capable of holding a patient who weighs up to 770 pounds or 349 kilograms.

CIGARETTES

Women who smoke during the pregnancy increase the risk of preterm labor, placental abruption, a baby with a low birth weight, fetal hypoxia, and criminal or deviant behavior in their children (Roush, 2006; Pratt, McGloin, & Fearn, 2006). Counseling and support from the midwife or physician may help a pregnant woman quit smoking (Roush, 2006). Helping her partner quit smoking may also help the patient quit smoking (Gage, Everett, & Bullock, 2007). The transdermal nicotine patch is also safe for use during pregnancy. The by-product of nicotine metabolism, cotinine, was much lower in women who wore the patch than the cotinine found in nonpregnant adults who smoked (Wright et al., 1997). If your patient is a smoker, ask her when she last smoked a cigarette and record it in the notes. Look for signs of fetal hypoxia such as tachycardia, or absent or minimal long-term variability or fewer accelerations.

Documentation example: Patient reports she last smoked two cigarettes within the last two hours. FHR 160 with minimal variability, no accelerations, no decelerations. Positioned on right side. Oxygen applied at 10 liters/minute with tight-fitting face mask. Dr. Fumes notified of FHR and actions. Contractions every 2 to 3 minutes x 50–80 seconds, moderate. 5/85%/−1.

COCAINE AND OTHER ILLEGAL DRUGS

Cocaine use increases the risk of preterm labor, low birthweight, and placental abruption. Often, cocaine users are also cigarette smokers. The average age of cocaine and/or heroin users was 29.4 years but the average age of marijuana users was 23.4 years. Cocaine/heroin users generally also use multiple illicit drugs (Shieh & Kravitz, 2006). Women who undergo cocaine withdrawal during labor may need to be restrained to stay in the bed and deliver their baby. There must be a physician's order for the restraints. Review your hospital's restraint policy and notify your charge nurse or supervisor that you will be applying restraints. Be sure the bed is in its lowest position and stay with the patient. You should also keep the side rails up.

CULTURE

Care should be individualized and sensitive, with an open and inquiring attitude about cultural beliefs and behaviors (Cooper, Grywalski, Lamp, Newhouse, & Studlien, 2007). The woman's admission for labor and birth may be her first exposure to the health care system. Beliefs and practices related to childbirth are part of culture and they will be different between the Western and non-Western cultures. To understand the patient's expectations and desires, you may need to use a translator or translation service. Record the name of the translator in the medical records.

Be sensitive to the patient's unique needs. You will need to determine who will make decisions, the patient or a member of her family. Note dietary preferences for hot or cold food, or no preference. Note if she is a vegetarian. Identify her comfort with eye contact and touch. If you learn of her desires for her infant son's circumcision, or infant feeding, or customs related to clothing or praise for the newborn, discuss those with the postpartum nursing staff when you give your report. To learn more about the psyche, spirituality, and the cultural dimensions of care, see chapter 10.

DEPRESSION

Pregnant women should avoid taking Paxil (paroxetine, an antidepressant), because it increases the risk of fetal heart defects. The intrapartal nurse needs to gather information related to maternal behavior and characteristics to appreciate their potential impact on the mother and her child during labor and birth. Depression before childbirth increases the risk of postpartum depression.

DIABETES

Pregnancy increases the risk of diabetes because it creates a state of insulin resistance and reduced sensitivity to the action

Exhibit 2.3: Body mass index calculation.

$$BMI = \frac{weight\ (kg)}{height^2\ (m^2)} \qquad BMI = 703 \times \frac{weight\ (lb)}{height^2\ (in^2)}$$

BMI (kg/m²)	19	20	21	22	23	24	25	26	27	28	29	30	35	40
Height (in.)	Weight (lb.)													
58	91	96	100	105	110	115	119	124	129	134	138	143	167	191
59	94	99	104	109	114	119	124	128	133	138	143	148	173	198
60	97	102	107	112	118	123	128	133	138	143	148	153	179	204
61	100	106	111	116	122	127	132	137	143	148	153	158	185	211
62	104	109	115	120	126	131	136	142	147	153	158	164	191	218
63	107	113	118	124	130	135	141	146	152	158	163	169	197	225
64	110	116	122	128	134	140	145	151	157	163	169	174	204	232
65	114	120	126	132	138	144	150	156	162	168	174	180	210	240
66	118	124	130	136	142	148	155	161	167	173	179	186	216	247
67	121	127	134	140	146	153	159	166	172	178	185	191	223	255
68	125	131	138	144	151	158	164	171	177	184	190	197	230	262
69	128	135	142	149	155	162	169	176	182	189	196	203	236	270
70	132	139	146	153	160	167	174	181	188	195	202	207	243	278
71	136	143	150	157	165	172	179	186	193	200	208	215	250	286
72	140	147	154	162	169	177	184	191	199	206	213	221	258	294
73	144	151	159	166	174	182	189	197	204	212	219	227	265	302
74	148	155	163	171	179	186	194	202	210	218	225	233	272	311
75	152	160	168	176	184	192	200	208	216	224	232	240	279	319
76	156	164	172	180	189	197	205	213	221	230	238	246	287	328

of insulin (American College of Obstetricians and Gynecologists, 2005b). And diabetes significantly increases the risk of a poor birth outcome. Screening for diabetes usually takes place between 24 and 28 weeks of gestation. The screening test requires the woman to ingest a solution that contains 50 grams of glucose. One hour later her blood will be drawn. If her glucose is 140 mg/dL or higher (7.8 mmol/L), she will need a 100-gram, 3-hour glucose tolerance test (GTT).

The diagnosis of gestational diabetes will be made based on the results of the GTT. If two of the four plasma glucose values are abnormal, she will be diagnosed with gestational diabetes. The four abnormal plasma glucose values are: greater

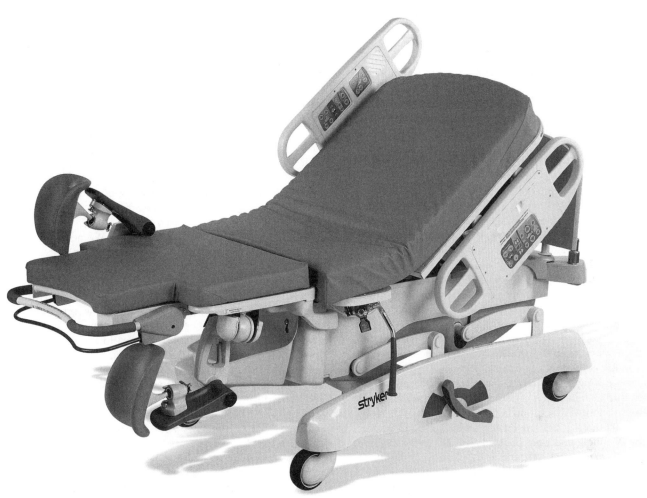

Figure 2.1: Fully equipped birthing bed designed for general patient care use. The standard configuration is 475 pounds. With all options and accessories, the bed weighs 525 pounds. Maximum patient weight (safe working load) suggested for this bed is 500 pounds (227 kilograms). (Reproduced with permission of Stryker Corporation, Portage, MI.)

than 105 mg/dL fasting, greater than 190 mg/dL at 1 hour, greater than 165 mg/dL at 2 hours, and greater than 145 mg/dL at 3 hours (American Diabetes Association, 1999). When a woman is diagnosed with gestational diabetes, diet therapy may be prescribed for at least 2 weeks before insulin is prescribed. However, if her fasting glucose is above 95 mg/dL, insulin may be prescribed after only 1 week of dietary therapy (McFarland, Langer, Conway, & Berkus, 1999).

Gestational diabetes occurs in approximately 4% of all pregnant women in the United States. In some ethnic groups, this level is as high as 14% (Kahn, Davies, Lynch, Reynolds, & Barbour, 2006). For example, Hispanic American, Native American, Asian American, African American, and Pacific Islanders have a higher prevalence of diabetes than non-Hispanic White women (American Diabetes Association, 1999). Women who are overweight or obese also have an increased risk for developing gestational diabetes.

Gestational diabetes increases the risk of fetal macrosomia, neonatal hypoglycemia, hypocalcemia, polycythemia, and jaundice (American Diabetes Association, 1999). The incidence of spina bifida and anencephaly increases when women have diabetes or are obese. Daily folic acid supplements reduce the risk of these neural tube defects (Case, Ramadhani, Canfield, Beverly, & Wood, 2007).

Women with diabetes are at risk for hypoglycemia and hyperglycemia. Signs of maternal hypoglycemia may include cold sweats, irritability, dizziness, blurred vision, confusion, headache, tremors or twitching, lethargy, tingling of the tongue and/or lips, palpitations, slurred speech, inability to speak (aphasia), and loss of consciousness. These signs should be immediately reported to the physician. A fingerstick blood glucose should be obtained. If the woman is conscious and the blood glucose is less than 60 mg/dL, the physician may order an IV of 5% dextrose or 10% dextrose in water, or 4 ounces of orange juice or apple juice. If she is confused or agitated and the fingerstick glucose is less than 60 mg/dL, an immediate serum blood glucose is usually obtained and the physician should be immediately notified. An intravenous dextrose solution should be administered. The fingerstick blood glucose should be repeated 10 minutes and 1 hour after initiating the intravenous infusion. Changes in maternal behavior should be recorded. If the woman is comatose or seizing, an immediate serum blood glucose should be obtained, the physician should be notified immediately, an intravenous line should be initiated, and a minimum of 50 mL of 50% dextrose will probably be ordered for stat administration. After 10 minutes, the fingerstick glucose should be reassessed. If there is no improvement, another 25 mL of the 50% glucose solution may be ordered for IV push stat. Assessments may be performed at 15-minute intervals until the patient is stable. Assess maternal vital signs, the level of consciousness, fingerstick glucose, and signs and symptoms of hypoglycemia.

Signs of maternal hyperglycemia include thirst, hunger, frequent urination, blurry vision, and high blood sugar. Assess the fingerstick glucose and follow physician orders for insulin. Usually a sliding scale has been ordered. If there are sliding scale insulin orders, administer insulin and notify the physician of your assessments and actions. Continue to evaluate your patient after the administration of insulin and document changes in her condition.

Diabetes during labor may be managed differently. For example, if an insulin drip is ordered, you may be administering an intravenous (IV) solution of 0.9% sodium chloride (100 mL) with 100 units of regular insulin added to the solution. Label the IV tubing and fluid bags. In addition to the insulin infusion, you may be asked to infuse 5% dextrose in lactated Ringer's solution as a backup solution. Other fluids or medication will probably be administered in a solution of lactated Ringer's or 0.45% normal saline. Endocrinologists may order the continuous use of an insulin pump during labor or there may be orders for insulin on a sliding scale. You will continue to monitor glucose using a glucose monitoring device. Vital signs should be assessed and recorded at a minimum of every hour, or more frequently, based on the patient condition. Review the results of any laboratory tests and report findings promptly to the physician. Document your actions, drugs given, and any patient teaching.

Signs of ketoacidosis may include shortness of breath, a fruity odor on the breath, ketones in the urine, dry or flushed skin, nausea, vomiting, abdominal pain, and confusion. Loss of consciousness is also possible. Notify the physician of any of these signs. If possible, dip the urine to assess ketones.

DOMESTIC VIOLENCE

Physical or mental abuse is a major concern, especially when the pregnant woman is younger than 18 years of age (Marasinghe & Amarasinghe, 2007). Abuse occurs most frequently prior to 18 weeks of gestation (Connolly, Katz, Bash, McMahon, & Hansen, 1997).

Domestic violence has also been called spouse abuse, battering, or intimate partner violence. Whichever name is used, the woman is the victim of an individual with whom she has had an intimate or romantic relationship (Allen, 2005). Domestic violence is a pattern of behaviors exhibited by the partner to establish power and control, and may include physical abuse, sexual abuse, emotional abuse, economic abuse, threats, isolation, pet abuse, intimidation, stalking, kidnapping, false imprisonment, use of children to maintain fear and power over the woman, and often combinations of these behaviors (Allen, 2005).

Violence against pregnant women affects 1 in 100 (1%) to 1 in 5 (20%) women (American College of Obstetricians and Gynecologists, 1998; Huzel & Remsburg-Bell, 1996). If these women seek prenatal care, a screening questionnaire may help identify women who have been victims of domestic violence (Yost, Bloom, McIntire, & Leveno, 2005). Women who are verbally abused have a greater incidence of babies with a low birth weight. Physical abuse increases the risk of neonatal death (Yost, Bloom, McIntire, & Leveno, 2005). To elicit honest responses, questions about abuse must be asked in private, between the provider and the patient only. It is important to express the belief that abuse is not the woman's fault and to ensure her confidentiality. Documentation of the abuse is critical, including photographs of injuries, if possible. These photographs should be taken only with the woman's permission. Education about community resources should be offered. The period during labor and birth is not the time or place to encourage her to leave her partner. Your goal is to provide her with a safe environment where she can undergo labor and deliver her child.

To determine if a woman has been the victim of abuse, it will be necessary to interview her alone. You will need to ask about violence when you gather information related to her social history. A key question to ask her is: "Have you been hit, punched, or otherwise hurt by someone within the past year?" You will need to follow up with, "If so, by whom?" and "Do you feel safe in your current relationship?" You might also ask, "Is a partner from a previous relationship making you feel unsafe now?" You should assess her for stress in her relationship, safety, and what happens if she disagrees with her partner. Ask her if she has been hurt and if her friends or family know. If she is in danger, determine if she has a safe place to go in case of an emergency. You may need to work to obtain a consultation with a social worker or counselor so she can discuss her situation and develop a plan.

Sexual assault was experienced by 68% of battered and physically abused women in a study conducted in Texas. Sexual assault often occurs concurrently with physical assault. Battered women have a high level of posttraumatic stress and are more likely to terminate their pregnancies than women who were not sexually abused. Posttraumatic stress may manifest as depression with symptoms of sleep disturbances and hypervigilance (McFarlane et al., 2005). Stress is related to poor pregnancy outcomes and low infant birth weight (Curry

Durham, Bullock, Bloom, & Davis, 2006). Hispanic women had higher posttraumatic stress disorder test scores than African American women or White women (McFarlane et al., 2005).

The abuser is generally possessive and jealous, and tends to be controlling of everyday family activities (Allen, 2005). Unfortunately, even with psychosocial interventions, there may be no overall improvement in maternal health or the incidence of low birth weight.

You should suspect abuse if the woman presents with multiple injuries. Women who suffer from battered woman's syndrome often feel overwhelming guilt and depression, loss of appetite, and insomnia. The abuser often has low self-esteem, anger, depression, and paranoia (Allen, 2005).

Always knock before entering the patient's room. If you cannot communicate in the language the patient understands, find a translator. It should not be a family member. Prior to asking sensitive questions, introduce yourself by name and licensure and maintain eye contact. The woman should be in street clothes when questions are asked, and her privacy must be maintained. Childhood sexual abuse screening questions may include, "Have you ever been forced to have sex?" or "What age were you when you first had intercourse?" or "How was it growing up in your house?" or "Did anyone ever touch you in a way that was uncomfortable?" or "As a child, were you ever abused physically, emotionally, or sexually?" Respond with affirmation and acceptance in a calm, nonjudgmental, empathetic manner. Statements such as "You are not to blame for what has happened" or "You have done nothing wrong" are supportive. It has been suggested that documentation of her abuse history should occur with her permission and that there should be an offer to refer her to agencies, therapists, or literature. If she has been a victim of childhood sexual abuse, touch may be viewed as invasive, intrusive, or noxious. Therefore, it is important to ask her how she would like to be cared for, especially during labor. She may want to wear undergarments during labor or have a stuffed animal or favorite blanket with her. She will need support to maintain control, education to understand sensations and experiences during the labor and birth process, and acknowledgement of her perceptions (Hobbins, 2004).

Some women who present at the hospital are labeled as "frequent fliers." They may present once a week or more often. Rather than judge them, it is important to determine what continues to bring them into the hospital, especially when they are not in labor. Perhaps some of these women are the victims of domestic violence. It will be important to ask them (without their partner around), "Do you feel safe at home?" or "Have you been hit recently in the abdomen or head?" Other questions you can ask are, "Within the past year have you been hit, slapped, kicked, or otherwise physically hurt by anyone?" You can ask "Have you ever been emotionally or physically abused by your partner or someone important to you?" Other questions to ask include, "Within the last year, has anyone forced you to have sex?" or "Are you afraid of your partner or anyone you know?" If you have a patient who does not speak English, it is important to find a translator. These questions in Spanish include: "¿En el año pasado, alguien le ha golpedo, pateado o herido fisicamente?," "¿Ha sido usted abusada emocionalmente o fisicamente por su pareja o por alguna persona importante para usted?," "¿En el año pasado, alguien le ha forzado a tener relación sexual?," and "¿Tiene usted miedo de su parejo o de alguien a quien usted conoce?"

Physical abuse signs may not be evident. If she has back pain, for example, in the lower back or near a kidney, think retroperitoneal bleed. This can be caused by blunt trauma. Is she pale, diaphoretic, with a systolic blood pressure below 100 mm Hg and a pulse above 100 beats per minute? She may be in hypovolemic shock. What is the mean arterial pressure? It should be between 70 and 100 mm Hg. If it is less than 60 mm Hg, there will be inadequate blood flow to her brain, heart, kidneys, and the uterus (Wagner, Johnson, & Kidd, 2006). The fetus will show you signs that she is bleeding before she does. Is the fetus tachycardic? Are there decelerations? If the maternal organs become ischemic, she may suffer from multiple organ dysfunction and even death. Share the information you gain with the physician and expect an immediate evaluation if you suspect internal bleeding. Expect the physician to order either a computed tomography (CT) scan or ultrasound of the abdomen or even surgery, such as a stat cesarean section. Consult members of your chain of command if the maternal or fetal status is deteriorating and/or there is not a prompt physician response. Be sure a type, screen, and complete blood count were drawn, especially when you suspect internal bleeding. If she is bleeding into the retroperitoneal space and/or in shock, her fetus is at risk of dying from uterine ischemia. She must have a large-bore intravenous catheter, that is, an 18- or 16-gauge catheter. If you have difficulty inserting the catheter, obtain help from another skilled nurse or an anesthesia provider. Continue to monitor the fetus closely. Although a retroperitoneal bleed is a physician diagnosis, your ability to elicit information about being hit recently or experiencing trauma in her pelvic area may be a life-saving question. Ask the patient about any recent falls, and get the details of when and where the fall occurred. Share the information with the physician.

FIBROIDS

If the ultrasound reports are in the prenatal chart, note the presence of fibroids (leiomyomas) and their location. If they are behind the placenta, for example, retroplacental, there is an increased risk of an abruption (Rice, Kay, & Mahony, 1989). If they are in the lower segment of the uterus, they may act as an obstruction to fetal descent and vaginal delivery. Fibroids also increase the risk of fetal malpresentation, preterm delivery, and cesarean section (Klatsky, Tran, Caughey, & Fujimoto, 2008).

HEMORRHAGE: DETERMINE THE RISKS

You should first assess your patient's blood type and her history of blood transfusions. If she has a history of transfusions, ask her when and why she received a transfusion. For example, after a motor vehicle accident she might have received several units of blood and blood products. After a transfusion, some women develop antibodies that cross the placenta and cause fetal hemolysis. The tendency to bleed, on the other hand, may be inherited. To anticipate a possible postpartum hemorrhage, ask the nulliparous woman's mother, if she is present, if she had any unusual bleeding after giving birth, or if she needed to receive a transfusion. Some causes of bleeding are genetic, such as Von Willebrand's disease or a Factor 8 or 9 deficiency. There is a myth that women with red hair bleed more heavily after delivery or have a higher risk of hemorrhage. This is not true. They may bruise more often than women with black or dark-brown hair, but they have normal coagulation tests (Liem, Hollensead, Joiner, & Sessler, 2006).

Risk factors for hemorrhage during pregnancy include trauma, placenta previa, and placental abruption. Abruption may be related to intrauterine growth restriction, a placental infarction, or trauma. Trauma occurs in approximately 7% of all pregnancies and trauma includes falls, burns, motor vehicle accidents, and physical abuse and battery (Huzel & Remsburg-Bell, 1996). After a motor vehicle accident, uterine activity and the fetal heart rate will be monitored. If you note frequent contractions and even uterine irritability (small contractions with little to no time between them), with or without abnormal vital signs or pain, this may be evidence of a placental abruption. Report your findings to the midwife or physician.

Other risk factors for postpartum hemorrhage include pre-eclampsia, multiple gestation (for example, a twin pregnancy), Asian ethnicity, Hispanic ethnicity, and nulliparity (Combs, Murphy, Laros Jr., 1991). Other factors include a past history of postpartum hemorrhage, a second stage of labor longer than 1 hour, a forceps delivery, and incomplete expulsion of the placenta, that is, placental tissue remains in the uterus (Henry, Birch, Sullivan, Katz, & Wang, 2005). Women who have labor lasting longer than 12 hours, women with a baby weighing more than 4,000 grams, and women who had a fever in labor also have an increased risk for postpartum hemorrhage. Women with Von Willebrand's disease or who have a Factor 8 or 9 deficiency also have an increased risk of hemorrhage.

You must report abnormal vital signs such as maternal tachycardia or hypotension to the physician immediately. Include your observations such as pallor, any vaginal bleeding, shortness of breath, or other unusual findings. Confirm there is a patent intravenous line. Determine who is available to obtain blood and blood products. Determine if there are any contraindications for blood administration, such as the religious beliefs of the patient. Is she a Jehovah's Witness? Work with the certified nurse midwife or physician to create a plan of care if she needs blood and refuses. For an in-depth discussion of postpartal hemorrhage, see chapter 3.

HERBS

Some herbs should never be used during pregnancy. For example, goldenseal has oxytocin-like actions, and dong quai, ephe-dra, chaste tree, and black or blue cohosh are uterine stimulants. Chamomile tea, known as yerba buena, is an antispasmodic and may be taken as a sedative for insomnia. When zinc is consumed at higher than the recommended daily allowance (15 mg/day), there is an increased risk of premature birth and stillbirth (Born & Barron, 2005). If a woman is contracting and is preterm, it is especially important to assess her herb use. Document herb use in the medical record.

Ginger (zingiber officinale) has been used as a therapy to treat nausea and vomiting during pregnancy and it may be safe and effective. Adverse effects of ginger include headache, diarrhea, abdominal discomfort, drowsiness, heartburn, and reflux (Borrelli, Capasso, Aviello, Pittler, & Izzo, 2005). Some physicians suggest that one cannot assume dietary supplements are safe for the embryo or fetus and that it is imprudent, and possibly unethical, to conduct research related to ginger or other herbs (Marcus & Snodgrass, 2005). However, in six studies when ginger was used as a dietary supplement or a spice, there were no adverse effects on pregnancy outcomes (Schwertner, Rios, & Pascoe, 2006). More research appears to be needed to determine if ginger and ginger root powders and extracts are safe during pregnancy.

Another adverse effect of some herbs is bleeding. Garlic and ginseng inhibit aggregation of platelets and ginkgo biloba is a vascular relaxant that also causes reduced platelet aggregation and increases bleeding time (Burnham, 1995; Dasgupta, 2003; Gilbert, 1997; Greenspan, 1983; Rose, Croissant, Parliament, & Leven, 1990).

> **Documentation example**: Patient reports use of chamomile tea today. Also admits to use of blue cohosh last week and to taking 30 mg of zinc supplements daily for the last month. Contracting every 2 minutes for 60 to 70 seconds, mild to moderate.

Infections and Sexually Transmitted Diseases

Sexually transmitted diseases that are untreated pose a risk to the infant. For example, gonorrhea, chlamydia, trichomoniasis, hepatitis B and C, herpes, syphilis (*T. pallidum*), and human immunodeficiency virus (HIV) can be transmitted to the fetus.

Chlamydia

Chlamydia is a sexually transmitted infection and the most commonly reported infectious disease in the United States (Ravin, 2007). If untreated, women develop pelvic inflammatory disease (PID) and may become infertile. Untreated chlamydia infection may result in preterm delivery and neonatal infection.

Group B Streptococcus

Group B streptococcus (GBS) is the most common cause of infections and death in newborns (Gavino & Wang, 2007; Kim, Page, McKenna, & Kim, 2005). It is also known as genital strep (Group B) or beta hemolytic streptococcus, Group B. It is found in the vagina, cervix, and rectum. The Centers for Disease Control and Prevention (CDC) released revised recommendations for GBS screening and prevention. They recommend all pregnant women be screened at 35 to 37 weeks of gestation for vaginal and rectal GBS colonization. If GBS is found in a patient's urine during the pregnancy, she should receive antibiotics during labor. If your patient previously gave birth to an infant who had GBS, she will need antibiotics during labor. If her GBS status is unknown at the time of labor, she should receive antibiotics during labor. In addition, antibiotics should be administered if the gestation is less than 37 weeks, the membranes rupture preterm, the membranes have been ruptured 18 or more hours, or she has a fever. Typically 5 million units of penicillin G is the initial dose, followed by 2.5 million units intravenously every 4 hours until delivery. Alternatively, the initial dose may be ordered as Ampicillin 2 grams intravenously followed by 1 gram every 4 hours until delivery (Alvarez, Williams, Ganesh, & Apuzzio, 2007; Schrag, Gorwitz, Fultz-Butts, & Schuchat, 2002).

Hepatitis B and C

Exposure to the hepatitis B virus is tested during prenatal care. Exposure to the hepatitis C virus is not usually tested during prenatal care. However, women who are infected with the hepatitis B virus are at an increased risk for infection with hepatitis C. Most infants who have hepatitis acquired it in utero from their mothers. Hepatitis C virus transmission may not be decreased by a cesarean section (McIntyre, Tosh, & McGuire, 2006). There is no vaccine for hepatitis C. There is a vaccine for hepatitis B. About 1 in 20 women who have the hepatitis C virus transmit it to their infant. These children may not develop liver problems until later in their childhood. Persons infected with hepatitis may develop liver fibrosis, cirrhosis, or even liver cancer. It is estimated that as many as 3% of pregnant women in Europe and North America have hepatitis C. The incidence is higher in substance abusers who inject drugs intravenously using contaminated needles (McIntyre, Tosh, & McGuire, 2006). Nurses who work in labor and delivery must follow universal precautions when they come in contact with any body secretions. Personal protective equipment, including gloves, should be worn prior to patient examinations in which you will be exposed to blood or body fluids.

Herpes Simplex Virus Type 2

Routine screening for herpes is not cost-effective and is not a routine part of prenatal care (Thung & Grobman, 2005). However, at the first prenatal visit, a woman should be asked if she or her partner has genital herpes, which is caused by herpes simplex virus type 2 (HSV-2). For HSV-2 positive women, drugs such as acyclovir, to suppress outbreaks, may be prescribed. A laboratory test is used to identify the presence of this virus (Morrow & Brown, 2005).

More than 25% of adults in the United States are infected with HSV-2. When pregnant woman who had HSV-2 were given valacyclovir to suppress the infection after 36 weeks of gestation, there was less recurrence of genital herpes. In addition, the need for a cesarean section decreased (Sheffield et al., 2005).

Some women may have a primary genital herpes infection at the time they present in labor and delivery. Therefore, it will be important to look for lesions when her perineal area is exposed. Provide privacy when asking about genital herpes as sometimes the woman's partner is unaware that she has this infection. When women with a history of HSV-2 present during labor, they should be asked about lesions or active outbreaks. It is important to create a trusting atmosphere without the partner present when asking about these lesions. In some cases, an occlusive clear dressing will be applied over the lesion.

Human Immunodeficiency Virus

The number of childbearing women and adolescent girls who have human immunodeficiency viruse (HIV) has increased from 14% in 1992 to 22% in 2003. HIV infection is due to heterosexual exposure in 80% of women and girls who have the disease. While it is not the standard of care, the Centers for Disease Control and Prevention (CDC) in the United States recommend rapid HIV testing in labor and delivery (Tyer-Viola, 2007). Some women and girls with known HIV avoid prenatal care due to fear of discrimination. Therefore, it is imperative that nurses set aside any prejudices or fear they may have and provide respectful, dignified care to all of their patients.

HIV screening is not mandated in most states of the United States. However the CDC recommends voluntary HIV screening as a routine part of medical care for patients aged 13 to 64 years (Hellwig, 2007). HIV transmission to the fetus may occur by microtransfusion of maternal blood across the placenta or during labor or delivery (Cibulka, 2006). Approximately 39 million people worldwide were living with AIDS at the end of 2004. Known HIV-infected women will be taking antiretroviral (ARV) drugs such as Retrovir or AZT (zidovudine) or Viramune (nevirapine). Usually more than one antiretroviral drug will be prescribed. Typically women with HIV may take Combivir (lamivudine and zidovudine). These are nucleoside analog reverse transcriptase inhibitors. All antiretroviral drugs can be toxic and they cross the placenta (Cibulka, 2006). Toxicity can damage the nerves, muscles, heart, and pancreas, and usually lead to lactic acidosis. The patient may have hemolysis, elevated liver enzymes, and a low platelet count, which mimics HELLP syndrome of severe preeclampsia (Lachat, Scott, & Relf, 2006).

Delivery is usually planned as an elective cesarean section. However, if that plan is refused, antiretroviral drugs will be administered during labor. One regimen is to administer zidovudine intravenously (2 mg/kg) over the first hour, then 1 mg/kg/hour until delivery. Zidovudine might also be ordered as 600 mg by mouth at the onset of labor and 300 mg by mouth every 3 hours until delivery. Zidovudine is often given with lamivudine (3TC) 150 mg by mouth at the onset of labor and

150 mg by mouth every 12 hours until delivery (Lachat, Scott, & Relf, 2006). If your patient has HIV or AIDS, invasive procedures should be avoided to minimize fetal exposure to maternal blood. You should also avoid artificial rupture of membranes, the application of a fetal spiral electrode, fetal scalp sampling, vacuum extraction, and the application of forceps (Lachat, Scott, & Relf, 2006).

Some women have HIV but do not know they are infected. Acute HIV infection often produces symptoms of a nonspecific infectious illness resembling mononucleosis, and the patient may not know she has been infected. Unfortunately, most women learn about their HIV infection when their child is diagnosed (Norman & Leonard, 2005). Therefore, universal precautions should be practiced by all health care workers to prevent disease exposure.

Listeria

Listeriosis is an infection caused by eating food contaminated with *Listeria monocytogenes*. Pregnant women are more likely than a member of the healthy general population to contract this disease (Moos, 2006). Listeria grows in soil, wood, decaying matter, and is found in the refrigerator, especially if it is set at more than 40 degrees Fahrenheit. The freezer should be set at 0 degrees Fahrenheit or lower. Listeriosis increases the risk of miscarriage and premature delivery. Signs and symptoms of listeriosis are fever, chills, muscle aches, diarrhea, and upset stomach. Some women or their fetuses die from this infection. To avoid exposure to listeria, pregnant women should not eat hot dogs, luncheon meats, bologna, or other deli meats unless they are reheated until they are steaming hot. They should avoid eating refrigerated pâté, meat spreads from a meat counter, or refrigerated seafood, such as salmon, trout, whitefish, cod, tuna, or mackerel as they can harbor listeria. Fish should be cooked or be from a can. Unpasteurized milk is a source of listeria. Salads made in a store, such as a ham salad, chicken salad, egg salad, tuna salad, or seafood salad can be a source of listeria. Soft cheese, such as feta, queso blanco, queso fresco, brie, camembert, blue-veined cheeses, and panela must be pasteurized to avoid exposure to listeria (see www.fsis.usda.gov). Cheeses such as mozzarella, pasteurized processed cheese slices and spreads, cream cheese, and cottage cheese are safe to eat (Moos, 2006).

Syphilis

Women with a positive Venereal Disease Reference Laboratory (VDRL) titer should be treated for syphilis. Treatment with penicillin may cause a Jarisch-Herxheimer reaction with fever, chills, muscle aches, headache, and even hypotension within 2 to 24 hours. During that time, contractions, fetal distress, and fetal death have been reported (Klein, Cox, Mitchell, & Wendel Jr., 1990). Therefore, if the patient is in your unit, monitor her, her contractions, and the fetal heart rate closely during and after antibiotics are administered. Report abnormal findings to the midwife or physician. If she is allergic to penicillin, erythromycin or another antibiotic may be prescribed.

Even if she receives antibiotics, the infant may still be born with congenital syphilis (Sheffield et al., 2002).

Toxoplasma gondii

Toxoplasma gondii increases the risk of preterm birth, premature rupture of the membranes, and low-birth-weight infants (Simhan et al., 2007). Pregnant women should avoid cats and cat litter as the cat can excrete oocysts (zygotes) of *Toxoplasma gondii*, which can then be transmitted from mother to fetus. Congenital toxoplasmosis, a parasitic infection of the fetus, occurs only when the mother is infected with the parasite for the first time. Transmission of this parasite increases with gestational age. If the mother contracts the *Toxoplasma gondii* infection, there will be no overt symptoms. The infant may develop lesions in the eyes and brain. Prenatal treatment may not prevent maternal–child transmission (The Systematic Review on Congenital Toxoplasmosis (SYROCOT) Study Group, 2007).

URINARY TRACT INFECTIONS, CHORIOAMNIONITIS, AND CEREBRAL PALSY

If available, use diagnostic reagent strips for urinalysis to assess the presence of glucose, bilirubin, ketones, specific gravity, blood, pH, protein, urobilinogen, nitrite, and/or leukocytes. Test results may provide insight related to your patient's carbohydrate metabolism, kidney and liver function, acid-base balance, and the presence of a urinary tract infection (UTI). Note any verbal complaints about burning when she urinates and observe for any blood in the urine.

There is an established relationship between a UTI during pregnancy and the risk of the infant having mental retardation and developmental delay (McDermott, Callaghan, Szwejbka, Mann, & Daguise, 2000). This does not mean that every mother who has a UTI during pregnancy will have an infant with brain damage. However, maternal infection during pregnancy increases the risk of brain damage when the fetus experiences the fetal inflammatory response syndrome (FIRS). Researchers have found that there is a fourfold increased risk of a child with cerebral palsy when there was a UTI during pregnancy versus no UTI (Polivka, Nickel, & Wilkins Jr., 1997). Infant brain damage can occur even when the woman takes antibiotics.

> **Documentation example:** Urine positive for protein and blood, negative for ketones. No burning or pain with urination. Dr. Babiesarus notified.

Preterm and term infants who were exposed to a maternal infection at the time of delivery had a threefold increased risk of developing cerebral palsy (Neufeld, Frigon, Graham, & Mueller 2005). In addition, Wu and Colford (2000) performed a meta-analysis and found chorioamnionitis was a risk factor for both cerebral palsy and periventricular leukomalacia. Cystic periventricular leukomalacia in preterm infants was related to a maternal urinary tract infection when patients were admitted with a diagnosis of preterm labor (Spinillo et al., 1998).

TRIAGE

Triage is the place to evaluate a patient and her fetus. Registered nurses who work in a triage setting will need to be competent enough to assess the patient, identify problems, determine her acuity, and communicate with personnel to meet the patient's needs (Mahlmeister & Van Mullem, 2000). In triage, midwives, nurse practitioners, physician's assistants, and physicians diagnose and make management decisions to admit, deliver, or discharge the patient. Occasionally, triage will be used to evaluate gynecologic patients or postoperative or postpartum patients (Ciranni & Essex, 2007). Sometimes triage units include a separate fetal assessment area and a holding area where versions and other procedures are performed (Angelini, 2006).

Typical patients in an obstetric triage unit include women who report decreased fetal movement, term and preterm labor, women who present after trauma, premature or spontaneous rupture of membranes, pregnancy-induced hypertension, infections, deep vein thrombosis, dehydration, complaints of shortness of breath, chest pain, and gastrointestinal disease (Jenkin-Capiello, 2000). The data you collect will be critical to assisting the midwife or physician so that he or she can make an accurate diagnosis and avoid unnecessary procedures or surgery.

Triage is an area designated for outpatient services (Ciranni & Essex, 2007). Triage is also defined as a visual assessment and acuity assignment by a qualified health care provider for the purpose of identifying obstetrical emergency or life-threatening problems. Federal law in the United States related to the Emergency Medical Treatment and Active Labor Act (EMTALA), Title 42, Part 489.20 requires that a log be maintained in the emergency department for pregnant women, 20 weeks or more, who are sent to the obstetrics department for their screening. This is called the "central log." However, if a pregnant woman bypasses the emergency department, there should be a log kept in the triage area or in the obstetrics department. Do you know where the log is? Do you know who enters data into the log? It is computerized?

When a woman presents to triage, a medical screening examination should be performed to determine if an emergency medical condition exists. She must be stabilized when an emergency medical condition exists, and the physician must certify that there are benefits of transfer that outweigh the risks (Angelini & Mahlmeister, 2005). Once screened, her acuity must be determined. Acuity has been categorized as follows:

Category I patients have life-threatening problems, such as diabetic ketoacidosis, seizures, preterm labor, or decreased fetal movement. One to 2% of pregnancies are complicated with an obstetrical emergency (Clements, Flohr-Rincon, Bombard, & Catanzarite, 2007).

Category II patients may be dehydrated, have a fever, or be in active labor. They may be uninjured. When nulliparous women presented to the hospital in the latent phase of labor, their risk of a cesarean section increased from 6.7% to 14.2%. They also had double the odds for an arrest of the active phase of labor, oxytocin use, insertion of an intrauterine pressure catheter and/or a fetal spiral electrode, and almost a threefold increase in chorioamnionitis (Bailit, Dierker, Blanchard, & Mercer, 2005). The cause of these outcomes was not determined. However, if nulliparous women are in the hospital in early labor and their screening in triage reveals maternal and fetal well-being, it may be best to send them home with instructions to return when they are in active labor.

Category III patients do not need urgent care. For example, they may have a urinary tract infection or need a nonstress test or a scheduled procedure such as an induction. Determine if your hospital has a policy or procedure for triage and how various patient conditions are categorized.

Clinical example of an incomplete admission assessment following suspected trauma: A nulliparous woman presented to labor and delivery at 29 weeks of gestation after she had fallen down 7 stairs 3 1/2 hours prior to her arrival. She had no pain, no vaginal bleeding, no uterine tenderness, and no contractions. She had an abraded right knee, a tender right shoulder, and an active fetus. She did not fall on her abdomen. A brief fetal monitor tracing revealed a heart rate in the 80 to 90 beats per minute range. Maternal vital signs were not recorded. Without obtaining an admission strip or applying a pulse oximeter to continuously monitor the maternal rate while the fetal rate was recorded, a second-year resident scanned the abdomen to locate the fetal heart. The resident did not evaluate the fundal placenta for an abruption, did see the fetal heart rate beating at a rate in the 80 to 90 bpm range, did not look for fetal movement, and called another second-year resident. That second-year resident agreed with the resident who performed the ultrasound, and they both decided to call for an immediate cesarean section. They did not call the in-hospital obstetrician for a second opinion, and they did not wait for the attending obstetrician to arrive. The nurse did not suggest they get a longer tracing or report that there was fetal movement. They performed the cesarean section. The baby was born with high Apgar scores and was diagnosed with an arrhythmia. Second-degree heart block is the most common fetal bradyarrhythmia. The most common dysrhythmia is premature atrial contractions (PACs). The neonate was diagnosed with premature atrial contractions with some blocked PACs. Because the baby was premature there was an intracranial bleed, and the child now has mild cerebral palsy.

In some hospitals, women who are not in labor and not dilated will be sent home. In other settings, she will be asked to walk for an hour or two and her cervix will be rechecked.

It is a myth that walking will speed up dilation. Researchers reviewed the findings of the very best studies (randomized controlled trials). They pooled the data from seven of these studies, which included 2,166 women, and could find no evidence that an upright position or walking reduced the duration of the first stage of labor or the number of cesarean sections (Souza, Miquelutti, Cecatti, & Makuch, 2006).

INFORMED CONSENT

The purpose of the informed consent process is to help patients understand their diagnoses and recommended treatment, potential complications, and treatment options. A signed informed consent is not required for tests such as a nonstress test. However, it is required for invasive procedures such as a cesarean section. In an emergency, state law may allow a physician or physicians to decide to perform surgery without a written consent.

The process of obtaining informed consent is an expression of respect for the patient who has a moral and legal right to bodily integrity, self-determination, and to the support of her freedom within a caring relationship (American College of Obstetricians & Gynecologists, 2005a). This information is given by physicians or midwives and should be documented by them in the medical record. Women should make an informed decision to have a trial of labor after a cesarean section. Some women may be given a booklet to read about vaginal birth after cesarean (VBAC). Patients may have a higher knowledge level after reading the booklet (Shorten, Shorten, Geogh, West, & Morris, 2005). Your duty as a nurse is to determine who informed them of the potential complications and options, and that they understand the plan of care.

Nurses need to confirm that this process took place. They need to know their patient's desires, concerns, and fears. Prior to beginning any procedure that can increase maternal and/ or fetal risk, there also must be evidence of a well-oxygenated fetus. The midwife or physician will document what they did and that the woman understood the risks and benefits of the procedure. For example, the risk of uterine rupture significantly increases when there is less than 2 years between the prior cesarean section and the birth of the current baby. Review the prenatal record to determine the date of her last cesarean section and to see if she received informed consent information from the physician, midwife, or nurse practitioner. If not, ask the physician or midwife to come to the bedside to talk to your patient and to obtain informed consent for the induction or augmentation. This is a high-risk situation and your responsibility is to help your patient make a well-informed decision about her care.

DETERMINE RISK FACTORS

High-risk women have an increased risk of injury and death. The most common causes of maternal death worldwide are infection, hemorrhage, pregnancy-induced hypertension, obstructed labor, and unsafe abortion (Callister, 2005). All types of analgesia and anesthesia are related to an increased risk of

Exhibit 2.4: Examples of some risk factors during pregnancy.

- Diabetes
  - Prepregnancy
  - Gestational
- Hypertension
  - Prepregnancy
  - Gestational
- Thrombophilia (tendency to clot)
- Infections
- Prior preterm labor and/or birth
- History of a poor pregnancy outcome
- Vaginal bleeding during the pregnancy
- Infertility treatment and pregnancy
- Prior cesarean section (cesarean delivery) or previous uterine surgery
- Breech or other noncephalic presentation
- History of prolonged labor
- History of precipitous labor (< 3 hrs during 1st stage)
- Premature rupture of the membranes

fetal acidemia, especially if there is maternal hypotension and/ or respiratory depression (Bonnet, Bruyère, Moufouki, De la Dorie, & Benhamou, 2007). Exhibits 2.4, 2.5, and 2.6 illustrate some of the risk factors that increase the risk of injury to the mother and her infant. Obstructed labor is related to the failure of the fetus to move through the pelvis. To anticipate problems with labor progress, you will need to know your patient's height, weight or body mass index, and an estimated fetal weight. In addition, it is important to know if her pelvis is adequate for a vaginal birth. Find the entry in the prenatal records for clinical pelvimetry. Is the pelvis gynecoid or are there abnormalities?

The day of the week may also be related to an increased risk of injury. It was found that the risk of neonatal death was higher on the weekend possibly due to lower hospital staffing and reduced availability of service (Hamilton & Restrepo, 2003).

Routine episiotomy was found to be no longer advisable in the year 2000 because it contributed to trauma, pain, and suffering (Eason & Feldman, 2000). When it is needed, it does allow faster delivery of the baby's head. Therefore, the midwife or physician will need to decide when it is needed. The use of forceps or a vacuum extractor increases the risk of trauma to the fetus (see Exhibit 2.6).

ASSESS PARITY

Sometimes a woman may not be honest in front of a spouse or partner about prior pregnancies. Therefore, confirm the

Exhibit 2.5: Examples of some labor and delivery risk factors.

• Premature rupture of the membranes

• Induction

• Augmentation

• Nonvertex presentation

• Clinical chorioamnionitis (with fever)

• Meconium staining of the amniotic fluid

• Fetal intolerance of labor and in utero resuscitative measures

• Epidural or spinal anesthesia during labor

• Uterine rupture

• Episiotomy or perineal laceration

Exhibit 2.6: Examples of delivery risk factors.

• Forceps

• Vacuum extractor

pregnancy history in private. It is important to have an accurate history because the duration of labor is related to parity. It is also related to cervical dilatation at the time of admission, the time of rupture of the membranes, professional support, and the use of analgesia (Gross, Hecker, Matterne, Guenter, & Keirse, 2006). Parity reflects the times a woman has given birth to a fetus or fetuses (such as twins) who are 20 or more weeks of gestation with a weight of 400 to 500 grams or more (Bai, Wong, Bauman, & Mohsin, 2002; Beebe, 2005). Parity is not based on the number of babies delivered. For example, delivering one baby who was 23 weeks of gestation categorizes the woman as a gravida 1 para 1. If she delivered twins at 36 weeks, she would be classified as a gravida 1, para 1. Even if the infant was stillborn, that adds to the count or parity.

To help understand the number of births of preterm and term infants, miscarriages or elective abortions, and living children, a system has been devised for parity (P) followed by the letters T-P-A-L. $G_5P_{3-1-0-2}$ means the woman has been pregnant 5 times, had 3 infants at term, 1 who was preterm, no miscarriages or abortions, and 2 living children. Parity is important in planning care since a G_2P_1 often has a faster labor than a G_1P_0.

ASSESS THE ONSET OF LABOR

Normal labor is also called labor eutocia. Labor eutocia occurs between 37 and 42 completed weeks of pregnancy and progresses steadily until there is a vaginal delivery of a fetus in a

vertex presentation. There is a wide variation of opinions on when labor begins. For purposes of this book, labor begins when there are regular contractions (e.g., 5 minutes apart or closer) with a change in the dilatation of the cervix.

To determine if there has been a change in the cervix, review the prenatal record. What was her last dilatation? If you can't find the prenatal record, ask her what her exam was the last time she was at the office. If she had no prenatal care, you will have to determine if she is in labor based on her uterine activity and cervical examination.

Labor can be plotted (see Figures 2.2 and 2.3). The latent phase begins with a change of the cervix and ends when the labor curve begins to ascend. The active phase is known retrospectively from this point of maximum slope or steep incline on the dilatation graph until 10 centimeters. The active phase of labor may begin at 3, 4, or 5 centimeters. The next chapter explains how to evaluate labor using a labor curve.

INTIMATE PIERCINGS

Part of the initial assessment when a woman presents to labor and delivery includes a sterile speculum examination or a vaginal examination to assess the dilatation and effacement of the cervix and the fetal station. When the woman is exposed, you may note an intimate piercing in the clitoral hood. The piercing can lift and retract the clitoral hood and should not obstruct the "exit route" for the baby. The piercing may be horizontal or vertical. Occasionally, the labia minora has a horizontal piercing as well as a horizontal piercing of the clitoral hood. It is less common for women to have a fourchette piercing.

Body piercing breaches the skin, cartilage, or mucous membrane to insert an object, usually jewelry. Genital piercing refers to piercing of the genitalia. Often this is done with a hollow, lancet-point needle that is 12 to 16 gauge. Jewelry that is gold, stainless steel, platinum, niobium, or titanium may be placed once the hole is made.

Female genital piercing of the clitoral hood has been reported to increase sexual desire. More than half of the women with this intimate piercing are between the ages of 19 and 29 years and 76% are White and heterosexual. Forty-five percent of the women studied had a college degree or some college education. Most of the jewelry women wore in this study was made of stainless steel. Some of it was made of titanium or 18-karat gold (Millner, Eichold II, Sharpe, & Lynn, Jr., 2005).

Nipple piercings with nipple rings increase the risk of infection and may cause breast milk to be ejected from the tract created by the piercing (Armstrong, Caliendo, & Roberts, 2006). Women also pierce their abdomens. Removal of these unique pieces of adornment will be easier if you stabilize the piece of jewelry with a hemostat prior to their removal.

KNOW THE BABY: ASSESS THE PAST AND CURRENT FETAL STATUS

It is rare to have a copy of a prenatal record with all the prenatal visits recorded. Therefore, to appreciate the size of

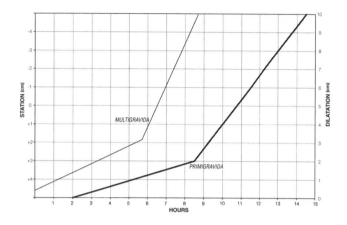

Figure 2.2: Labor curve of multigravida and primigravida women.

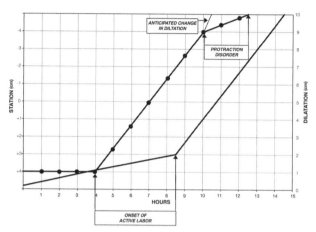

Figure 2.3: Labor curve of a primigravida woman who was not overweight (bottom line) and labor curve of an obese (300 pound) primigravida woman (top line). Note her protraction disorder (slower than normal rate of cervical dilation) near the end of labor and the early onset of her active phase of labor.

the fetus, you may need to measure the fundal height or palpate the fetus through the abdomen to estimate the fetal weight. Is the fetus preterm or term?

To "know the baby" you need to know past heart rates. What fetal heart rates were recorded at each visit? When you apply the fetal monitor or auscultate the rate is the rate similar to those recorded in prenatal record? Can you access any nonstress tests? They can provide additional information about the baby's normal heart rate. For example, if the fetal heart rate (FHR) was near 130 or 140 beats per minute (bpm) during the pregnancy, yet on admission the FHR is in the 160s without accelerations, that's an abnormal finding for that baby. Any abnormalities should be reported to the midwife or physician. In this example, assessment of maternal vital signs may provide clues as to the cause of the tachycardia. If she has an elevated pulse (greater than 100 bpm) and an elevated temperature, there may be an intrauterine infection.

ADMISSION TEST

A low-risk woman may not need to be monitored with the electronic fetal monitor. However, when monitoring is chosen as the surveillance method, the fetal heart rate and uterine activity tracing for the first 20 to 30 minutes has been called a labor admission test. It is a screening test for fetal compromise and will be used to decide to admit or discharge the woman. This initial tracing of the fetus has no impact on women who are low risk. However, it may increase the chance that the women will receive continuous electronic fetal monitoring or other interventions, such as epidural analgesia (Blix, Reinar, Klovning, & Øian, 2005).

Fetal heart rate long-term variability without accelerations is not a good predictor of good or adverse fetal outcomes (Berkus, Langer, Samueloff, Xenakis, & Field, 1999). Spontaneous accelerations discriminate the nonacidotic fetus from the acidotic fetus and are reassuring (Berkus, Langer, Samueloff, Xenakis, & Field, 1999). Fetal asphyxia may be associated with

a FHR rate that has absent to minimal baseline (long term) variability and/or late decelerations and/or prolonged decelerations. Variability was defined as fluctuations in the baseline FHR and was classified based on the amplitude of the peak to trough in beats per minute. Absent variability was a flat or undetectable amplitude and minimal was less than 6 bpm wide (Low, Victory, & Derrick, 1999). If you note absent to minimal long-term variability, late decelerations, or prolonged decelerations in the first 30 minutes of monitoring, notify the midwife and/or physician promptly and ask to evaluate the mother and fetus.

PERFORM A HEAD-TO-TOE ASSESSMENT

If time permits, perform a head-to-toe assessment (see Exhibit 2.7). Assess her skin for warmth, turgor, lacerations, contusions, abrasions, or wounds. Look for a rash, pallor, or cyanosis. Perform a respiratory assessment, noting the shape and symmetry of chest excursion. Listen to breath sounds. Note any cough, the color and consistency of sputum, and the presence of pain when she breathes. Perform a cardiovascular assessment. Palpate the radial pulse and note the rate and rhythm. Assess the blood pressure and heart sounds. Do you see any jugular vein distension or edema? Perform a gastrointestinal assessment. Note the condition of her teeth, gums, and mucous membranes. When did she eat last and what did she eat? Is she constipated or does she have diarrhea? Does she have nausea or vomiting? Assess her urine. What is its color and odor? Does she have flank pain? Assess the fundal height, estimate fetal weight, and assess for any vaginal discharge or bleeding. Perform a neurologic assessment. Note her level of consciousness, orientation, speech, behavior, pupil size and

Exhibit 2.7: Essential items to assess (initial admission database).

Directions: Check if present and/or write comments about your findings in the lines provided.

Item Assessed		Date/Time	Present	Details
Head				
☐	Level of consciousness			
☐	Headache		☐ yes ☐ no	
☐	Dizziness		☐ yes ☐ no	
☐	Blurred vision		☐ yes ☐ no	
☐	Wears contacts or glasses		☐ yes ☐ no	
☐	Facial edema		☐ yes ☐ no	
☐	Other:		☐ yes ☐ no	
Chest				
☐	Epigastric pain		☐ yes ☐ no	
☐	Other:		☐ yes ☐ no	
Heart				
☐	Rate (beats per minute)			
☐	Rhythm (regular or irregular)			
☐	Capillary refill and site assessed		☐ yes ☐ no	
☐	Arms, edema		☐ yes ☐ no	
☐	Legs, edema		☐ yes ☐ no	
☐	Other:		☐ yes ☐ no	
Lungs				
☐	Respiratory rate			
☐	Breath sounds			
☐	Left upper			
☐	Left lower			
☐	Right upper			
☐	Right lower			
☐	Other:			

(continued on next page)

Exhibit 2.7: *(continued)*.

Item Assessed	Date/Time	Present	Details
Abdomen			
☐ Nausea		☐ yes ☐ no	
☐ Vomiting		☐ yes ☐ no	
☐ Pain near or over liver		☐ yes ☐ no	
☐ Contractions		☐ yes ☐ no	
☐ Fetal movement		☐ yes ☐ no	
☐ Fetal heart rate		☐ yes ☐ no	
☐ Tender abdomen		☐ yes ☐ no	
☐ Distention		☐ yes ☐ no	
☐ Other:		☐ yes ☐ no	
Genitourinary			
☐ Vaginal discharge: color, amount, odor		☐ yes ☐ no	
☐ Pain (describe site, location, level, intermittent or constant)		☐ yes ☐ no	
☐ CVA tenderness (with the side of your fist, tap over kidneys)		☐ yes ☐ no	
☐ Other:		☐ yes ☐ no	
Skin			
☐ Scars		☐ yes ☐ no	
☐ Tattoos		☐ yes ☐ no	
☐ Piercings		☐ yes ☐ no	
☐ Warmth		☐ yes ☐ no	
☐ Dry vs. diaphoretic		☐ yes ☐ no	
☐ Other:		☐ yes ☐ no	
Psychosocial and Spiritual			
☐ History of depression and medications		☐ yes ☐ no	
☐ Support person			
☐ Coping		☐ yes ☐ no	
☐ Pain perception		☐ yes ☐ no	
☐ Birth plan		☐ yes ☐ no	

Exhibit 2.8: Some facts, signs and symptoms possibly related to dehydration.

1. Rapid (recent) weight loss

2. Dry eyes

3. Dry mouth

4. Abnormal vital signs
   A. pulse greater than 100 beats per minute
   B. systolic blood pressure less than 100 mm Hg, or a drop in systolic blood pressure of 20 or more mm Hg when position is changed
   C. temperature of 100.4° F or higher (fever)

5. Small amount and concentrated urine

6. A history of urinary tract infections

7. Functional decline with dizziness or confusion

8. Elevated blood urea nitrogen (BUN)

9. Elevated sodium (may be low if she is taking a diuretic)

10. BUN/creatinine ratio greater than 25:1 (American Medical Directors Association, 2001)

Exhibit 2.9: Amount of liquid to record for intake (1 ounce = 30 mL).*

Large paper cup	240 mL
Hot foam cup	180 mL
Coffee cup	200 mL
Cream	15 mL
Tablespoon	15 mL
Milk carton	240 mL
Soup bowl or cup	180–220 mL
Gelatin (Jello)	90–100 mL
Ice Cream/Sherbet	60 mL
Popsicle	90 mL
Water pitcher	900 mL

*Amount may vary based on your supplies.

reaction, muscle strength, gait and posture, vision and hearing, and headache or dizziness. Assess her musculoskeletal system. Does she have a normal range of motion, or any cramps, tingling, spasms, deformities, or amputations?

ASSESS HYDRATION AND DEHYDRATION

Hydration affects the duration of labor. A well-hydrated woman should have a shorter labor than a dehydrated woman. When nulliparous women received 125 mL/hour of crystalloid, 26% had labors lasting more than 12 hours compared with 13% of women who received 250 mL/hour (Garite, Weeks, Peters-Phair, Pattillo, & Brewster, 2000).

Dehydration is not just too little body fluid: it also includes an electrolyte deficiency. Dehydration is related to maternal fatigue, which may have an impact on her pain tolerance and her ability to push her baby out. During labor it is suspected that a dehydrated uterus will not contract well, and may even result in poor labor progress. Therefore, it is important that the nurse recognize the signs and symptoms of dehydration and report them to the certified nurse midwife or physician as soon as possible so that treatment may be promptly initiated. (See Exhibit 2.8 for signs and symptoms of dehydration.)

Every woman in labor should have her intake and output recorded on every shift. Oral intake and intravenous intake are the most common in labor and delivery. Output should include urine and any bleeding or amniotic fluid. Usually urine

is measured and bleeding and amniotic fluid is described. However, blood usually weighs about 1 gram per milliliter, as does amniotic fluid or water. Clots can be weighed on the linen protector. After weighing a dry linen protector (often called a Chux), and deducting that weight, the amount of blood loss can be estimated.

Documentation example: Fundal massage s/p cesarean section. Clot passed and weighed. Estimated clot size, 220 mL. Reported finding to Dr. Red. Additional oxytocin ordered and 20 U added to 500 mL at 200 mL/hour.

Documentation example: Patient voided 200 mL amber urine. Drinking water. Reports contractions feel stronger at this time.

THE DANGERS OF REHYDRATION

Vomiting can precede dehydration and rehydration with intravenous fluids may be ordered. Treatment of dehydration has been separated into two phases: a rehydration phase and a maintenance phase. It may take some time to achieve normal hydration status. However, intravenous solutions should be administered with care as fluid overload during labor can lead to hyponatremia and water intoxication resulting in coma and death (Borcherding & Ruchala, 2002) (see Exhibit 2.10). For example, an isotonic solution such as lactated Ringer's solution may be a better choice of fluids than a hypotonic solution such as 5% dextrose in water. It is particularly dangerous to administer oxytocin in a hypotonic solution, especially over a 24-hour period because there is an increased risk of water intoxication.

ASSESS MATERNAL VITAL SIGNS

Abnormal maternal vital signs are often related to pathologic conditions. It is important to promptly report abnormal vital

Exhibit 2.10: Signs and symptoms of hyponatremia.

Early

- Apathy
- Weakness
- Nausea
- Vomiting
- Headache

Advanced

- Unresponsiveness
- Hallucinations
- Urinary incontinence
- Pulmonary edema

Severe

- Seizures
- Respiratory arrest
- Coma
- Permanent brain damage
- Death

signs to the midwife or physician whenever you detect them. Exhibit 2.11 suggests time intervals between assessments. Centigrade is the same as the Fahrenheit temperature minus 32 degrees, then multiplied by 5/9. Fahrenheit temperature is the centigrade temperature multiplied by 9/5, plus 32 degrees.

Documentation example: Maternal temp 100.8°, Dr. Feever notified of fever and fetal heart rate in the 170s. Maternal heart rate 120–130 bpm. Changed IV antibiotic to 1 gram Ampicillin now. Oxygen by tight-fitting face mask at 10 L/min. Skin warm to the touch. Sponge bath given and cool washcloth now on forehead. Amniotic fluid clear, half of linen protector saturated. No foul odor. Peri care done. Antipyretic discussed with physician. Plan of care discussed with physician, including possible cesarean section since exam is 5/80%/0. Physician discussed possible cesarean section with patient.

MATERNAL TACHYCARDIA

A maternal pulse that persists at a rate greater than 100 bpm is tachycardia. The midwife and/or physician should be notified of tachycardia. Tachycardia has many causes. The elevation may be due to a viral or bacterial infection related to chorioamnionitis, a urinary tract infection, or an upper respiratory infection. The fetal heart rate should be assessed when there is maternal tachycardia. Abnormalities should also be reported to the midwife and/or physician.

Tachycardia might also be related to maternal fear, pain, or endogenous epinephrine, or it might be related to amphetamine use or an arrhythmia such as supraventricular tachycardia. Tachycardia may also be related to an occult hemorrhage.

A rapidly beating heart can perform inefficiently. In the case of a woman in labor, it poses a risk for fetal hypoxia due to decreased cardiac output and blood flow to the uterus. It may also be related to less oxygen delivery to maternal tissues and a feeling of being out of breath.

SINUS TACHYCARDIA

The most common type of tachycardia is sinus tachycardia, which is the body's normal reaction to fever, dehydration with hypovolemia, hypovolemic shock, or blood loss. If the patient is bleeding, sinus tachycardia would be a compensatory response to try to maintain adequate blood flow and blood pressure. This type of sinus tachycardia has also been called reflex tachycardia.

On an electrocardiogram, sinus tachycardia is reflected by the narrow QRS complexes. Diagnosis and treatment require identification of the underlying cause. Therefore, before you call the physician, complete a quick evaluation of her temperature, pulse, blood pressure and respiratory rate, complaints such as chest pain or shortness of breath, level of consciousness, agitation or restlessness, bleeding, or diaphoresis, and discuss your assessments with the anesthesia provider (for postoperative patients) and/or the obstetrician. Your assessments should help him or her decide the best treatment plan, which should be directed at alleviating or treating the cause of the sinus tachycardia.

ATRIAL FIBRILLATION

Although this is one of the most common cardiac arrhythmias, it is not common in laboring women. Palpate the pulse. It may exceed 150 bpm. If it is irregular and fast, there may be an arrhythmia. The electrocardiogram would include wide QRS complexes.

AV NODAL REENTRANT TACHYCARDIA

AV nodal reentrant tachycardia (AVNRT) is the most common reentrant tachycardia. The QRS complex will be narrow and is best treated with drugs such as Sotalol or adenosine. Therefore, after you gather data such as the regularity and rhythm of the palpated and/or auscultated maternal pulse, notify the physician. When a woman has AVNRT, her fetus usually remains well oxygenated. Be prepared to order an electrocardiogram (ECG) when an arrhythmia is suspected.

AV REENTRANT TACHYCARDIA

AV reentrant tachycardia (AVRT) is an arrhythmia that requires an accessory pathway in the heart to maintain the abnormal rate. AVRT may involve orthodromic conduction in which

Exhibit 2.11: Vital signs and amniotic fluid assessments during spontaneous labor — basic guidelines.

Intact membranes, no infection suspected	Temperature q 4 hours
Ruptured membranes	Temperature q 2 hours
Ruptured membranes, suspect infection	Take temperature more frequently. Discuss labor and delivery plan of care with provider. Report temperature elevations.
Maternal heart rate every hour, or more frequently if tachycardic (> 100 bpm)	Report tachycardia.
Blood pressure every hour during the active phase of labor (between contractions)	Report systolic 140 mm Hg or more. Report diastolic 90 mm Hg or more. Report systolic < 90 mm Hg.
Respirations	Report 12/minute, consider discontinuation of magnesium sulfate. Report < 12/minute, discontinue magnesium sulfate. Assess reflexes.
Amniotic fluid	Provide perineal care with soap and water every 1 to 2 hours. Assess and record the color, amount, and odor of amniotic fluid.
Documentation example:	98°–110/68–72 bpm–20/min. Half of Chux saturated with clear, nonfoul fluid. Peri care done.

Exhibit 2.12: Suggested additional assessments when there is maternal tachycardia.

1. Vital signs including blood pressure, palpation of the radial pulse. Is it thready or weak?
2. Does the patient have shortness of breath?
3. SpO$_2$

Evidence of

1. Bleeding (vaginal or elsewhere)
2. Is the patient dehydrated (lethargic, dry mouth and tongue; rapid or shallow breathing; cool, clammy skin; blotchy skin at the knees and elbows; anxious, restless, thirsty; constipated, in discomfort, drowsy, sunken eyes without tears, confused, in a stupor, feverish)?
3. Does the patient have an infection? What is the white blood count; the odor of the amniotic fluid?
4. Is the patient anemic? What are the hemoglobin and hematocrit?

the SA nodal impulse travels down the AV node to the ventricles and back up to the atria through the accessory pathway. In that case, the QRS complex on the ECG will be narrow.

Antidromic condition occurs when the impulse travels down the accessory pathway and up to the atria through the AV node. In that case the QRS complex will be wide and often mimics ventricular tachycardia on the ECG. Antiarrhythmics will not be ordered when there is AVRT because they may, paradoxically, increase conduction across the accessory pathway and worsen the situation.

JUNCTIONAL OR VENTRICULAR TACHYCARDIA

You will rarely see these types of tachycardia because junctional tachycardia, which originates in the AV junction, may be a sign of digitalis toxicity. Ventricular tachycardia (VT or V-tach) is a common and often lethal complication of a myocardial infarction.

The physician will decide the best treatment of tachycardia. It is the nurse's duty to provide him or her with enough data to make the best patient-centered decisions. Your correct assessment and clear communication is therefore vital.

BLOOD PRESSURE DURING LABOR AND DELIVERY

Automatic blood pressure devices underestimate the systolic pressure and overestimate the diastolic pressure (Rebenson-

Piano, Holm, Foreman, Kirchhoff, 1989). Therefore, when you are assessing the blood pressure of a hypertensive woman, it may actually be higher than the reading shown on the automatic device. Automated sphygmomanometer readings are lower than mercury sphygmomanometer readings (Myers, McInnis, Fodor, & Leenen, 2008).

The initial vital signs should be assessed with the woman in a sitting position since the blood pressure in the office or clinic setting is usually taken with the patient seated. If she is admitted with a diagnosis of pregnancy-induced hypertension or preeclampsia, you will have assessed the blood pressure in a similar position as that used when the midwife or physician made the diagnosis.

Inform the midwife or physician of new-onset hypertension. Hypertension decreases uterine perfusion and increases the risk of fetal hypoxia. It is not uncommon for women to have an elevation of their heart rate and blood pressure when they are pushing to deliver. Use your judgment and report significant changes in maternal vital signs to the midwife and/or physician. Carefully monitor the fetus during the second stage. As women become tachycardic and accelerate their heart rate during contractions and pushing in the second stage of labor, vigilance is needed to be sure the fetus, not the woman, is monitored.

> **Documentation example**: Received patient from clinic. Reported headache above her eyes and around the top of her head since 10:00 a.m. Blood pressure in a sitting position was 138/68. Lying on left side, right arm, it was 142/92. Lying on right side, left arm, it was 148/90. Bilateral patellar reflexes 3+, denied blurred vision or epigastric pain.

ASSESS DEEP TENDON REFLEXES

Hyperreflexia is a result of central nervous system irritability, which may occur as a result of vasospasm during preeclampsia. Deep tendon reflexes (DTRs) are used to determine the need to start, adjust, or stop the magnesium sulfate infusion (Nick, 2004). The risk of magnesium sulfate toxicity is myoneural junction paralysis, respiratory arrest, and cardiac arrest.

Figures 2.4 and 2.5 illustrate the assessment of the biceps reflex and the patellar reflex. To elicit the biceps reflex, the thumb nail or just above the nail is tapped while the thumb presses on the tendon. To elicit the patellar reflex, the tendon just below the knee cap is tapped with the reflex hammer.

Reflexes are rated as absent (0), small with a trace response or decreased normal (1 or 1+), the lower range of normal or a normal response (2 or 2+), the upper range of normal or hyperreflexia (3 or 3+), and greater than normal or hyperreflexia with or without clonus (4 or 4+).

> **Documentation example**: Bilateral patellar reflexes 3+. Complains of headache and blurred vision. Physician notified.

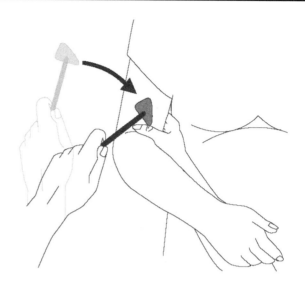

Figure 2.4: Biceps reflex assessment.

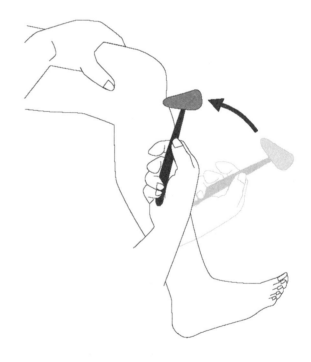

Figure 2.5: Patellar reflex assessment.

CLONUS

"Clonus" is a word derived from Greek, meaning violent, confused motion. Clonus might appear as small spontaneous twitching or large motions that may be initiated by assessment

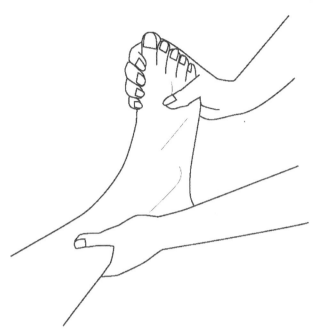

Figure 2.6: Assessment of clonus. Press the ball of the foot briskly towards the patient's head (dorsiflex the foot).

of a reflex. It is most common in the ankles. To test for clonus, rapidly dorsiflex the foot by pushing on the ball of the foot (see Figure 2.6). Sustained clonus of 5 beats or more is abnormal. Notify the physician immediately when you observe any clonus. Also inform the physician of her reflexes. He or she may order a magnesium sulfate infusion, especially if the woman has pregnancy-induced hypertension or preeclampsia. The doctor will probably come to the bedside to evaluate the patient.

> **Documentation example**: Bilateral biceps reflexes 2+, patellar reflexes 3+, 1 beat of clonus left foot, no clonus right foot. Findings reported to Dr. Nerviosa.

ASSESS PAIN

Assess the woman's discomfort and describe it based on location, quantity, and quality (or her perception). Is there any pain? Is it mild? Does it distress her? Is it excruciating? An entire chapter in this book is devoted to pain and its assessment and treatment.

IF TIME PERMITS, CONTINUE TO COLLECT DATA

Labor and delivery nurses perform a comprehensive collection of data that is needed to determine the appropriate, patient-centered plan of care. They may delegate tasks to licensed practical or licensed vocational nurses, depending on their state's Nurse Practice Act, rules, and regulations. To organize

data collection, you can think of the many "Ps" for the patient in labor. A nurse researcher identified 13 "Ps" when she reviewed content of women's birth stories (VandeVusse, 1999). They included the powers, passenger, and passageway or passage first identified by Dr. Jeffcoate in 1950, who discussed a second stage of labor delay. There was also the maternal psyche and positioning. Dr. VandeVusse also added the "P" of physiology and other sensations women reported that were involuntary during labor, such as vomiting and large muscle shaking. When women vomit they probably release an antidiuretic hormone, also known as vasopressin (Rowe, Shelton, Helderman, Vestal, & Robertson, 1979). Vasopressin can cause uterine contractions. Some women vomit, contract more, and dilate quickly. When a woman vomits, you may want to check dilatation after you clean up the mess.

Other "Ps" Dr. VandeVusse (1999) identified were childbirth preparation, the psychology of the mother, the professional provider of care, people who were not part of the medical staff, politics in a social context, the place of birth, and procedures. You will find that your patient may ask you to keep certain family members out of the labor room. You may need to play "visitor police" at times to keep unwanted people from entering the labor room or to keep the visitors to a minimum. If you do not do this, you may not be able to reach the bedside to provide needed care or to perform your assessments. Your work should always be directed at providing care for the most important "P," your patient.

CONCLUSIONS

Assessment identifies patient needs, helps the obstetric provider determine a proper diagnosis, and is the foundation of the plan of care. The plan of care should also be based on the woman's risk factors. It should change as her needs change. Triage is an area designated for outpatient services and assessment. Nurses need to be as complete as possible in their collection of data to avoid a misdiagnosis by the physician or midwife and unnecessary treatment or surgery. Women should have an opportunity to learn the risks and benefits of invasive procedures so that they can make an informed choice. Occasionally, an emergency prevents a formal informed consent procedure. In the absence of emergency surgery, nurses must continue to be vigilant in their care and treat conditions such as dehydration. They need to report abnormal findings to the midwife or physician so that the plan of care can change as the patient's needs change.

REVIEW QUESTIONS

True/False: Decide if the statements are true or false.

1. Lack of transportation is the primary reason women do not seek prenatal care.
2. Domestic violence may affect one in three pregnant women.
3. Invasive procedures, such as the application of a spiral electrode, increase the risk of HIV transmission.

4. Urinary tract infections and pyelonephritis during pregnancy are associated with an increased risk of mental retardation and developmental delay in infants.
5. The triage unit may be where women who have a gynecologic, postoperative, or postpartum complication are evaluated.
6. Cocaine withdrawal during labor may require the use of restraints.
7. If a pregnant woman's glucose screening test is greater than 100 mg/dL, she will need a 3-hour glucose tolerance test because she may have diabetes.
8. Dehydration is a water deficiency, not an electrolyte deficiency.
9. Atrial fibrillation is common in pregnant women.
10. An automated blood pressure device estimates higher blood pressures than a mercury sphygmomanometer.

References

Alkazaleh, F., Seaward, G., Ryan, G., Malik, A., & Farine, D. (2001). Maternal age and its relationship to cesarean section rate—a longitudinal study over 15 years. *American Journal of Obstetrics and Gynecology, 185*(6), S107.

Allen, M. C. (2005). *Domestic violence: The Florida requirement* (pp. 13–24). Sacramento, CA: CME Resource.

Alvarez, J. R., Williams, S. F., Ganesh, V. L., & Apuzzio, J. J. (2007). Duration of antimicrobial prophylaxis for group B streptococcus in patients with preterm premature rupture of membranes who are not in labor. *American Journal of Obstetrics and Gynecology, 197*(4), 390.e1–390.e4.

American College of Obstetricians and Gynecologists. (1998). Obstetric aspects of trauma management. *ACOG Educational Bulletin* Number 251. Washington, DC: Author.

American College of Obstetricians and Gynecologists. (2005a). Maternal decision making, ethics, and the law. ACOG Committee Opinion Number 321. *Obstetrics & Gynecology, 106*(5), 1127–1130.

American College of Obstetricians and Gynecologists. (2005b). Pregestational diabetes mellitus. Clinical Management Guidelines for Obstetrician-Gynecologists Number 60. *Obstetrics & Gynecology, 105*(3), 675–685.

American Diabetes Association. (1999). Gestational diabetes mellitus. *Diabetes Care, 22*(Suppl. 1), S74–S76.

Angelini, D. J. (2006). Obstetric triage: State of the practice. *Journal of Perinatal and Neonatal Nursing, 20*(1), 74–75.

Angelini, D. J., & Mahlmeister, L. R. (2005). Liability in triage: Management of EMTALA regulations and common obstetric risks. *Journal of Midwifery and Women's Health, 50*(6), 472–478.

Armstrong, M. L., Caliendo, C., & Roberts, A. E. (2006). Pregnancy, lactation, and nipple piercings. *AWHONN Lifelines, 10*(3), 210–217.

Bai, J., Wong, F. W. S., Bauman, A., & Mohsin, M. (2002). Parity and pregnancy outcomes. *American Journal of Obstetrics and Gynecology, 186*(2), 274–278.

Bailit, J. L., Dierker, L., Blanchard, M. H., & Mercer, B. M. (2005). Outcomes of women presenting in active versus latent phase of spontaneous labor. *Obstetrics and Gynecology, 105*(1), 77–79.

Beazley, D., Sundell, T., Patters, M., Carr, T., Blankenship, A., & Mercer, B. (2001). Correlation of periodontal disease, risk factors, and perinatal outcomes in high-risk population. [Abstract]. *American Journal of Obstetrics and Gynecology, 185*(6), S146.

Beebe, K. R. (2005). The perplexing parity puzzle. *AWHONN Lifelines, 9*(5), 394–399.

Berkus, M. D., Langer, O., Samueloff, A., Xenakis, E. M. J., & Field, N. T. (1999). Electronic fetal monitoring: What's reassuring. *Acta Obstetricia et Gynecologica Scandinavica, 78*(1), 15–21.

Blix, E., Reinar, L. M., Klovning, A., & Øian, P. (2005). Prognostic value of the labour admission test and its effectiveness compared with auscultation only: A systematic review. *British Journal of Obstetrics and Gynaecology, 112*, 1595–1604.

Bonnet, M. P., Bruyère, M., Moufouki, M., De la Dorie, A., & Benhamou, D. (2007). Anaesthesia, a cause of fetal distress? [Abstract]. *Annales francaises d'anesthèsie et de rèanimation, 26*(7–8), 694–698.

Borcherding, K. E., & Ruchala, P. L. (2002). Maternal hyponateremia. *AWHONN LIfelines, 6*(6), 514–519.

Born, D., & Barron, M. L. (2005). Herb use in pregnancy. What nurses should know. *American Journal of Maternal/Child Nursing, 30*(3), 201–208.

Borrelli, F., Capasso, R., Aviello, G., Pittler, M. H., & Izzo, A. A. (2005). Effectiveness and safety of ginger in the treatment of pregnancy-induced nausea and vomiting. *Obstetrics & Gynecology, 105*(4), 849–856.

Braveman, P., Marchi, K., Egerter, S., Pearl, M., & Neuhaus, J. (2000). Barriers to timely prenatal care among women with insurance: The importance of prepregnancy factors. *Obstetrics & Gynecology, 95*(6, Part 1), 874–880.

Burnham, B. E. (1995). Garlic as a possible risk for postoperative bleeding. *Plastic Reconstructive Surgery, 95*(1), 213–219.

Callister, L. C. (2005). Global maternal mortality: Contributing factors and strategies for change. *American Journal of Maternal/Child Nursing, 30*(3), 185–194.

Case, A. P., Ramadhani, T. A., Canfield, M. A., Beverly, L., & Wood, R. (2007). Folic acid supplementation among diabetic, overweight, or obese women of childbearing age. *Journal of Obstetric, Gynecologic, and Neonatal Nursing, 36*(4), 335–341.

Chauhan, S. P., Magann, E. F., Carroll, C. S., Barrilleaux, P. S., Scardo, J. A., & Martin Jr., J. N. (2001). Mode of delivery for the morbidly obese with prior cesarean delivery: Vaginal versus repeat cesarean section. *American Journal of Obstetrics and Gynecology, 185*(2), 349–354.

Cibulka, N. J. (2006). Mother-to-child transmission of HIV in the United States. *American Journal of Nursing, 106*(7), 56–64.

Ciranni, P., & Essex, M. (2007). Better care, better bottom line. *Nursing for Women's Health, 11*(3), 275–281.

Clements, C. J., Flohr-Rincon, S., Bombard, A. T., & Catanzarite, V. (2007). OB team stat: Rapid response to obstetrical emergencies. *Nursing for Women's Health, 11*(2), 194–199.

Combs, C. A., Murphy, E. L., & Laros Jr., R. K. (1991). Factors associated with postpartum hemorrhage with vaginal birth. *Obstetrics & Gynecology, 77*(1), 69–76.

Cooper, M., Grywalski, M., Lamp, J., Newhouse, L., & Studlien, R. (2007). Enhancing cultural competence: A model for nurses. *Nursing for Women's Health, 11*(2), 148–159.

Connolly, A., Katz, V. L., Bash, K. L., McMahon, M. J., & Hansen, W. F. (1997). Trauma and pregnancy. *American Journal of Perinatology, 14*(6), 331–336.

Cragin, L., & Kennedy, H. P. (2006). Linking obstetric and midwifery practice with optimal outcomes. *Journal of Obstetric, Gynecologic, and Neonatal Nursing, 35*(6), 779–785.

Curry, M. A., Durham, L., Bullock, L., Bloom, T., & Davis, J. (2006). Nurse case management of pregnant women experiencing or at risk for abuse. *Journal of Obstetric, Gynecologic, and Neonatal Nursing, 35*(2), 181–192.

Dasgupta, A. (2003). Review of abnormal laboratory test results and toxic effects due to use of herbal medicines. *American Journal of Clinical Pathology, 120*, 127–137.

Eason, E., & Feldman, P. (2000). Much ado about a little cut: Is episiotomy worthwhile? *Obstetrics & Gynecology, 95*(4), 616–618.

Ecker, J. L., Chen, K. T., Cohen, A. P., Riley, L. E., & Lieberman, E. S. (2001). Increased risk of cesarean delivery with advancing maternal age: Indications and associated factors in nulliparous women. *American Journal of Obstetrics and Gynecology, 185*(4), 883–887.

Gage, J. D., Everett, K. D., & Bullock, L. (2007). A review of research literature addressing male partners and smoking during pregnancy. *Journal of Obstetric, Gynecologic, and Neonatal Nursing, 36*(6), 574–580.

Garite, T. J., Weeks, J., Peters-Phair, K., Pattillo, C., & Brewster, W. R. (2000). A randomized controlled trial of the effect of increased intravenous hydration on the course of labor in nulliparous women. *American Journal of Obstetrics and Gynecology, 183*(6), 1544–1548.

Gavino, M., & Wang, E. (2007). A comparison of a new rapid real-time polymerase chain reaction system to traditional culture in determining group B streptococcus colonization. *American Journal of Obstetrics and Gynecology, 197*, 388.e1–388.e4.

Gilbert, G. J. (1997). Ginkgo biloba [Letter to the editor]. *Neurology, 48*, 1137.

Green, L. A., & Froman, R. D. (1996). Blood pressure measurement during pregnancy: Auscultatory versus oscillatory methods. *Journal of Obstetric, Gynecologic, and Neonatal Nursing, 25*(2), 155–159.

Greenberg, M. B., Cheng, Y. W., Sullivan, M., Norton, M. E., Hopkins, L. M., & Caughey, A. B. (2007). Does length of labor vary by maternal age? *American Journal of Obstetrics and Gynecology, 197*, 428.e1–428.e7.

Greenspan, E. M. (1983). Ginseng and vaginal bleeding [Letter to the editor]. *Journal of the American Medical Association, 249*, 2018.

Gross, M. M., Hecker, H., Matterne, A., Guenter, H. H., & Keirse, M. J. N. C. (2006). Does the way that women experience the onset of labour influence the duration of labour? *British Journal of Obstetrics and Gynaecology, 113*, 289–294.

Groth, S. (2007). Are the Institute of Medicine recommendations for gestational weight gain appropriate for adolescents. *Journal of Obstetric, Gynecologic, and Neonatal Nursing, 36*(1), 21–27.

Gülmezoglu, A. M., Crowther, C. A., & Middleton, P. (2006). Induction of labour for improving birth outcomes for women at or beyond term. *Cochrane Library*, Issue 4.

Hamilton, P., & Restrepo, E. (2003). Weekend birth and higher neonatal mortality: A problem of patient acuity or quality of care? *Journal of Obstetric, Gynecologic, and Neonatal Nursing, 32*(6), 724–733.

Heffner, L. J., Elkin, E., & Fretts, R. C. (2003). Impact of labor induction, gestational age, and maternal age on cesarean delivery rates. *Obstetrics & Gynecology, 102*(2), 287–293.

Hellwig, J. P. (2007). Routine HIV screening recommended. *AWHONN Lifelines, 10*(6), 455–462.

Henry, A., Birch, M.R., Sullivan, E.A., Katz, S., & Wang, Y.A. (2005). Primary postpartum haemorrhage in an Australian tertiary hospital: A case-control study. *Australian and New Zealand Journal of Obstetrics and Gynaecology, 45*(3), 233–236.

Hobbins, D. (2004). Survivors of childhood sexual abuse: Implications for perinatal nursing care. *Journal of Obstetric, Gynecologic, and Neonatal Nursing, 33*(4), 485–497.

Huzel, P. S., & Remsburg-Bell, E. A. (1996). Fetal complications related to minor maternal trauma. *Journal of Obstetric, Gynecologic, and Neonatal Nursing , 25*(2), 121–124.

Jenkin-Capiello, E. (2000). Oh baby! *Nursing Management, 31*(2), 35–37.

Johnson, K. (2000). Short maternal height increases risk of dystocia cesarean. *Ob Gyn News.*.

Kahn, B. F., Davies, J. K., Lynch, A. M., Reynolds, R. M., & Barbour, L. A. (2006). Predictors of glyburide failure in the treatment of gestational diabetes. *Obstetrics & Gynecology, 107*(6), 1303–1309.

Kim, D. D., Page, S. M., McKenna, D. S., & Kim, C. M. (2005). Neonatal group B streptococcus sepsis after negative screen in a patient taking oral antibiotics. *Obstetrics & Gynecology, 105*(5, Part 2), 1259–1261.

Klatsky, P. C., Tran, N. D., Caughey, A. B., & Fujimoto, V. Y. (2008). Fibroids and reproductive outcomes: A systematic literature review from conception to delivery. *American Journal of Obstetrics and Gynecology, 198*(4), 357–366.

Klein, V. R., Cox, S. M., Mitchell, M. D., & Wendel Jr., G. D. (1990). The Jarisch-Herxheimer reaction complicating syphilotherapy in pregnancy. *Obstetrics & Gynecology, 75*, 375–379.

Lachat, M. F., Scott, C. A., & Relf, M. V. (2006). HIV and pregnancy: Considerations for nursing practice. *American Journal of Maternal/Child Nursing, 31*(4), 233–242.

LaCoursiere, D. Y., Bloebaum, L., Duncan, J. D., & Varner, M. WA. (2005). Population-based trends and correlates of maternal overweight and obesity, Utah 1991–2001. *American Journal of Obstetrics and Gynecology, 192*, 832–839.

Liem, E. B., Hollensead, S. C., Joiner, T. V., & Sessler, D. I. (2006). Women with red hair report a slightly increased rate of bruising but have normal coagulation tests. *Anesthesia and Analgesia, 102*, 313–318.

Low, J. A., Victory, R., & Derrick, E. J. (1999). Predictive value of electronic fetal monitoring for intrapartum fetal asphyxia with metabolic acidosis. *Obstetrics & Gynecology, 93*(2), 285–291.

Luke, B. (1998). Maternal weight, body mass index, and cesarean delivery [Letter to the editor]. *American Journal of Obstetrics and Gynecology, 179*(2), 564.

Mahlmeister, L., & Van Mullem, C. (2000). The process of triage in perinatal settings: Clinical and legal issues. *Journal of Perinatal and Neonatal Nursing, 13*(4) 13–31.

Mahony, R., Foley, M. E., Daly, L., & O'Herlihy, C. (2005). Obstetric outcome of second delivery following first delivery of a macrosomic infant (> 4.5 kg). [Abstract #545]. *American Journal of Obstetrics and Gynecology, 193*.

Maloni, J. A., Cheng, C.-Y., Liebl, C. P., & Maier, J. S. (1996). Transforming prenatal care: Reflections on the past and present with implications for the future. *Journal of Obstetric, Gynecologic, and Neonatal Nursing, 25*, 17–23.

Marasinghe, J. P., & Amarasinghe, A. A. W. (2007). Reliability of a preventability model in maternal death and morbidity needs further assessment [Letter to the editor]. *American Journal of Obstetrics and Gynecology, 440*. DOI: 10.1016/j.ajog.2007.06.087.

Marcus, D. M., & Snodgrass, W. R. (2005). Effectiveness and safety of ginger in the treatment of pregnancy-induced nausea and vomiting. *Obstetrics & Gynecology, 106*(3), 640.

McDermott, S., Callaghan, W., Szwejbka, L., Mann, H., & Daguise, V. (2000). Urinary tract infections during pregnancy and mental retardation and development delay. *Obstetrics & Gynecology, 96*(1), 113–119.

McFarland, M. B., Langer, O., Conway, D. L., & Berkus, M. D. (1999). Dietary therapy for gestational diabetes: How long is long enough? *Obstetrics & Gynecology, 93*(6), 978–982.

McFarlane, J., Malecha, A., Watson, K., Gist, J., Batten, E., Hall, I., & Smith, S. (2005). Intimate partner sexual assault against women: Frequency, health consequences, and treatment outcomes. *Obstetrics & Gynecology, 105*(1), 99–108.

McIntyre, P. G., Tosh, K., & McGuire, W. (2006). Caesarean section versus vaginal delivery for preventing mother to infant hepatitis C virus transmission. *Cochrane Database of Systematic Reviews,* Issue 4. Art No.: CD005546. doi: 0.1002/14651858.CD005546.pub2.

Miller, D. A. (2005). Is advanced maternal age an independent risk factor for uteroplacental insufficiency. *American Journal of Obstetrics and Gynecology, 192,* 1974–1982.

Millner, V. S., Eichold II, B. H., Sharpe, T. H., & Lynn Jr., S. C. (2005). First glimpse of the functional benefits of clitoral hood piercings. *American Journal of Obstetrics and Gynecology, 193,* 675–676.

Moos, M.-K. (2006). Listeriosis: How nurses can prevent the preventable. *AWHONN Lifelines, 10*(6), 498–501.

Morrow, R. A., & Brown, Z. A. (2005). Common use of inaccurate antibody assays to identify infection status with herpes simplex virus type 2. *American Journal of Obstetrics and Gynecology, 193,* 361–362.

Myers, M. G., McInnis, N. H., Fodor, G. J., & Leenen, F. H. (2008). Comparison between an automated and manual sphygmomanometer in a population survey. *American Journal of Hypertension,* doi:10.1038/ajh.2007.54.

Norman, J. C., & Leonard, J. M. (2005). HIV/AIDS: Epidemic update for Florida. *CME Resource, 131*(2), 27–64.

Neufeld, M. D., Frigon, C., Graham, A. S., & Mueller, B. A. (2005). Maternal infection and risk of cerebral palsy in term and preterm infants. *Journal of Perinatology, 25*(2), 108–113.

Nick, J. M. (2004). Deep tendon reflexes, magnesium, and calcium: Assessments and implications. *Journal of Obstetric, Gynecologic, and Neonatal Nursing, 33*(2), 221–230.

Payne, P. A., & Martin, E. J. (2002). Caring for the laboring woman. In E. J. Martin (Ed.), *Intrapartum management modules* (pp. 128–183). Philadelphia: Lippincott Williams & Wilkins.

Perez-Delboy, Shevell, T., Cleary, J., Smok, D., & Simpson, L. (2002). Increasing rates of cesarean deliveries in the past two decades. *American Journal of Obstetrics and Gynecology, 187*(6), S107.

Polivka, B. J., Nickel, J. T., & Wilkins III, J. R. (1997). Urinary tract infection during pregnancy: A risk factor for cerebral palsy? *Journal of Obstetric, Gynecological and Neonatal Nursing, 26*(4), 405–413.

Pratt, T. C., McGloin, J. M., & Fearn, N. E. (2006). Maternal cigarette smoking during pregnancy and criminal/deviant behavior: A Meta-analysis. *International Journal of Offender Therapy and Comparative Criminology, 50*(6), 672–690.

Price, S., Lake, M., Breen, G., Carson, G., Quinn, C., & O'Connor, T. (2007). The spiritual experience of high-risk pregnancy. *Journal of Obstetric, Gynecologic, and Neonatal Nursing, 36*(1), 63–70.

Ravin, C. R. (2007). Preventing STIs. Ask the questions. *Nursing for Women's Health, 11*(1), 88–91.

Rebenson-Piano, M., Holm, K., Foreman, M. D., & Kirchhoff, K. T. (1989). An evaluation of two indirect methods of blood pressure measurement in ill patients. *Nursing Research, 38*(1), 42–45.

Rice, J. P., Kay, H. H., & Mahony, B. S. (1989). The clinical significance of uterine leiomyomas in pregnancy. *American Journal of Obstetrics and Gynecology*, 160(5, Part 1), 1212–1216.

Rose, K. D., Croissant, P. D., Parliament, C. F., & Levin, M. B. (1990). Spontaneous spinal epidural hematoma with associated platelet dysfunction from excessive garlic ingestion: A case report. *Neurosurgery*, 26, 880–882.

Roush, K. (2006). Helping patients quit smoking. *American Journal of Nursing*, 106(7), 71.

Rowe, J. W., Shelton, R. L., Helderman, J. H., Vestal, R. E., & Robertson, G. L. (1979). Influence of the emetic reflex on vasoporessin release in man. *Kidney International*, 16(6), 729–735.

Samuels-Kalow, M. E., Funai, E. F., Buhimschi, C., Norwitz, E., Perrin, M., Calderon-Margalit, R. (2007). Prepregnancy body mass index, hypertensive disorders of pregnancy, and long-term maternal mortality. *American Journal of Obstetrics and Gynecology*, 197, 490.e1–490.e6.

Schrag, S., Gorwitz, R., Fultz-Butts, K., & Schuchat, A. (2002). Prevention of perinatal group B streptococcal disease. *MMWR Recommendations and Reports*, 51(RR11), 1–22. Retrieved August 15, 2007. Available: http://www.cdc.gov/mmwr/preview/mmwrhtmL/rr5111a1.htm

Schug, S. A. (2001). Patient satisfaction: Politically correct fashion of the nineties or a valuable measure of outcomes? *Regional Anesthesia and Pain Medicine*, 26(3), 93–195.

Schwertner, H. A., Rios, D. C., & Pascoe, J. E. (2006). Variation in concentration and labeling of ginger root dietary supplements. *Obstetrics & Gynecology*, 107(6), 1337–1343.

Sheffield, J. S., Hill, J., Laibl, V., Hollier, L. M., Sanchez, P., & Wendel, G. D. (2005). Valacyclovir suppression to prevent recurrent herpes at delivery: A randomized controlled trial. *American Journal of Obstetrics and Gynecology*, 105(4 Suppl), 5S.

Sheffield, J. S., Sánchez, P. J., Morris, G., Maberry, M., Zeray, F., McIntire, D. D. (2002). Congenital syphilis after maternal treatment for syphilis during pregnancy. *American Journal of Obstetrics and Gynecology*, 186, 569–573.

Sheiner, E., Shoham-Vardi, I., Hershkovitz, R., Katz, M., & Mazor, M. (2001). Infertility treatment is an independent risk factor for cesarean section among nulliparous women aged 40 and above. *American Journal of Obstetrics and Gynecology*, 185, 888–892.

Shi, M., Wehby, G. L., & Murray, J. C. (2008). Review on genetic variants and maternal smoking in the etiology of oral clefts and other birth defects. *Birth Defects Research. Part C, Embryo Today*, 84(1), 16–29.

Shieh, C., & Kravitz, M. (2006). Severity of drug use, initiation of prenatal care, and maternal-fetal attachment in pregnant marijuana and cocaine/heroin users. *Journal of Obstetric, Gynecologic, and Neonatal Nursing*, 35(4), 499–508.

Shorten, A., Shorten, B., Geogh, J., West, S., & Morris, J. (2005). Making choices for childbirth: A randomized controlled trial of a decision-aid for informed birth after cesarean. *Birth*, 32(4), 252–261.

Shy, K., Kimpo, C., Emanuel, I., Leisenring, W., & Williams, M. A. (2000). Maternal birth weight and cesarean delivery in four race-ethnic groups. *American Journal of Obstetrics and Gynecology*, 182(6), 1363–1370.

Simhan, H. N., Anderson, B. L., Krohn, M. A., Heine, R. P., Martinez de Tejada, B., Landers, D. V. (2007). Host immune consequences of asymptomatic *Trichomonas vaginalis* infection in pregnancy. *American Journal of Obstetrics and Gynecology*, 196(1), 59–60.

Souza, J. P., Miguelutti, M. A., Cecatti, J. G., & Makuch, M. Y. (2006). Maternal position during the first stage of labor: A systematic review. *Reproductive Health*, 3, 10.

Spinillo, A., Capuzzo, E., Stronati, M., Ometto, A., De Santolo, A., & Acciano, S. (1998). Obstetric risk factors for periventricular leukomalacia among preterm infants. *British Journal of Obstetrics and Gynaecology*, 105(8), 865–871.

Stotland, N. E., Haas, J. S., Brawarsky, P., Jackson, R. A., Fuentes-Afflick, E., & Escobar, G. J. (2005). Body mass index, provider advice, and target gestational weight gain. *Obstetrics & Gynecology*, 105(3), 633–638.

Stotland, N. E., Washington, E., & Caughey, A. B. (2007). Prepregnancy body mass index and the length of gestation at term. *American Journal of Obstetrics and Gynecology*, 197, 378–380. doi: 10.1016/j.ajog.2007.05.048.

Suplee, P. D., Dawley, K., & Bloch, J. R. (2007). Tailoring peripartum nursing care for women of advanced maternal age. *Journal of Obstetric, Gynecologic, and Neonatal Nursing*, 36(6), 616–623.

Taylor, C. R., Alexander, G. R., & Hepworth, J. T. (2005). Clustering of U.S. women receiving no prenatal care: Differences in pregnancy outcomes and implications for targeting interventions. *Maternal and Child Health Journal*, 9(2), 125–133.

The Systematic Review on Congenital Toxoplasmosis (SYROCOT) Study Group. (2007). Effectiveness of prenatal treatment of congenital toxoplasmosis: A meta-analysis of individual patients' data. *Lancet*, 369, 115–122.

Thung, S. F., & Grobman, W. A. (2005). The cost-effectiveness of routine antenatal screening for maternal herpes simplex virus-1 and –2 antibodies. *American Journal of Obstetrics and Gynecology*, 192, 483–488.

Tyer-Viola, L. A. (2007). Obstetric nurses' attitudes and nursing care intentions regarding care of HIV-positive pregnant women. *Journal of Obstetric, Gynecologic, and Neonatal Nursing*, 36(5), 398–409.

Usta, I. M., Zoorob, D., Abu-Musa, A., Naassan, G., & Nassar, A. H. (2008). Obstetric outcome of teenage pregnancies compared with adult pregnancies. *Acta Obstetricia et Gynecologica*, 87, 178–183.

VandeVusse, L. (1999). The essential forces of labor revisted: 13Ps reported in women's stories. *MCN: American Journal of Maternal/Child Nursing*, 24(4), 176–184.

Vergnes, J.-N., & Sixou, M. (2007). Preterm low birth weight and maternal periodontal status: A meta-analysis. *American Journal of Obstetrics and Gynecology*, 196, 35.e1–135.e7.

Wagner, D. W., Johnson, K., & Kidd, P. S. (2006). *High acuity nursing* (4th ed.). Upper Saddle River, NJ: Pearson, Prentice Hall.

Walker, L. O. (1996). Predictors of weight gain at 6 and 18 months after childbirth: A pilot study. *Journal of Obstetric, Gynecologic, and Neonatal Nursing, 25*(1), 39–48.

Ward, K., Argyle, V., Meade, M., & Nelson, L. (2005). The heritability of preterm delivery. *Obstetrics & Gynecology, 106*, 1235–1239.

Wax, J. R. (2007). Trends in state/population-based Down syndrome screening and invasive prenatal testing with introduction of first trimester combined Down syndrome screening, South Australia 1995–2005. *American Journal of Obstetrics and Gynecology, 196*(4), 285–286. doi: 10.1016/j.ajog.2007.01.042.

Wilson, B. L. (2007). Assessing the effects of age, gestation, socioeconomic status, and ethnicity on labor inductions. *Journal of Nursing Scholarship, 39*(3), 208–213.

Wood, M. R., Kettinger, C. A., & Lessick, M. (2007). Knowledge is power. How nurses can promote health literacy. *Nursing for Women's Health, 11*(2), 178–188.

Wu, Y. W., & Colford Jr., J. M. (2000). Chorioamnionitis as a risk factor for cerebral palsy: A meta-analysis. *Journal of the American Medical Association, 284*(11), 1417–1424.

Wright, L. N., Thorp Jr., J. M., Kuller, J. A., Shrewsbury, R. P., Ananth, C., & Hartmann, K. (1997). Transdermal nicotine replacement in pregnancy: Maternal pharmacokinetics and fetal effects. *American Journal of Obstetrics and Gynecology, 176*(5), 1090–1094.

Yost, N. P., Bloom, S. L., McIntire, D. D., & Leveno, K. J. (2005). A prospective observational study of domestic violence during pregnancy. *Obstetrics & Gynecology, 106*(1), 61–65.

Young, T. K., & Woodmansee, B. (2002). Factors that are associated with cesarean delivery in a large private practice: The importance of prepregnancy body mass index and weight gain. *American Journal of Obstetrics and Gynecology, 187*, 312–320.

Zamorski, M. A., & Biggs, W. S. (2001). Management of suspected fetal macrosomia. *American Family Physician, 63*, 302–306.

3

Phases and Stages of Labor

They are able because they think they are able.

—Virgil

THE FIRST STAGE OF LABOR

Labor has been divided into four stages (see Exhibit 3.1). The first stage of labor has two phases: the latent phase and the active phase. It has also been divided into three parts: early labor, active labor, and transition. For a nulliparous woman, the latent phase begins when the firm, closed cervix softens, and the external os or opening of the cervix increases in diameter. The change in the os will be accompanied by regular contractions that occur approximately every 5 minutes. Multiparous women, who often have a slight opening of the cervical os before the onset of labor, begin the first stage of labor with a change in dilatation and regular contractions. The first stage of labor ends at 10 centimeters (cm) of dilatation.

The latent phase was considered to be prolonged when it lasted 20 or more hours in nulliparous women and 14 or more hours in multiparous women (Friedman, 1978). The change between the latent phase and the active phase can only be seen when a labor curve or graph is plotted (see Figure 3.1).

CATEGORIES OF THE FIRST STAGE

The first stage of labor has also been arbitrarily divided into three parts based on dilatation: early labor (1 to 3 cm), active labor (4 to 7 cm), and transition (8 to 10 cm). The category of active labor is not the same as the active phase of labor. Active labor is based on dilatation while the active phase of labor is determined when a labor curve or graph is plotted. It is evident with the change in the slope of the graph. The beginning of the active phase is at the point where the slope of the labor graph increases. For example, in Figure 3.1, the active phase began near 2 cm in the primigravida woman and near 3 cm in the multigravida woman.

BENEFITS OF PLOTTING A LABOR GRAPH

A labor graph creates a visual image to help you determine if there is normal or abnormal labor progress. The labor graph has also been called a labor curve, partogram, or cervicograph. Without plotting a labor graph, you will need to think about the woman's dilatation and evaluate the change in the cervix over time. Exhibit 3.2 reflects the contractions during the first stage of the labor of a nulliparous woman who had a drug-free labor that ended in a normal spontaneous vaginal delivery (NSVD). Her cervix dilated almost 1 cm per hour.

THE DURATION OF THE FIRST STAGE OF LABOR

Normal labor (from 0 to 10 cm) should last 9 to 12 hours in nulliparous and multiparous women (Cesario, 2004; Studd, 1975). However, 19 hours to dilate from 0 to 10 cm for nulliparous women, and 14 hours for multiparous women, may still end with good neonatal outcomes (Albers, 1999; Albers, Schiff, & Gorwoda, 1996). When labor (0 cm to delivery) lasts less than 3 hours, it is called a precipitous labor.

Exhibit 3.1: Stages of labor.

STAGE 1: Onset of labor to 10 cm.
STAGE 2: 10 cm to birth of the baby.
STAGE 3: Birth of the baby to delivery of the placenta.
STAGE 4: Delivery of the placenta until recovery is finished (usually 2 hours).

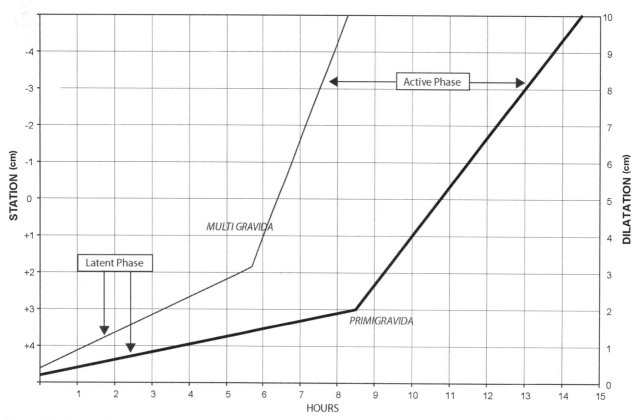

Figure 3.1: Generic labor graph. Note the time in hours at the bottom of the graph, and the station and dilatation at the sides. Station is measured in centimeters above and below the ischial spines.

Exhibit 3.2: Normal, drug-free labor in a nulliparous woman with a term gestation (derived from the medical records of an actual patient).

TIME	CONTRACTION FREQUENCY	DURATION	STRENGTH	DILATATION/STATION
0700–0800	every 4–5 minutes	not noted	not noted	2 cm
1200–1300	every 4, 3–4, and 4–6 min.	60 seconds	moderate	
1300–1400	every 3–6, 3, 3–4 minutes	60 seconds	moderate	7 cm/0 station
1400–1500	every 3–5 minutes	60+ seconds	moderate	
1500–1600	every 5, 4–5 minutes	60 seconds	moderate	9 cm
1600–1700	every 3–4, 4, 5 minutes	60 seconds	moderate	10 cm at 1630
1700–1800	every 1–3, 3, 2–4 minutes	60 seconds	moderate	
1812	delivered			

The rule of thumb is to expect women to dilate about 1 cm per hour once the active phase of labor begins, or the woman is dilated 4 cm (in active labor). Women may dilate faster than 1 cm per hour. Researchers studied 1,329 nulliparous women in spontaneous labor. They found the time between 4 to 10 cm averaged 5.5 hours (Zhang, Troendle, & Yancey, 2002). In another study, researchers found that nulliparous women who were at least 3 cm dilated and 100% effaced, or 4 cm and 75% effaced with 2 or more contractions every 10 minutes, dilated even faster at 1.4 cm per hour. Multiparous women dilated 1.8 cm per hour (Rouse, Owen, Savage, & Hauth, 2001). Therefore, it is reasonable for you to expect your patient to dilate 1 cm per hour once active labor begins or she has reached 4 cm.

Normal active labor (4 to 10 cm) should last 5 to 8 hours in nulliparous women and 5 to 6 hours in multiparous women.

While this is less than 1 cm per hour in a nulliparous woman, it is near 1 cm per hour in a multiparous woman. In 1955, Dr. Emanuel Friedman published his findings of 500 primigravid women who had an average active phase of labor of 4.9 hours (Pitkin, 2003). Active labor (4 to 10 cm) averaged 7.7 hours in nulliparous women and 5.6 hours in multiparous women who were managed by certified nurse midwives and who did not have an epidural. The average duration of the second stage of labor (10 cm to delivery) was 53 minutes in nulliparous women and 17 minutes in multiparous women (Albers, Schiff, & Gorwoda, 1996).

PROTRACTED, SLOW LABOR PROGRESS

Abnormal labor is called a protraction disorder or an arrest disorder. A protraction disorder is characterized by slow dilatation and/or slow fetal descent. Protraction and arrest disorders are easy to recognize if you plot a labor graph. Exhibit 3.3 illustrates a woman who was induced with an amniotomy and an oxytocin infusion. Factors that increased her risk for a cesarean section were her age (39 years) and her high body mass index (228 pounds, 5 feet 4 inches tall). She also had gestational diabetes. Overweight and obese women are likely to have an oxytocin induction and/or augmentation, and a longer first stage of labor than women of normal weight (Vahratian, Zhang, Troendle, Savitz, & Siega-Riz, 2004). In the case illustrated in Exhibit 3.3, the cesarean section was needed because the fetus was remote from delivery (0 station) and there was an abnormal (nonreassuring) and worsening fetal heart rate pattern.

Unlike Exhibit 3.2, where there was a change from 2 to 10 cm between 0700 and 1630, in Exhibit 3.3, the change from 2 to 5 cm occurred in the same amount of time, yet dilatation stopped after 1815 (6:15 p.m.). There was also an arrest of dilatation, which appears as a flattening of the labor curve. This labor had a protraction and an arrest disorder. When dilatation is unchanged for two or more hours during the active phase of labor, an arrest of labor or arrest disorder is diagnosed. An arrest of labor despite 200 Montevideo units,

Exhibit 3.3: Nulliparous woman at 38 weeks with an abnormal first stage of labor, oxytocin augmentation, and a diagnosed protraction disorder with an abnormal fetal heart rate pattern.	
Time	Dilatation/Effacement/Station
0700	2 cm/85% effaced/–2
1200	3/90%/0
1430	4–5/100%/0
1615	5/100%/0
1815	6/100%/0
2015	6/100%/0

a generally recognized level of adequate uterine activity, increases the risk of complications such as chorioamnionitis, shoulder dystocia, and endometritis (Greenberg et al., 2006). In a normal labor, fewer vaginal examinations are needed. Long labors increase the risk of an ascending infection and chorioamnionitis due to multiple vaginal examinations after the rupture of the membranes.

RECOGNIZE AND REPORT ABNORMALITIES

A normal pregnancy does not predict normal labor, and normal labor does not predict a normal delivery. Therefore, it is unreasonable to promise a woman she will have a normal labor and delivery. A reasonable goal for obstetric health care personnel is a safe delivery for both the mother and her child (Ness, Goldberg, & Berghella, 2005). Labor and delivery nurses play a vital role in reaching that goal. They can prevent harm by recognizing and reporting abnormal labor findings early so that the physician or certified nurse midwife can modify the plan of care. After you report abnormal dilatation progress or descent, expect the midwife or physician to come to the bedside and evaluate the woman and the fetal size, presentation, and position. The new plan of care may include procedures such as an amnioinfusion, an operative vaginal delivery, or a cesarean section.

PROTRACTION DISORDERS
Definition
A protracted active phase of labor is present when dilatation changes less than 1.2 cm per hour in the nulliparous woman and less than 1.5 cm per hour in the multiparous woman (Martin, 2002). Protracted dilatation often occurs between 4 and 6 cm in overweight and obese women. For example, the time that elapsed between 4 and 10 cm averaged 7.5 hours for overweight women and 7.9 hours for obese women, but only 6.2 hours for normal weight women. Obese women also had an almost twofold increased risk for a cesarean delivery (Vahratian et al., 2004). The strength of contractions during the first and second stages of labor is similar in both obese women and normal weight women (Buhimschi, Buhimschi, Malinow, & Weiner, 2001). Therefore, the protraction may be due to the size of the passenger and the fit in the passageway.

A protraction disorder is easy to recognize if your patient is still undelivered and contracting when you return to work the next day! Imagine your nulliparous patient was 5 centimeters when you left work after a 12-hour shift. You return to work the next day and she is still in the labor room contracting. You should be questioning why she is not yet delivered, how her fetus is tolerating labor, the length of time since the membranes ruptured, and whether there are any signs of infection. You should also review the current plan of care.

Discuss your concerns with the charge nurse, midwife, and/or physician. An effective charge nurse will accept ownership for the outcomes of care provided by the entire patient care team. They are expected to assume an active role in help-

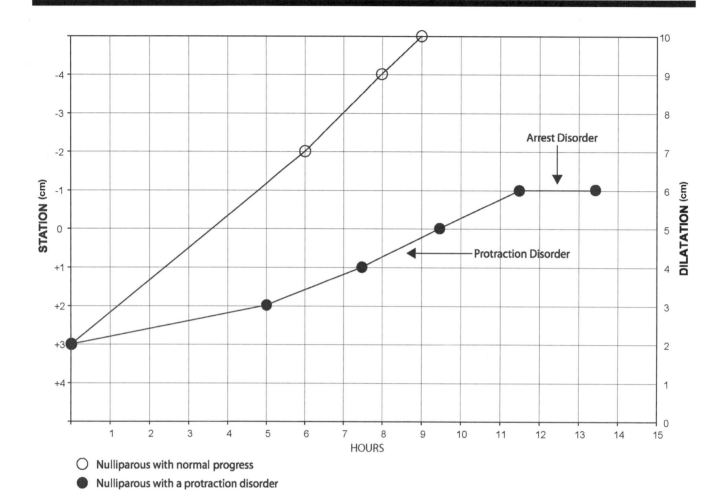

Figure 3.2: Normal and abnormal labor dilatation-based data from Exhibits 3.2 and 3.3. Station is not recorded on this example, but dilatation is recorded using open and closed circles.

ing you resolve patient problems (Mahlmeister, 1999). When you discuss your concerns about a protraction and/or arrest disorder, expect the midwife or physician to evaluate the fetal size, presentation, and position. If he or she is not immediately available and you do the assessment, be sure to record the presence of caput (swelling) and/or molding (overlapping sutures). If you can determine the fetal position, record it as well. If you cannot tell if the formerly vertex fetus has a fetal butt or head presenting due to the amount of swelling you feel, think "cesarean section"! With that amount of caput, it will only get worse as the fetus descends, increasing the risk of brain trauma.

Causes

Protraction disorders may be due to a problem with the powers (functional dystocia) or problems with the passenger-passage-way fit (mechanical dystocia). Sometimes, there is both functional and mechanical dystocia. When you note a protraction

disorder, ask yourself several questions. Could there be a fetal malposition or fetal macrosomia? What are the frequency, duration, and strength of contractions? What are the color, amount, and odor of the amniotic fluid? Is there amniotic fluid? The lack of fluid may slow descent. Is there meconium present where the fluid was clear before? Could the cord be wrapped around the baby preventing the baby from descending? Plot and review the labor graph or have the computer create one, if that is possible. Review the medical record. Review the maternal height, weight, and estimated fetal weight. Do you think the baby will safely pass through the birth canal? Discuss your concerns with your charge nurse, the midwife and/or the physician.

FUNCTIONAL VERSUS MECHANICAL DYSTOCIA

"Dystocia" is derived from the Greek language and means "difficult labor." There are three types of dystocia: functional dystocia, which is related to ineffective powers; mechanical dystocia, which is related to the passenger and passageway; and emotional dystocia, which is related to the woman's psyche.

Functional Dystocia

Functional dystocia has been called uterine dystocia. Functional dystocia exists when the powers do not work well. Examples of functional dystocia are uterine inertia, abnormal uterine contractions, or prolonged labor. Functional dystocia is related to the interval between births. As the interval between deliveries increases, the incidence of functional dystocia increases (Bao-Ping et al., 2006).

Mechanical Dystocia

Mechanical dystocia occurs when the baby is too big for the pelvis, has a malpresentation, or is malpositioned (American College of Obstetricians and Gynecologists, 2003). Mechanical dystocia and protraction disorders may also be related to fetal malpresentation, such as an occiput posterior or occiput transverse position. Mechanical dystocia may also be related to an obstruction such as an overfull bladder or a large fibroid in the lower segment of the uterus. A soft cervix prior to administration of oxytocin is critical to avoid mechanical dystocia caused by a firm, unripe cervix.

If you suspect mechanical dystocia may be slowing dilatation or descent, palpate the bladder. Ask the patient to urinate or empty it as needed if you have a standing order to catheterize. If you do not have a standing order, discuss the need for catheterization with the midwife or physician and request an order to do so.

If the bladder is already empty, yet the fetus is not descending or has caput at a high station, review the prenatal records for the pelvic type. What is the estimated fetal weight? Is there a note from an ultrasound related to fibroids in the lower segment of the uterus? Could a fibroid be blocking the exit? Notify the physician or midwife and ask them to evaluate the fetopelvic relationship. They will need to determine if the fetal head is asynclitic, deflexed, occiput transverse, or occiput posterior. There may even be a face presentation. Based on their evaluation, expect the plan of care to change.

Emotional Dystocia

High epinephrine levels related to inordinate fear may cause emotional dystocia and ineffective contractions (Simkin & Ancheta, 2005). Fear reduction may improve uterine activity to reduce functional dystocia. Providing analgesia and anesthesia as requested and when appropriate may decrease emotional distress and help the patient cope with labor.

HYPERVENTILATION MAY INCREASE EMOTIONAL DISTRESS

Women who are frightened and in pain often hyperventilate. They will breathe faster and/or deeper than normal. Hyperventilation potentially reduces the carbon dioxide concentration in their blood causing hypocapnia and respiratory alkalo-sis. Symptoms of respiratory alkalosis include: numbness or tingling in the hands, feet, and lips; dizziness; headache; slurred speech; and feeling faint. Coach the patient to slow her breathing. You may need to establish eye contact with her, touch her on her arm, and say to her, "breathe with me" in order to help her establish a normal breathing pattern. Sometimes it helps her slow her breathing if she breathes into a small brown paper bag. Unfortunately, it is rare to find a paper bag, let alone a brown paper bag, in labor and delivery settings. You can also ask her to cup her hands over her nose and mouth and breathe slower.

CAN DYSTOCIA BE PREVENTED?

Dystocia is the most common reason for a cesarean section. Therefore, if it could be prevented, perhaps the risk of cesarean section would decrease. Functional dystocia is not improved by eating and drinking early in labor (Tranmer, Hodnett, Hannah, & Stevens, 2005). Artificial rupture of the membranes and administration of oxytocin may prevent functional dystocia (Ness, Goldberg, & Berghella, 2005). However, these procedures do nothing to shrink the baby or enlarge the pelvis, and therefore have no impact on mechanical dystocia. So, even if the powers are working well, the baby may be too big to pass through the pelvis.

There will be days where no one is in spontaneous labor and everyone is receiving an infusion of oxytocin. Some hospitals even have nurses designated as members of the "pit crew," who initiate the oxytocin infusion prior to 6:00 a.m., and a "delivery crew," who arrives in the afternoon to assist the primary nurse with the delivery. Laboring in a hospital increases the risk of a cesarean delivery when women arrive early in labor (Holmes, Oppenheimer, Walker, & Wen, 2001). Laboring in a hospital also increases the risk of invasive procedures such as an intravenous catheter, artificial rupture of membranes, parenteral analgesia and/or neuraxial analgesia or anesthesia, placement of a spiral electrode or intrauterine pressure catheter, amnioinfusion, and delivery by forceps or a vacuum extractor. This is called the "cascade of interventions." Epidural anesthesia is related to protracted dilatation for women of any parity, including grandmultiparous women (P_5 or greater) (Gurewitsch et al., 1999).

Shoulder dystocia is more common when labor is protracted or there is an arrest of dilatation for two or more hours in the active phase of labor (Rouse, Owen, Savage, & Hauth, 2001). You should always be ready for a shoulder dystocia in these cases. Keep your charge nurse and/or supervisor informed of the impending vaginal delivery. Let them know you may be calling for help before or after you encounter a shoulder dystocia because you will need someone to perform McRoberts' maneuver while you provide suprapubic pressure or vice versa.

There are only two exit routes. If dystocia prevents delivery through the vagina, a cesarean section will be necessary. Delivery by cesarean section affects a woman's perception of her childbirth experience. When a word such as "failed" is used, she may feel like she was a failure. Unfortunately, physicians' discharge summaries often list final diagnoses that may include words such as "failed induction" or "failure to progress." A study of 1,661 women who had delivered their first baby by cesarean section found they were distressed by the following: the lack of communication related to their need for surgery; their fear of surgery; a feeling they missed out on the birth; a feeling they lacked a good bonding experience; and other emotions of disappointment, failure, or regret (Porter, van Teijlingen, Yip & Bhattacharya, 2006). It is critical that labor and delivery nurses show compassion for these women because many of them had a birth plan that was not fulfilled.

BIRTH PLANS ARE WISH LISTS

A woman's birth plan is a communication tool. Women and their significant others often take a lot of time thinking about their needs and what they would like their childbearing experience to include. They use a birth plan as a way to be heard. Birth plans, like living wills, can help everyone understand the woman's desires for her childbearing experience (Philipsen & Haynes, 2005). The birth plan is also a way for her to participate in the decisions related to childbearing. It can be thought of as a wish list. It should be used to aid communication and cooperation between the patient and the health care team (Simkin, 2007). Unfortunately, plans, like wish lists, may not end with the desired outcome. Birth plans cannot prevent cesarean sections when dystocia occurs. When the delivery will be by cesarean section, you might say to the patient, "I'm sorry we could not complete your birth plan" or "I know you had a plan for a vaginal birth. I'm sorry that we can't meet your expectations."

THE SECOND STAGE OF LABOR

The second stage of labor begins with complete dilatation of the cervix (10 cm) and ends with birth of the infant. In countries such as Canada or the United Kingdom, as well as the northeastern United States, "fully dilated" or "fully" means dilatation of 10 cm. In the remaining United States, it is more common to hear "completely dilated" or "complete" to describe dilatation of 10 cm.

The second stage of labor is a time for a one-to-one nurse/patient ratio. Inform the charge nurse that you will need to attend to your patient until she delivers and that you would like another nurse to watch your other patient(s). If your patient is nulliparous, do not begin pushing until she is fully or completely dilated and has an urge to push. Pushing prematurely increases the risk of fetal and maternal injury. If there is premature pushing, there will be a significant decrease in fetal oxygen delivery. Pushing prior to complete cervical dilatation may also cause the cervix to swell and make a vaginal delivery impossible.

Documentation example: Patient in bathtub. SVE by CNM Easybirth. 10 cm and 0 station. Pushing in tub with constant attendance by this nurse. FHR 142 bpm

by auscultation with Doppler. Maternal heart rate is 92 bpm.

Documentation example: Oxytocin discontinued. Patient encouraged to rest between contractions and to continue to push with contractions. Contractions are strong and every 2 to 3 minutes × 60 to 90 seconds. Family members at bedside. Voided large amount of yellow urine on linen protector. +1 to +2/5.

By documenting +2/5 you indicate that you use a 5-cm scale for station below the ischial spines. A linen protector may also be called a Chux, blue pad, or soaker in different countries.

THE TWO PHASES OF THE SECOND STAGE OF LABOR

The second stage of labor, like the first stage, has two phases: the latent phase and the active phase (Roberts, 2002, 2007). An upright position is best in the latent phase of the second stage. In the latent phase there is no strong expulsive urge because of insufficient pressure on the rectum and perineal tissues. Asking a woman to push at this time would increase her risk of exhaustion and therefore is ill-advised. Instead, consider passive descent of the fetus (Fraser & Cooper, 2003).

PASSIVE DESCENT VERSUS EARLY PUSHING

Passive descent is also known as laboring down or delayed pushing. Early pushing is the process of encouraging a woman to begin pushing immediately after she is found to be 10-cm dilated. Passive descent or laboring down means pushing efforts should not be encouraged and contractions alone should help the baby descend. Delayed pushing may delay delivery. Delaying pushing for more than 1 hour was associated with an increased risk of injury to the anal sphincter (Donnelly et al., 1998). Therefore, you must be vigilant and assess descent at least once an hour. Arrest of descent requires two vaginal examinations spaced at least 1 hour apart. If there is no progress, the diagnosis is "arrest of descent" (Cohen & Friedman, 1983).

Be sure passive descent is a reasonable option because delivery may be delayed with passive descent. Confirm that there are no signs of infection such as fever, and that the fetus is tolerant without an abnormal or nonreassuring fetal heart rate pattern. There also should be stable maternal vital signs and a normal temperature if passive descent occurs. If both the fetal heart rate and maternal vital signs are normal, she is probably a low-risk patient. In that case, assess and record the fetal heart rate every 15 minutes during this time.

When the patient has regional anesthesia, it is a good idea to assess the perineum every 15 minutes or more often because the fetus may descend and deliver under the sheets! Watch the patient's face. Note her body language. Even a grimace suggests progress is being made. She may say, "I feel different," or you may hear flatus or see a little stool. Look for more amniotic fluid being expressed or hair on the fetal head. Obviously, grunts, groans, and moans, and even screams suggest birth is imminent. During this time, if you need to move the ultrasound lower on the abdomen to keep the fetal heart rate on the monitor, that is an indirect sign of descent. Be sure to call the midwife or physician to the bedside in a timely manner.

PASSIVE DESCENT WITH AN EPIDURAL

One protocol for passive descent allows the primigravid woman to rest 2 hours and the multigravid woman to rest 1 hour before pushing commences. Using this protocol, it was found that women who had an epidural and a second stage of 4.9 hours still had neonates with similar Apgar scores and arterial cord pH values as women who immediately began to push at 10 cm (Hansen, Clark, & Foster, 2002). Women in their study did not have a known fetal anomaly, multiple gestation, a nonvertex fetus, a fetus less than 37 weeks or more than 42 weeks, pregnancy-induced hypertension, heart disease, or insulin-dependent diabetes. If your patient has any of these factors, there is no known research that supports delayed pushing, so be careful about who you select for delayed pushing.

Another protocol for passive descent required nulliparous women who had an epidural in place to rest 2 or more hours or until there was an irresistible urge to push or the fetal head was visualized (the perineum was inspected every 15 minutes), or there was a medical indication to shorten the second stage of labor (Fraser et al., 2000). In their study, Fraser and colleagues compared 936 women in the delayed pushing group with 925 women in the early pushing group. These women were from 12 medical centers in the United States, Canada, and Sweden. Ninety percent of women in the delayed pushing group were pushing within 1 1/2 hours, with 16.6% pushing in less than 1 hour. The second stage of labor for all but 10% lasted a maximum of 314 minutes in the delayed pushing group, and 248 minutes in the early pushing group. Actual pushing time was less when pushing was delayed (68 minutes compared with 175 minutes median, or the 50th percentile). In addition, the first stage of labor median (the 50th percentile) was 9.25 hours in the delayed pushing group, and 9.7 hours in the early pushing group. Women who delayed pushing had a twofold increase in fever, but the researchers did not attribute fever to infection. There were more abnormal umbilical cord venous and arterial pH values in the delayed pushing group (4.5%) than in the early pushing group (1.5%). An abnormal venous pH value was defined as less than 7.15. An abnormal arterial value was defined as less than 7.10. Fraser and colleagues (2000) also found there were fewer difficult deliveries when pushing was delayed 2 or more hours. There were fewer cesarean sections, midpelvic deliveries, and low pelvic deliveries with rotation. There were more spontaneous vaginal deliveries. Women from both groups similarly felt they were exhausted because of the pushing, and 40.4% in the early pushing group versus 31.4% in the delayed pushing group felt they

pushed a long time. Delayed pushing best helped women whose fetus was in an occiput transverse or occiput posterior position and women with a fetal station above +2 (using a 0 to +5 scale). There was no difference in the number of neonates who had complications between the groups.

Intrapartal fever is related to the duration of the rupture of membranes, epidural anesthesia, parity, histologic chorioamnionitis (on the placental pathology report), and the number of vaginal examinations (Greves, Curtin, Florescue, Metlay, & Katzman, 2007). Fever is also an independent risk factor related to neonatal encephalopathy, cerebral palsy, and death (Impey et al., 2008). When you note a maternal temperature elevation, especially when you note she has a fever, promptly notify the midwife or physician.

Seven studies related to passive descent were evaluated by Brancato, Church, and Stone (2008). They found that when women with an epidural did not immediately begin to push, they had an increased chance for a spontaneous vaginal delivery, fewer operative vaginal deliveries, pushing time decreased an average of 11 minutes, and their first stage of labor increased an average of 42 minutes. The second stage of labor increased an average of 14 minutes. Epidural anesthesia alone increased the risk of a midforceps delivery or vacuum extraction delivery but not the risk of a cesarean section or operative vaginal delivery for dystocia (Halpern, Leighton, Ohlsson, Barrett, & Rice, 1998).

FERGUSON'S REFLEX

When the fetus descends, dilates the vagina, and puts pressure on the pelvic floor there is a strong urge to push. This is called Ferguson's reflex. Dr. James Ferguson from Toronto experimented with rabbits and found that stretching their uterine horns, cervixes, and vaginas increased uterine activity and augmented the secretion of oxytocin from the posterior pituitary gland. He postulated that this same reaction might occur in humans. Even though it has never been proven to be true, Ferguson's reflex became part of the obstetric nomenclature (Ferguson, 1941).

CLEAR THE PATHWAY

An empty bladder and bowel will help maximize the diameter of the passageway. Is your patient's bladder empty? If not, catheterize her if ordered, or ask her to try to empty her bladder. Record the time the bladder was emptied and the color and amount of urine.

She will empty her rectum. Have four or five washcloths available for perineal care and to create warm moist compresses (if she will be able to feel the heat) to help your patient focus on the location to direct pushing efforts. For nulliparous women who feel their overwhelming and strong contractions during the second stage, they may have difficulty focusing on pushing down towards the rectum and perineum. If you apply a warm, moist towel or washcloth to the perineum, the pressure helps the woman focus and the washcloth can be used to sweep away any "evidence of progress" she expels from her rectum. If she has flatus, to avoid embarrassment, you can also mention that that too is "evidence of progress."

THE ACTIVE PHASE OF THE SECOND STAGE

Normally, the active phase of the second stage is associated with an involuntary, overwhelming urge to push with each contraction (Fraser & Cooper, 2003). Once pushing begins, passive descent is no longer an option. Contractions with pushing compress the placenta and cord to a point where oxygen delivery to the fetus is compromised. If the fetus has an abnormal fetal heart rate when active pushing begins, expect it to get worse. A hypoxic fetus prior to active pushing has an increased risk of decompensation due to the additional decrease in blood flow and oxygen delivery during this phase of the second stage of labor (Bakker & van Geijn, 2008). To enhance fetal oxygenation, oxytocin should be discontinued prior to this phase of the second stage of labor. If contractions space out or become unusually weak, oxytocin may be given to strengthen contractions and to increase their frequency. However, the fetus must demonstrate the lack of acidosis, such as the presence of accelerations.

NATURAL CHILDBIRTH

Women who labor, push, and deliver without analgesia or anesthesia have a natural childbirth. And while birth may be a natural process, it is certainly not pain free. Women who labored and delivered without analgesia will tell you they had intense, unrelenting pain. Nurses can assist the woman during this pain-filled birthing process by encouraging her to "listen to her body," respond to her own bearing-down reflexes, and rest between contractions (Gennaro, Mayberry, & Kafulafula, 2007). Often, when women push without the benefit of analgesia or anesthesia, they may vocalize their pain using colorful language or obscenities. If she appears to be out of control, work with her to help her refocus her energy towards pushing. You might say, "I know it hurts. Let's try to get you comfortable and redirect your energy" or "Screaming is directing your energy towards the ceiling. Let's try to redirect it down towards your bottom and push your baby out." Assist her in finding her position of comfort. It may be on her left side or her right side. Pushing does not have to be in a lithotomy position. Let her be the best judge of when and how to push. Do not encourage breath holding. Once she regains control, it is helpful to speak as little as possible. Distractions deplete energy. Limit distractions and noise in the room during this critical phase of the birthing process.

Observe her position in the bed. She may need to be assisted to bring herself up in the bed. You may need to lower the head of the bed, especially near the end of the second stage when you anticipate delivery of a large baby. At that point, it is helpful to encourage her to push straight ahead. It may be helpful to use the squat bar or stirrups to rest her legs, especially if she is a large woman.

If, close to the time of delivery the midwife or physician are called out of the room to attend to another patient in another department or another room, ask him or her who the back-up physician is or whom to call in their place. Call the charge nurse or supervisor to the room. Ask them to help you locate another midwife or physician who will deliver your patient's baby.

PITFALLS AND PERILS OF THE SECOND STAGE
Breath Holding

The risk of fetal hypoxia increases when women hold their breath and push (Bloom, Casey, Schaffer, McIntire, & Leveno, 2006; Simpson & James, 2005). If women hold their breath 10 seconds or longer, their faces may seem discolored. Some people call this "purple pushing." Normally, when women are not coached, they hold their breath only 5 to 6 seconds. Breath holding while someone counts to 10 decreases fetal oxygen delivery and only decreases the second stage of labor an average of 13 minutes (Bloom et al., 2006). Therefore, women can hold their breath and push, but breath holding should not last more than 5 to 6 seconds at a time.

What Not to Say

When women are in excruciating pain and are laboring or pushing without having had any analgesia or anesthesia, it is inappropriate to say, "You have done it once before, you can do it again." Help her find a position of comfort. This may be on "all fours" if she is having severe lower back pain, or on one of her sides. Another chapter in this book illustrates positions for labor and birth.

It is best not to say, "All women poop in labor" or "When you poop it will help the baby come out" or "That's just a little bowel movement." All of these comments can embarrass the woman and distract her from the hard work of pushing her baby out. If they expel gas and look embarrassed, just say, "That's a sign of progress!"

> **Documentation example**: Stooling with pushing. Perineal care done.

> **Documentation example**: FHR 140/minute. Perineum bulging with pushing. Dr. Delivery at bedside.

FUNDAL STABILIZATION DURING AMNIOTOMY

Fundal stabilization is the application of gentle fundal pressure with one or two hands in the labor room to keep the fetal head from moving out of the pelvis during an amniotomy. Fundal stabilization is accepted nursing practice. However, the application of fundal pressure prior to delivery (Kristeller maneuver) in an attempt to expedite delivery is not accepted nursing practice (Maryland Board of Nursing, 1999 correspondence). If fundal stabilization and an amniotomy occur when the fetus is at a high station, there is a risk of an umbilical cord prolapse or prolapse of an arm or leg. Prolapse of an

---

> **Exhibit 3.4: What to do and not do during the second stage of labor.**
>
> **DO**
>
> 1. Position her in her position of comfort and/or to help the baby move into an occiput anterior position.
> 2. Lower the head of the bed, use the McRoberts' maneuver, and ask her to "push straight ahead" when you anticipate the birth of a large or very large baby.
> 3. Stay in the room 100% of the time (one-to-one care) and leave only when another RN relieves you.
> 4. Observe family members who may be overly tired especially the father of the baby—we don't want anyone to pass out.
> 5. Use a cool, wet washcloth to keep the patient's face, chest, and arms cool (PRN).
> 6. Use warm, moist towels or washcloths on the perineum (and clean PRN) to help her focus on the location to push.
> 7. Assess and record the fetal heart rate at intervals based on the level of risk.
>
> **DON'T**
>
> 1. Begin pushing prior to 10-cm dilatation.
> 2. Push when there is an anterior lip, especially in a nulliparous woman.
> 3. Use fundal pressure.

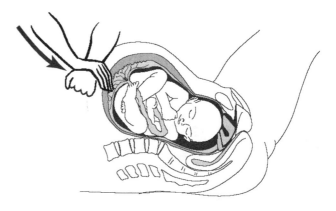

Figure 3.3: Fundal pressure is potentially harmful with no proven benefits. Do not perform this procedure during the second stage.

> **Exhibit 3.5: The dangers of fundal pressure.**
>
> | | |
> |---|---|
> | Maternal | Perineal trauma |
> | | Anal sphincter damage |
> | | Uterine rupture |
> | Fetal | Fractures |
> | | Nerve damage (for example, Erb's palsy) |
> | | Brain damage |

arm or leg can cause a compound presentation. Compound presentations are discussed in another chapter of this book.

If you are concerned about the risk of cord or limb prolapse because the fetus is at a high station, discuss your concerns outside of the patient's room with the midwife or physician before the procedure. Perhaps they will reconsider the amniotomy and postpone it until the fetus descends deeper into the pelvis.

> **Documentation example**: Dr. Imareadynow at bedside. Requested fundal stabilization. Fundal stabilization provided by this nurse. 2/50%/−3. Artificial rupture of membranes. Fluid clear, linen protector saturated, normal odor.

FUNDAL PRESSURE (KRISTELLER MANEUVER) DURING THE SECOND STAGE OF LABOR

Pressure on the uterine fundus towards the vagina with the aim of expediting delivery is known as the Kristeller maneuver or fundal pressure (see Figure 3.3) (Verheijen, Raven, & Hofmeyr, 2006). There is no confirmed benefit of fundal pressure during the second stage of labor (Merhi & Awonuga, 2005).

In the past, it was believed that fundal pressure increased intrauterine pressure and therefore increased the expulsive force to expedite delivery. However, fundal pressure did not shorten the second stage of labor and it increased the incidence of maternal and fetal injury (see Exhibit 3.5) (Association of Women's Health, Obstetric and Neonatal Nurses, 2000; Buhimschi, Buhimschi, Malinow, Kopelman, & Weiner, 2002; Verheijen, Raven, & Hofmeyr, 2008).

Fundal pressure prior to delivery of the fetus may cause a shoulder dystocia, increase the risk of neonatal brachial plexus injury and fractures, and increase the risk of asphyxia and neonatal death (Simpson & Knox, 2001). If the fetal head is out and shoulder dystocia is diagnosed, never perform fundal pressure (Buhimschi, Buhimschi, Malinow, Kopelman, & Weiner, 2002). Perform and document McRoberts' maneuver with suprapubic pressure to help free up the anterior shoulder and deliver the baby (see Figure 3.4).

MONITORING DURING THE SECOND STAGE OF LABOR

The Uterus

As much as we would like to think our manual palpation of uterine contractions is somewhat accurate in determining contraction strength, it is not (Arrabal & Nagey, 1996). Even if you think the contractions are moderate in strength, they may actually be strong. Evidence of the strength of contractions is the descent of the fetus when there is no other evidence

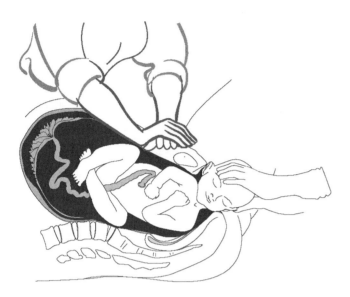

Figure 3.4: Suprapubic pressure helps dislodge the anterior shoulder when there is a shoulder dystocia. Lower the head of the bed and perform a McRoberts' maneuver prior to application of suprapubic pressure.

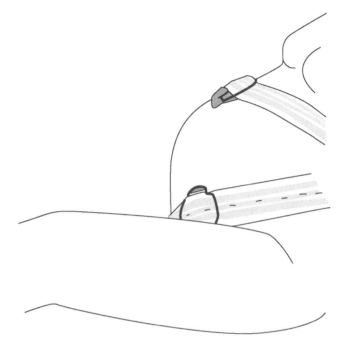

Figure 3.5: Placement of ultrasound transducer low on the abdomen during pushing with a fetus whose tip of the skull is at the level of the ischial spines (0 station).

of fetopelvic disproportion. If an intrauterine pressure catheter is in the uterus at the onset of active pushing, it is often removed and contractions are assessed by palpation for the duration of the labor. At the onset of active pushing, some physicians prefer that you deflate the indwelling urinary catheter balloon but not remove the catheter until you are sure the baby is descending. You may also remove the indwelling urinary catheter when women begin to push to avoid possible injury to the bladder or urethra. However, if her pushing is ineffective or if the fetus fails to descend, you will be inserting another indwelling urinary catheter for the cesarean section.

Documentation example: Pushing with contractions every 2 to 3 minutes.

Documentation example: Contractions q 2 to 3 minutes and strong. Encouraged to push with, not between, contractions.

The Fetus

As the baby moves down the "birth canal," your placement of the ultrasound transducer or fetoscope should also move downward. If the fetus is vertex, the transducer should be close to the pubic bone near the groin (see Figure 3.5). Continue to lower the transducer as the baby descends. You may need to place it in the groin area and angle it up towards the fetus or place it above the pubic bone and angle it down towards the fetus. Sometimes holding it will be better than using the belts because of the need to maintain an angle that allows for

monitoring of the fetal heart rate. If you are unable to maintain the fetal heart rate pattern using an ultrasound transducer, consider the application of a spiral electrode. If you cannot apply the spiral electrode, ask the midwife or physician to apply the electrode and tell them that you are unable to obtain adequate information using the external ultrasound.

Monitoring the maternal pulse may not help you differentiate the maternal rate pattern from the fetal rate pattern . Fetal monitors that print the maternal heart rate continuously on the paper and have a coincidence detection feature will help you differentiate the maternal from the fetal rate. If you do not have a maternal pulse oximeter for the fetal monitor, place the second ultrasound transducer over the maternal heart. It will record her pulse continuously and allow you to compare images. If there is an overlap, you are not monitoring the fetus. Continue to reposition the ultrasound transducer low on the abdomen until you capture the fetal heart rate and it is distinctly different from the maternal heart rate.

You should become familiar with the spiral electrode and cables that your hospital has purchased. Ask an experienced nurse to explain their use and read the manufacturer's instructions printed on the package. It has been recommended that the spiral electrode not be applied to the fetal face, fontanels, or genitalia, or when there is placenta previa. It has been recommended that the spiral electrode not be used in the presence of genital infections such as herpes, syphilis, gonorrhea, human immunodeficiency virus (HIV), or acquired immune deficiency syndrome (AIDS).

When a woman has a history of group B streptococcus, the midwife or physician will need to weigh the risks and benefits of the data they will gain from application of the electrode with the chance of neonatal transmission. Early onset (within the first 7 days of life) group B streptococcal neonatal septicemia and death related to group B streptococcal infection was associated with low birth weight, preterm birth, chorioamnionitis, intrapartum fever, premature rupture of membranes, a positive cerebral spinal fluid culture, and invasive fetal scalp electrode (spiral electrode) monitoring, even when antibiotics were administered during labor (Adair et al., 2003; Gill, Sobeck, Jarjoura, Hillier, & Benedetti, 1997). Adair and colleagues (2003) found the spiral electrode was associated with a twofold increase (double the risk) in neonatal group B streptococcal disease. The odds of neonatal death from group B streptococcal sepsis was eight times greater in infants who had a spiral electrode than in those who did not have a spiral electrode (Gill, Sobeck, Jarjoura, Hillier, & Benedetti, 1997).

The spiral electrode should not be used when the mother is a confirmed carrier of hemophilia or when it is not possible to identify the fetal presenting part. If your patient refuses the application of the spiral electrode, determine her reasons for refusal and notify the provider.

MATERNAL HEART RATE PATTERNS CAN MIMIC THE FETUS

When the maternal heart rate, instead of the fetal heart rate, is monitored during the second stage, you will not know the fetal condition. This can be life-threatening because the lack of knowledge creates a risk of fetal injury and death from unrecognized asphyxia. Some maternal heart rate patterns look nearly identical to the fetal heart rate pattern, especially when there is maternal tachycardia. To avoid misinterpretation, it is helpful to monitor the maternal heart rate either with a pulse oximeter, application of the maternal ECG leads for the fetal monitor, or placement of the other ultrasound (usually used for twin monitoring) over her heart. Look at the two images on the tracing. If they are nearly identical, you are not monitoring the baby! Readjust the ultrasound or apply a spiral electrode.

Although your protocol may only call for an assessment of the maternal pulse every half hour or hour during the second stage, it is a good idea to assess it more often and compare it with the rate reflected on the fetal monitor. Differences between the fetal and maternal heart rate include maternal heart rate decelerations (see Figure 3.7). Maternal heart rate decelerations occur during contractions but not usually between contractions. Maternal heart rate accelerations occur when women feel pain, especially during pushing in the second stage of labor (see Figures 3.6 and 3.8). It is common for women to be tachycardic during the second stage of labor due to pain (Murray, 2004). Maternal accelerations may appear as a large hill or as an increase in the rate that moves up and down in a similar fashion to the uterine contraction printout.

SETTING UP FOR DELIVERY

Vaginal birth in a hospital setting requires several items on the delivery table (see Exhibit 3.6).

Set up the delivery table using aseptic technique when your term nulliparous patient is 10-cm dilated and your multiparous patient is 7- or 8-cm dilated. Set up early with multiparous patients because their labor may progress rapidly and you need to be ready for the delivery. See Figure 3.9 for one example of the set-up for the delivery table. It is also helpful to remove the stoppers in the cord blood collection tubes and place them in the bottom of the medicine cup. You can also place a sterile towel in front of the basin. When you are finished, remove your gloves. Open the provider's package of gloves and using aseptic technique flip or lift them upward onto the sterile towel without contaminating them on the edges of the glove wrapper. Never cover the gloves with a towel as the provider will have a difficult time finding them.

> **Exhibit 3.6: Common items needed for delivery in a hospital.**
>
> 1. Basin for Placenta.
>   A. Consult the provider card or list to determine the glove size and preference.
>   B. Place drape, gloves, and sterile gown inside it.
> 2. Bulb syringe.
> 3. Hemostats (2).
> 4. Bandage scissors (for the cord).
> 5. Straight-bladed, blunt-ended pair of Mayo scissors (for the episiotomy).
> 6. Plastic cord clamp.
> 7. Medicine cup (usually for Lidocaine 1%, if requested).
> 8. Sterile syringe (will be added to the field if requested).
> 9. Radio-opaque sterile 4 × 4 gauze (10) (e.g., Raytex).
> 10. Sterile towels (6).
> 11. Tubes for cord blood collection (2).

IMMINENT DELIVERY

When your patient says, "The baby's coming" believe her! Look at the perineum. If the baby is crowning, immediately call for help, ask someone to call the obstetric care provider, put on gloves, grab a bulb syringe, and find a clean towel. When there is time, ask your helper to obtain warm blankets for the newborn. Stay close to the perineum and do not turn your back to set up the delivery table. Delivering the baby is more important than setting up for delivery.

Documentation example: Patient returned to bed from tub. Reported strong urge to push and was moaning and pushing, although encouraged not to push. Head crowning. Called for help. Head delivered and mouth

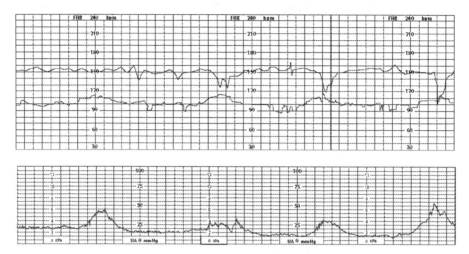

Figure 3.6: Maternal heart rate accelerations (on the lower heart rate printout) during the first stage of labor. There are variable decelerations in the fetal heart rate (on the upper printout). Paper speed is 3 cm/minute.

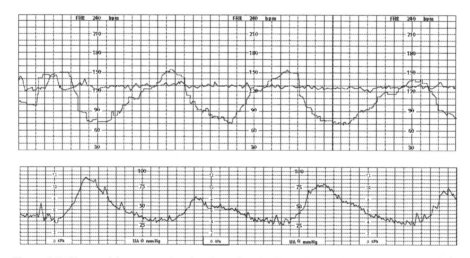

Figure 3.7: Maternal heart rate decelerations (on the lower heart rate printout) during the first stage of labor. Maternal decelerations may be related to a baroreceptor reflex that decreases the heart rate when blood pressure increases with contractions (Murray, 2004). Paper speed is 3 cm/minute.

and nose suctioned by nurse. Baby delivered and placed on mom's chest. Baby vigorous. Cord double clamped and cut. Physician arrived and delivered the placenta.

THE EPISIOTOMY

Episiotomy is a surgical incision in the perineum that facilitates the birth by enlarging the vaginal opening. If an episiotomy is performed with the first vaginal delivery, there is an increased risk of a laceration in subsequent deliveries (Alperin,

Krohn, & Parviainen, 2008). An episiotomy does not increase the risk of third- or fourth-degree tears or lacerations, but it does protect against periurethral, vaginal, and labial lacerations (Mikolajczyk, Zhang, Troendle, & Chan, 2008).

LACERATIONS AND HEMATOMAS

Tears and lacerations are graded as first, second, third, and fourth degree (see Exhibit 3.7). Third- and fourth-degree tears increase the risk of fecal incontinence that may persist long after the delivery.

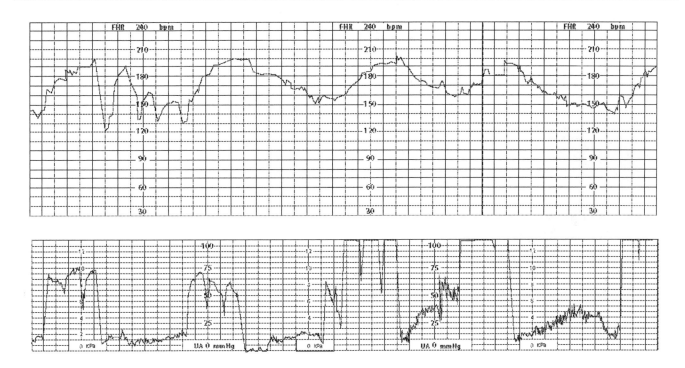

Figure 3.8: Second-stage maternal heart rate accelerations with baseline in the 140s to 150s. Paper speed is 3 cm/minute. Note that when women feel pain, they may begin to accelerate after the contraction has begun. Their accelerations last approximately the same duration as the contraction and pushing.

If there is an episiotomy or tear, you will be asked to add suture to the delivery table. You may need to add a needle holder, tissue forceps ("pickups"), and ring forceps ("rings"). Document on the delivery record the classification of the laceration, for example, first-degree laceration. This information should come directly from the provider. Superficial lacerations may not require any repair. During the repair of the laceration, assess the maternal blood pressure, pulse, and respirations, and record them on your recovery record. Once the laceration or episiotomy is repaired, assess the fundal height and massage the uterus. Superficial lacerations should begin to heal when the patient is no longer in a lithotomy position.

The occurrence of a vaginal hematoma may accompany vaginal delivery. Significant blood loss can occur. If the patient complains of pain in or near her vagina, look for a hematoma. A hematoma may begin as a swollen bruise that bulges from the vagina. The hematoma is the result of a bleeding vessel. You will need to look at the hematoma frequently for changes in its size. Notify the provider if you notice a hematoma that is enlarging. Sometimes it is helpful to measure the hematoma with a measuring tape.

WHEN THE PLAN OF CARE CHANGES: CESAREAN SECTION

Second-stage variable decelerations (see Figure 3.10) occur when the fetal head and cord are compressed as the woman pushes. To increase fetal oxygen delivery, discontinue the oxytocin infusion if there is one. Also, ask the patient to push with every other contraction. Do not encourage her to hold her breath longer than 5 to 6 seconds during contractions.

The depth and duration of the decelerations are related to fetal acid-base status and Apgar scores (Westgate et al., 2007). The fetal blood pressure decreases as the heart rate decreases. The drop in the fetal blood pressure increases the risk of fetal brain ischemia, especially during deep and/or prolonged decelerations.

Decelerations deepen or increase in their duration during the second stage. You may hear a physician say, "I don't want to section her until the baby declares itself." The fetus is totally dependent on the medical care team. To expect the fetus to announce that it needs to be delivered when there is a deteriorating heart rate is unreasonable. Discuss the plan of care with the physician. Call your charge nurse, team leader, or supervisor to the bedside. Show them the fetal heart rate pattern and share your concerns. Since you will need to remain at the bedside and be attentive to the needs of the mother and the fetus, your charge nurse can speak to the physician about the plan of care. Continue to closely monitor and document the fetal heart rate pattern and uterine contractions. The fetal heart rate pattern can quickly worsen, thus leaving little time to intervene (see Figure 3.11). Be prepared to move your patient quickly to the operating room for a cesarean section.

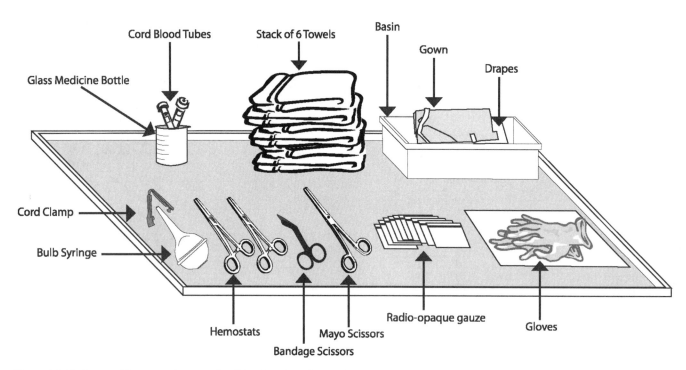

Figure 3.9: Delivery table set-up for a vaginal birth in a hospital setting. It is a good practice to account for each of the ten 4 × 4 radio-opaque gauze sponges after the delivery.

Labels in figure: Glass Medicine Bottle, Cord Blood Tubes, Stack of 6 Towels, Basin, Gown, Drapes, Cord Clamp, Bulb Syringe, Hemostats, Bandage Scissors, Mayo Scissors, Radio-opaque gauze, Gloves

---

Exhibit 3.7: Classifications of perineal lacerations.	
First degree:	Extends through the vaginal mucosa and perineal skin.
Second degree:	Extends through the perineal muscles.
Third degree:	Includes a perineal laceration involving the external anal sphincter.
Fourth degree:	Both the anal sphincter and the anal rectal mucosa are lacerated.

FETAL HEART RATE PATTERNS REQUIRING IMMEDIATE DELIVERY

One hour of abnormal fetal heart rate patterns significantly increases the risk of fetal injury. Variable decelerations or late decelerations and/or a baseline with absent to minimal variability (0 to 5 bpm) and the lack of accelerations can precede the birth of a neonate who has a low pH, low Apgar scores, metabolic acidosis, and asphyxia. These abnormal findings included low pH, metabolic acidosis, and a newborn 5-minute Apgar score of less than 7 (Low, Victory, & Derrick, 1999; Parer, King, Flanders, Fox, & Kilpatrick, 2006; Williams & Galerneau, 2003). Decelerations are not a prerequisite to asphyxiation at birth. There can simply be a baseline with absent or minimal variability that persists for 1 or more hours. Report

abnormal findings and request the immediate presence of the midwife or physician. Act to improve fetal oxygen delivery. Consider the most appropriate route of delivery. Notify your charge nurse or supervisor of the abnormal findings and your communication with the midwife or physician, and share your concerns.

> **Documentation example**: Bradycardia to 80 bpm. Patient placed on left side, oxytocin discontinued, physician called to the bedside STAT.

> **Documentation example**: Dr. Alwaysready at bedside. CRNA and OR tech notified by charge nurse. NICU high-risk team notified of impending cesarean section.

If any of the findings from Exhibit 3.8 are present, recognize, vocalize, act, and mobilize. Recognize the abnormal fetal heart rate pattern, bleeding, or abnormal uterine activity. Verbalize your concerns to other nurses and the provider. Act to protect your patients from harm by increasing fetal oxygenation, that is, change her position, discontinue the infusion of oxytocin, administer a drug to decrease uterine activity if ordered, provide oxygen with a tight-fitting face mask. Vocalize by calling for help. Call the anesthesia provider, surgeon, and pediatrician, or request another nurse to do so. The indwelling catheter can be inserted in the operating room. Shaving or clipping

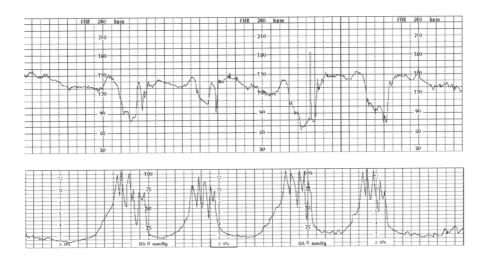

Figure 3.10: Second-stage (end-stage) variable decelerations are associated with fetal hypercarbia and hypoxia. Paper speed is 3 cm/minute.

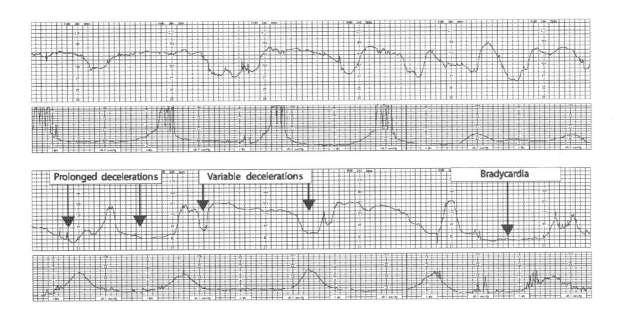

Figure 3.11: Abnormal second-stage fetal heart rate pattern. The top pattern has mostly nonperiodic (episodic) variable decelerations between contractions. The bottom pattern has prolonged decelerations, variable decelerations, and bradycardia that preceded the birth of an asphyxiated newborn. Paper speed is 3 cm/minute.

abdominal hair is not necessary prior to a cesarean section. Move your patient to the operating room and set her up for surgery. Recording the words "Crash C-section" sounds like a train wreck. It is better to write "To OR."

Documentation example: AROM by Dr. Caring for bloody fluid. FHR to 60 to 70 bpm. Anesthesia and NICU notified by charge RN. To OR #2 per birthing bed.

TERBUTALINE

Terbutaline (Brethine) may diminish uterine activity and result in improved fetal acid-base status (Patriarco, Viechnicki, Hutchinson, Klasko, & Yeh, 1987). Patriarco and colleagues' study of 11 women showed that 5 of the 11 who received terbutaline stopped contracting completely and the other 6 decreased their frequency of contractions. When the contractions stopped, late decelerations disappeared. When contrac-

Exhibit 3.8: Guidelines for delivery based on findings during labor.

Finding	Time to Deliver to Avoid Injury
SROM or AROM with bright red blood (think abruption or vasa previa—go to the OR immediately)	STAT
Late decelerations or prolonged decelerations before bradycardia with a suspected uterine rupture	10 minutes (Leung, 1993)
No prior deceleration, now prolonged deceleration with suspected uterine rupture	18 minutes (Leung, 1993)
Absent to minimal variability with variable or late or prolonged decelerations (when the FHR was previously normal)	60 minutes (Parer, King, Flanders, Fox, & Kilpatrick, 2006)

tions spaced out in all but one patient, the decelerations were less deep and less frequent. All of the women had "mild tachycardia" after the administration of terbutaline. The usual dose is 0.25 milligrams. Use a 1-mL syringe. Usually terbutaline is dispensed with 1 mg in each mL. In that case you will only be administering 0.25 mL, a very small amount. Terbutaline can be given subcutaneously or by slow IV push. Intravenous terbutaline is easier to administer if you pull some IV fluid into the syringe to create about 1 mL, then push it slowly into the IV port over 3 or more minutes. Assess and record the maternal and fetal heart rate after the drug is administered, and assess the maternal blood pressure if there is time. If you need to move quickly to the operating room, the anesthesia provider will assess the maternal vital signs.

DOCUMENTATION OF THE RESUSCITATION

At every delivery, you must be ready to resuscitate the newborn. Events that occur during the resuscitation should be documented. It helps to have a form to document the resuscitation (see Figure 3.12).

THE THIRD STAGE OF LABOR: DELIVERY OF THE PLACENTA

The third stage of labor begins with the birth of the baby and ends with delivery of the placenta. Active management of the third stage of labor should prevent postpartum hemorrhage. The three steps of active management of the third stage of labor include uterotonics, controlled cord traction, and uterine massage (Althabe et al., 2008; Geller, Adams, & Miller, 2007). Oxytocin is usually administered after the placenta is delivered. A slow IV push dose of 10 units of oxytocin resulted in

less postpartum blood loss than 10 units diluted in 500 mL of normal saline infused at 125 mL/hour (358 mL versus 424 mL) (Davies, Tessier, Woodman, Lipson, & Hahn, 2005). Oxytocin may also be injected into a large muscle, such as the vastus lateralis. A maximum of 40 units may be added to 1000 mL of intravenous fluid. However, the usual dose after delivery of the placenta is 10 to 20 units. Titrate the infusion to control the bleeding and to prevent uterine atony. If hemorrhage occurs, bimanual compression of the uterus may be needed. The midwife or physician will insert a gloved hand into the vagina while the other hand pushes on and compresses the uterine fundus (Geller, Adams, & Miller, 2007).

THE FOURTH STAGE OF LABOR: MATERNAL RECOVERY

The fourth stage of labor begins with delivery of the placenta and lasts approximately 2 hours. This is also called the "time of recovery." During recovery, the priorities during the first hour are airway, breathing, and circulation. If maternal and neonatal vital signs are stable and the neonate is not hypothermic, initiate breastfeeding if that is part of the patient's plan. Mothers are more likely to breastfeed their infants successfully when there is skin to skin contact rather than having the infant swaddled in blankets. Skin to skin contact also increases maternal attachment behaviors. There are no adverse effects of skin to skin contact (Caruna, 2008).

AIRWAY AND BREATHING

The frequency of vital signs during the immediate postpartum period may vary, but for a vaginal delivery the vital signs usually are monitored every 15 minutes for the first hour, every 30 minutes for the second hour, then once each shift. If your patient had a cesarean section, vital signs may be monitored more frequently. If the patient's condition is deteriorating, or if there is excessive vaginal bleeding or a change in her level of consciousness, then vital signs should be monitored more frequently and reported to the provider. A change in the level of consciousness requires the nurse to request a physician come to the bedside immediately and evaluate the patient.

CIRCULATION

If bleeding is not controlled within a few minutes after you begin the intravenous infusion of oxytocin (Pitocin or Syntocinon), 0.2 milligrams of methylergonovine maleate (Methergine) should be given to women who are not hypertensive. Intrarectal misoprostol (Cytotec) may be administered in addition to, or in place of, Methergine. Langenbach (2006) identified 22 studies of 30,017 women who received misoprostol after delivery of the placenta. The risk of postpartal hemorrhage was only 4% greater than when oxytocics were used. To treat postpartal hemorrhage, the dose of misoprostol (Cytotec) may range between 200 micrograms and 1000 micrograms. The drug is usually placed by the midwife or physician (Spratto & Woods, 2001). Because it is an inexpensive drug, its use is

DOCUMENTATION OF THE RESUSCITATION

Patient's Name_____

Date:_____ Time of Birth:_____ Gestation:_____weeks

Analgesia/Anesthesia: Analgesia type_____ Time of last dose_____
          ❑Epidural ❑General ❑Spinal

Gender: ❑Female   ❑Male

ICN(NICU) Team requested at_____

ICN (NICU) Team arrived at_____

INITIAL STEPS	TIME
DeLee Suction on delivery	
Tracheal suction for meconium	
Bulb suction	
Blow by O$_2$	
HR > 100 bpm	
Centrally pink	
O$_2$ discontinued	

ATTENDANTS

Obstetrician_____

Certified Nurse Midwife_____

Neonatal Care Provider_____

RN_____

RN_____

RRT_____

RRT_____

APGAR SCORES	1 MINUTE	5 MINUTES	10 MINUTES
Heart Rate			
Respiratory effort			
Tone			
Reflex irritability			
Color			
TOTAL			

TIME	ASSESSMENT	INTERVENTIONS/PERSONNEL	RESPONSE

Remarks:_____
_____
_____
_____

Signature/Title_____ Initials_____

Figure 3.12: Sample newborn resuscitation record.

Exhibit 3.9: Goals and expections for the fourth stage of labor.
• Stable vital signs, afebrile.
• Pain is controlled.
• Fundus is firm and midline.
• Lochia is not excessive.
• Perineum is swollen with an ice pack applied.
• Bladder is empty and/or nondistended.
• Patient has eaten and tolerated the diet.
• Bowel sounds are present.
• En face interaction with her baby (babies).

Exhibit 3.10: Common abbreviations during the fourth stage of labor (> means "more than" and < means "less than").

Fundus

F	Firm, FF = fundus firm
B	Boggy (be sure to document your actions for this)
U	Umbilicus
#/U	Location of fundus above the umbilicus
U/#	Location of fundus below the umbilicus
U/U	Fundus at the umbilicus

Lochia

S	Small amount of lochia (< 1/2 pad soaked in 15 minutes)
M	Moderate amount (> 1/2 pad and < 1 pad soaked in 15 minutes)
H	Heavy (saturated > 1 pad in 15 minutes)

Perineum

I	Intact
E	Edematous
G	Very edematous (grossly)
W	Well approximated
H	Hematoma

cost-effective, especially in countries that have financial limitations in their health care systems.

Another drug used by injection to treat uterine atony is carboprost tromethamine (Hemabate). The usual dose is 250 micrograms (not milligrams) injected into a muscle or directly into the uterus. A registered nurse may inject Hemabate into a muscle. A physician will inject Hemabate into the uterus during a cesarean section. The most common side effects of Hemabate are diarrhea and vomiting. So be sure to place a linen protector under the patient and have a basin ready after you administer Hemabate.

CARE DURING THE FOURTH STAGE

Care goals during the fourth stage of labor are listed in Exhibit 3.9. Common abbreviations used in charting during the fourth stage of labor are listed in Exhibit 3.10.

Every 15 minutes or more often during recovery, assess and record the patient's blood pressure, pulse, and respiratory rate. Determine and record the fundal height, its firmness, the amount of lochia, and the presence of blood clots (see Exhibit 3.10). While supporting the lower uterine segment, push hard on the uterine fundus toward the vagina to express clots that may have formed in the lower part of the uterus. If you do not push hard and large blood clots form, she can hemorrhage and the uterus can become boggy (see Figure 3.13). It is best to use two hands when you massage the fundus to prevent uterine inversion, one hand at the top of the fundus, and the other hand above the pubic bone holding the bottom of the uterus for stabilization.

Before you compress the fundus inform your patient of your plan. Ask her to take a deep breath and slowly exhale. As she exhales compress the fundus. Her abdomen should be less tense when she exhales.

Documentation example: FF 1/U, S, E. (This means the fundus was firm and found at one finger-breath above

the umbilicus with a small amount of lochia, with some perineal edema). Each hospital will have acceptable abbreviations for you to use. There is a list of common abbreviations in the Appendix.

Some hospitals document the location of the fundus as +1 U to mean 1 fingerbreadth above the umbilicus and –1 U to mean 1 fingerbreadth below the umbilicus. Sometimes the U precedes the number. For example, U –2 means the fundus was found two fingerbreadths below the umbilicus.

If you administered an intramuscular injection of Methergine during the second stage of labor, the effect will wear off in 3 hours (*Physicians' Desk Reference*, 2001). Most likely you will have transferred your patient's care to the postpartum nurse. If not, be extra vigilant and assess her uterus and lochia. Report drugs given during recovery, the estimated blood loss before and after drug use, and the current status of uterine bleeding (see Exhibits 3.11 and 3.12).

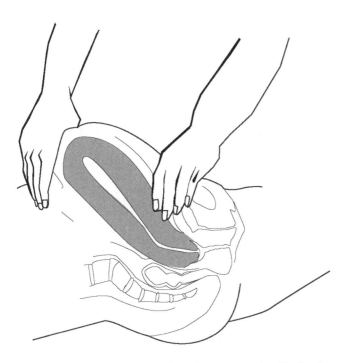

Figure 3.13: Two-handed technique for compressing the fundus to express clots the first two to three times after delivery (at a minimum every 15 minutes). The lower hand supports the lower segment of the uterus, while the upper hand pushes down toward the vagina to expel any clots that have formed.

> **Exhibit 3.11: Elements of the nurse-to-nurse report related to the mother.**
>
> - Patient's name, age, gravida, parity
> - Blood type/Rubella/Hep B/GBS status
> - Gender/Delivery Time
> - Vaginal/Spontaneous/Forceps/Vacuum Delivery
> - Cesarean/Bilateral Tubal Ligation
> - Episiotomy/Laceration/Degree/Repair
> - Anesthesia Type (epidural/spinal/general/local)
> - Duramorph or other medication used if intrathecal or spinal
> - Vital Signs/Fundus/Lochia/EBL
> - Abdominal dressing
> - I & O/Time of void/Catheter
> - Medications given (type/dose/time)
> - Medications due (type/dose/time)
> - Allergies
> - Cord blood collection
> - Lab work done/due
> - Significant prenatal history
> - Labor and delivery history

The transfer of care to the postpartum or mother–baby nurse will involve a nurse-to-nurse report also known as a patient hand-off communication. There are many formats for this communication process. Your hospital may use a checklist format or a fill-in-the-blank form to accomplish the patient report. Some hospitals require nurse-to-nurse communication on the telephone or face to face. Other hospitals may rely on faxed reports, but these reports increase the risk of communication failure if they are not read carefully. Regardless of the method of communication, a standardized approach for the transfer of information is a good idea. The report of the mother's labor, delivery, and recovery, and information related to the baby's first hours of life, are required for continuity of care and patient safety.

POSTPARTUM HEMORRHAGE

Postpartum hemorrhage (PPH) may be overt, with obvious vaginal bleeding and clots after a vaginal birth, or concealed, after a cesearean section. PPH has been defined as a blood loss of more than 500 mL within 24 hours of delivery (Airede & Nnadi, 2008; Burtelow et al., 2007).

Causes of Postpartum Hemorrhage

The most common cause of PPH is uterine atony (Geller, Adams, & Miller, 2007). Other causes of PPH include infection such as chorioamnionitis, retained placental tissue, and subinvolution of the placental implantation site as late as 12 days after delivery. Rare causes of a delayed postpartum hemorrhage include pseudoaneurysm of a uterine artery, arteriovenous malformations, and choriocarcinoma (Lausman, Ellis, Beecroft, Simons, & Shapiro, 2008).

Treatment Goals

The first goal will be to control or stop the bleeding (Kirkpatrick, Ball, D'Amours, & Zygun, 2008). Notify your charge nurse. If an anesthesia provider is available, call him or her to the bedside. The provider has learned that the traditional treatment for PPH is to administer 1 or more liters of crystalloid. Be prepared to start another intravenous line with at least an 18-gauge catheter. The bolus of 1 or more liters of crystalloid is called fluid resuscitation. Fluid resuscitation may actually increase blood loss because excess fluid dilutes clotting factors (Davies, Tessler, Woodman, Lipson, & Hahn, 2005). If uterine atony is causing the hemorrhage, drugs such as misoprostol (Cytotec) or methylergonovine maleate (Methergine) will be used to help the uterus become firm. This should decrease blood loss due to uterine atony (Baruah &

Exhibit 3.12: Elements of a nurse-to-nurse report for the newborn.

- Mother's name
- Gender of infant
- Delivery Time/type of delivery
- Resuscitation steps
- Weight, length/gestational age/assessment findings
- Apgars
- Vital signs
- Feeding type: breast/bottle/both
- Last feeding type/time
- I & O
- Labs done/due
- Routine medications given
- Other medications given/due (type/dose/time)
- Antibiotics that mother received
- Cord blood collected
- Significant prenatal history
- Labor & delivery history
- Provider notification of birth

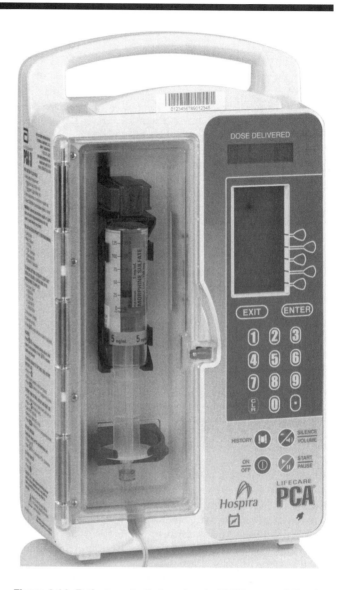

Figure 3.14: Patient-controlled analgesia (PCA) pump delivering morphine. This type of device is usually used after a cesarean section and it contains a syringe filled with a narcotic. (Reproduced with permission from Hospira Worldwide, Lake Forest, Illinois.)

Cohn, 2008). Every labor and delivery nurse must know where the medications are stored and have quick access to these life-saving drugs, as well as access to syringes and needles (see Exhibits 3.13 and 3.14).

The physician may order laboratory tests that include the prothrombin time (PT), partial thromboplastin time (PTT), fibrinogen, D-dimer, and a complete blood count. The results of these tests will help the physician decide the best treatment plan. For example, a 1-gram/dL drop in hemoglobin, or a 3% drop in the hematocrit, is equivalent to 1 unit of packed red blood cells or approximately 500 mL of whole blood (Gutierrez, Reines, & Wulf-Gutierrez, 2004).

MEASURE BLOOD LOSS

To further assist the midwife and/or physician in determining the treatment plan, you should measure and report all blood loss. One mL of blood weighs almost 1 gram. Weigh clots and subtract the weight of the dry pad or Chux. The estimated blood loss at the time of delivery, plus the additional blood loss you report, may cause the midwife or physician to order additional medications or may mean there is a need for surgery, such as a dilatation and curettage (D & C) or laparotomy.

DANGERS OF EXCESSIVE INTRAVENOUS FLUID

One bolus of intravenous solution is 500 mL or more. A preload bolus of intravenous fluid prior to neuraxial anesthesia does not prevent hypotension. Administration of a 500-mL bolus prior to an epidural and then supine positioning after the epidural was found to be related to a significant drop in the mean arterial pressure (MAP). This drop in blood pressure was not found if the patient was placed on her left side. Com-

pared with women who were placed on their left side, women in a supine position had a lower cardiac output (21%) and lower stroke volume (21%), higher systemic vascular resistance (50%), a similar heart rate, and a higher MAP (19%) (Danilenko-Dixon, Tefft, Cohen, Haydon, & Carpenter, 1996). Even a 2-liter preload of crystalloid did not prevent hypotension following spinal anesthesia (Chanimov, Gershfeld, Cohen, Sherman, & Bahar, 2006; Sharma, Gajraj, & Sidawi, 1997).

Aggressive restoration of intravascular volume by the infusion of a crystalloid solution may increase bleeding (Dagan,

Exhibit 3.13: Uterotonic medications (Baruah & Cohn, 2008; Mercier et al., 2008).

Brand Name	Generic Name	Usual Dose Range Expected	Response
Pitocin	Oxytocin	**10 to 20 units**	**Increased uterine tone**
	Route and onset:	IV: immediate	
	Dose:	5 to 10 units with delivery of the anterior shoulder and/or dilute 10 to 40 units in an intravenous solution and titrate to control bleeding, such as 60 mL/hour or 0.1 U/minute (Spratto et al., 2001)	
Methergine	Methylergono-vinemaleate	**0.2 mg**	**Increased rate, tone, and strength of contractions**
	Route and onset:	IM: 2 to 5 minutes IV: immediate	
	Contraindications:	high blood pressure or with vasoconstrictor medication	
	Side effects:	high blood pressure with headache or seizure, low blood pressure, palpitations, nausea, vomiting, diarrhea, foul taste, dizziness, ringing in the ears, hallucinations, sweating, chest pain, shortness of breath, blood in the urine, leg cramps, nasal congestion	
Cytotec	Misoprostol	**200 to 1,000 micrograms**	**Increased uterine tone**
	Route and onset:	Per rectum, 1 to 2 minutes	
	Contraindications:	allergies to prostaglandins	
	Side effects:	diarrhea, abdominal pain, nausea, headache	
Hemabate	Carboprost	**250 micrograms**	**Immediate**
	Route and onset:	IM or Intrauterine: immediate	
	Contraindications:	hypersensitivity to Hemabate Sterile Solution; acute pelvic inflammatory disease; patients with active cardiac, pulmonary, renal or hepatic disease	
	Side effects:	can cause bronchospasm, avoid use if patient has asthma, vomiting diarrhea, nausea, flushing or hot flashes, chills or shivering, coughing, headaches, endometritis, hiccough, severe cramps; consult the manufacturer's drug literature for additional information	
	Maximum dose:	total dose administered of carboprost tromethamine should not exceed 2 milligrams or 8 doses (50 to 90 minutes apart)	
Ergonovine	Ergometrine maleate	**0.2 mg**	**Tetanic contraction in 6 to 15 minutes**
	Route and onset:	IV or IM if history of hypertension	

Gabay, & Barnea, 2007; Lu et al., 2007). Intravenous fluids dilute the blood and may worsen tissue oxygenation and perfusion (Cavus et al., 2007). Excess intravascular fluid decreases the concentration of hemoglobin and oxygen delivery to the tissues (Gutierrez, Reines, & Wulf-Gutierrez, 2004). Crystalloids, such as lactated Ringer's solution, are poor plasma volume expanders (Sharma, Gajraj, & Sidawi, 1997). Yet, Advanced Trauma Life Support guidelines have called for aggressive crystalloid resuscitation starting with 2 liters of lactated Ringer's solution during surgery after trauma. The American College of Surgeons advised its members to administer 3 liters of crystalloid for every 1,000 mL of blood loss (Spaniol, Knight, Zebley, Anderson, & Pierce, 2007). If normal saline (0.9% sodium chloride) is rapidly infused, hyperchloremia and a reduction in plasma bicarbonate may occur, thus increasing the risk of metabolic acidosis (Reid, Lobo, Williams, Rowlands, &

Allison, 2003). Therefore, one should never administer a bolus of saline solution in a woman who is hemorrhaging. Excess intravenous fluid causes dilutional coagulopathy (Haas et al., 2008). Crystalloids dilute clotting factors and contribute to platelet dysfunction, thus decreasing their ability to create a clot, which results in increased bleeding (Haas et al., 2008; Tien, Nascimento Jr., Callum, & Rizoli, 2007). In addition, the excess fluid decreases blood viscosity and clots can be dislodged (Lee et al., 2007). Small volumes of colloids, such as hetastarch, may be a better choice than crystalloids such as lactated Ringer's solution for fluid resuscitation.

Tissue edema and pulmonary edema may occur following aggressive fluid administration, especially in women with abnormal kidney function. Unlike crystalloids, colloids increase oncotic pressure in plasma and reduce the likelihood of tissue edema (Kheirabadi et al., 2008). Crystalloids decrease colloid

Exhibit 3.14: Basic goals and principles related to the treatment of postpartum hemorrhage (MAP = mean arterial pressure).

1. Stop the bleeding: Administer uterotonic medications for uterine atony.
2. Replace (PRN or as ordered) volume and blood.
3. Limit crystalloid IV fluids to avoid hemodilution.
4. Hemodilution decreases the concentration of clotting factors and clot formation (dilutional coagulopathy) and the increase in MAP increases the risk of pulmonary edema.
5. Maintain an MAP of 60 mm Hg and/or a systolic BP of 90 mm Hg.
6. Assess airway, breathing, hourly urine output, BP, MAP, level of consciousness, respiratory rate, temperature, pulse, pulse pressure, capillary refill, and peripheral pulses.
7. Urine output should be ≥ 30 mL/hr.
8. Report findings to the provider.
9. Start additional IV PRN with normal saline.
10. Prepare to administer blood and blood products.
11. Monitor ECG, SpO$_2$, and BP as ordered.
12. High-flow oxygen PRN (10 L/min during labor, as ordered after delivery).
13. Laboratory tests: Complete (full) blood count, coagulation and cross-match studies.
14. Treat/avoid hypothermia. Use of forced-air warming blanket or warm blankets, warm intravenous solutions PRN. Never place warmed IV bags directly on patient's skin.
15. Administer blood and blood products as ordered.

osmotic pressure, which causes fluids to move out of the semi-permeable blood vessels into cells in the interstitium (Dagan, Gabay, & Barnea, 2007). This movement of water into the tissues can produce significant edema. Postpartum women may appear to have huge legs and swollen breasts, most likely because they were overloaded with fluid during their labors. It is important to avoid administering excessive crystalloid solutions such as lactated Ringer's or normal saline during labor, or as a treatment for postpartum hemorrhage. It is important to avoid administering a large volume of a dextrose-containing solution close to the time of delivery because it causes fetal hyperglycemia and an increase in insulin production. Soon after the umbilical cord is cut, the high level of insulin will cause neonatal hypoglycemia.

Prior to using any bolus of intravenous fluid, kidney function should be known. By keeping strict intake and output records during labor, you should be able to recognize abnormal kidney function. If the patient's urine output in the last 24 hours averages about 3,000 mL (or 125 mL/hour) her kidneys should be able to handle a 1- or 2-liter crystalloid bolus. If she has been diagnosed with severe preeclampsia and her 24-hour urine output averages 63 mL/hour (range of 30 to 136 mL/hour), she has a significant risk of developing pulmonary edema when an intravenous bolus is administered (Gilson, Kramer, Barada, Izquierdo, & Curet, 1998). Women who have preeclampsia have even more permeable blood vessels than women who do not have preeclampsia.

BALLOON COMPRESSION TO STOP THE BLEEDING

When the bleeding cannot be stopped with medications and uterine massage, vaginal packing with gauze or sterile towels may be needed (Schlicher, in press). Because the lower uterine segment is mostly connective tissue and not muscle, if the placenta had a low implantation, that area after delivery would not contract as well as the rest of the uterus after the delivery of the placenta. The open maternal vessels would tend to bleed more. If the bleeding does not decrease or if the fundus of the uterus is firm, but bleeding continues, the physician may elect to insert a tamponade device to apply direct pressure to the inside wall of the uterus.

If a tamponade device is inserted, an indwelling catheter should also be inserted into the bladder to keep it empty. The tamponade device may be created or purchased. Nigerian physicians created a tamponade device with a condom after it was cleaned in an antiseptic solution. They inserted a Foley catheter into the end of the condom, which was secured to the catheter with chromic catgut suture. The cervix was visualized with a speculum and the condom was inserted into the lower segment of the uterus. The condom was then filled with 300 to 500 mL of normal saline and the cervix was held together by "sponge-holding" forceps. The Foley catheter attached to the condom was clamped for 12 to 18 hours. Vaginal gauze packing was inserted and antibiotics were also administered (Airede & Nnadi, 2002). Another tamponade device is the Bakri postpartum balloon (see Figure 3.15).

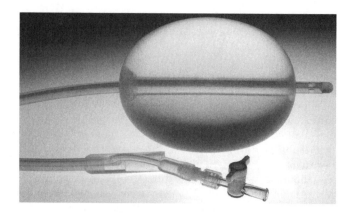

Figure 3.15: Photograph of the Bakri postpartum balloon (courtesy of Cook Urological, Spencer, Indiana).

Exhibit 3.15: Hemorrhagic shock (acute blood loss).

Advanced Trauma Life Support Classifications	Risks	Signs/Symptoms
CLASS I: 750 mL loss or 15% blood volume	Increased capillary permeability	CLASS I: blood volume restored within 24 hrs without transfusion
CLASS II: 750–1,500 mL loss or 15–30% blood volume	• Cerebral hypoperfusion • Myocardial hypoperfusion • DIC	CLASS II: • ↓ cardiac output • HR > 100 bpm • ↓ pulse pressure (↑ diastolic) • ↑ catecholaminas (↓ PVR) • ↑ respiratory rate • Pale, cool skin • Anxiety • ↓ urine output • Mild confusion • Irritability • Needs IVF, not necessarily blood transfusion
CLASS III: 1,500–2,000 mL or 30–40% loss (transfusion is needed)	• Hypoxemia • Hypotension	CLASS III: • HR > 120 bpm • Arrhythmia • ↓ BP • Respiratory distress • ↑ $PaCO_2$ • ↓ HCO_3 • ↓ PaO_2 • Significant ↓ in urine output • ↑ BUN and creatinine
CLASS IV: > 2,000 mL or > 40% loss LIFE THREATENING, PRETERMINAL	• Acidosis • Respiratory distress • Renal hypoperfusion	CLASS IV: • HR > 140 bpm • Severe hypotension • Narrow pulse pressure • ↑ Peripheral pulse • ↓ Urine output

SHOCK

Hemorrhagic shock occurs when a woman loses 1,500 to 2,000 mL (30 to 40%) of her blood volume (see Exhibits 3.15 and 3.16) (Kirkpatrick, Ball, D'Amours, & Zygun, 2008). Major obstetric hemorrhage is defined as a loss of 2,500 mL or more, the transfusion of 5 or more units of blood, or treatment for a coagulopathy (Wise & Clark, 2008). The clinical signs of shock include tachycardia (120 bpm or higher), a drop in systolic blood pressure (90 or lower), and/or a urine output of less than 15 mL/hour (Tien, Nascimento Jr., Callum, & Rizoli, 2007).

Shock injures cells (Shults et al., 2008). Organs such as the liver may be injured (Jarrar, Wang, Cioffi, Bland, & Chaudry, 2000). Lactic acid accumulates in the blood, which also damages tissue (Frankel et al., 2007). As a result of hypoxia, acidosis, and tissue injury, an inflammatory process occurs in which white blood cells (neutrophils) release reactive oxygen species known as free oxygen radicals or superoxides. These superoxides are toxic to cells because they impair cell antioxidant capacity, which leads to oxidative stress, apoptosis (cell death), and organ damage (Jarrar, Wang, Cioffi, Bland, & Chaudry, 2000; Yang, Zhao, & Reece, 2008; Zakaria, Campbell, Peyton, & Garrison, 2007).

After a vaginal delivery, bleeding is usually overt. After a cesarean section, however, bleeding may be overt or concealed. If bleeding is concealed and is intraabdominal, you should suspect that your patient is in shock if she becomes hypothermic or excessively hot, tachycardic (that is, her rate may be near 150 bpm), diaphoretic and/or agitated, she complains that she can't breathe or is short of breath, and/or is just not "with it." Call the obstetrician immediately to come to the bedside to evaluate your patient. She is probably in hypovolemic shock. Be sure you have intravenous access and be ready to administer blood and blood products. Because she is short of breath, you need to notify the anesthesia provider to evaluate her airway. Your charge nurse or supervisor should also be informed of your patient's status.

Diaphoresis
Diaphoresis is a sign of shock. Diaphoretic women sweat excessively. Check her pillow. Is it soaked? Assess her temperature. Touch her skin. Is it cool and clammy or warm? Document diaphoresis and her skin temperature.

Tachycardia
Tachycardia is a sign of shock. Sinus tachycardia is a stress response to the hypoxemia and hypoperfusion from blood loss. The patient's adrenal medulla will secrete epinephrine, which raises her heart rate. When the heart rate is tachycardic (over 100 bpm) her heart will pump less efficiently because there will be less time to relax between cardiac contractions. If the tachycardia lasts an extended period of time, the balance in her blood between oxygen and carbon dioxide carried by hemoglobin will change. Her tachycardic heart will consume more oxygen than before. Therefore, tachycardia should never be accepted as normal. Call the obstetrician and ask him or her to evaluate your patient immediately.

Decreased Blood Pressure
Decreased blood pressure is a sign of shock. Assess the patient's blood pressure. What was her blood pressure before delivery? What was her normal blood pressure when she was not in labor? If the systolic pressure has dropped 30%, she is hypotensive. Report your findings to the obstetrician. If the physician orders an immediate blood transfusion, enter the order as a "medical emergency," then call the blood bank and tell them you are sending them an order requesting blood for a medical emergency.

Decreased SpO$_2$
Shortness of breath is related to shock. Assess the patient's lung sounds and her respiratory rate. Apply a pulse oximeter. Apply oxygen with a tight-fitting face mask at 10 liters/minute. Sit her up. If she is having difficulty breathing or has shallow respirations, and she is tachycardic and her oxygen saturation drops to 90% or less, she may be near death. If she begins to kick and squirm, even when oxygen is on at 10 liters with a nonbreather mask, she may be near death. If she begins to foam at the mouth and her eyes roll back, she may be near

death. Your prompt assessments, actions, and communications with the obstetrician when there are abnormal vital signs can make the difference between life and death.

Call the Charge Nurse and the Obstetrician
Involve your charge nurse or supervisor in the care of your patient. You may need to call any obstetrician in the hospital to the bedside while someone else is calling the obstetrician who is not in the building. Once you reach an obstetrician, request a STAT hemoglobin and hematocrit (H & H) and an order to start a second intravenous (IV) line. Request an order for a blood transfusion. Call the laboratory and tell them you will need the H & H results STAT and send the request. Order the blood as a medical emergency (which is faster than STAT) and call the blood bank to let them know you need it immediately.

Before an emergency occurs, know the policy, procedure, and protocol to obtain blood and blood products, the location of the blood bank in your facility, and the form you will need to check out the blood and blood products.

Begin a Second Intravenous Line
Start a second intravenous line with a large-bore cannula, such as an 18-gauge catheter, and infuse normal saline to keep the vein open. Send a runner to the blood bank to pick up the blood. Your prompt assessments, communications, and actions could be the difference between life and death.

OTHER TYPES OF SHOCK
In addition to hemorrhagic shock (see Exhibit 3.16), there are three other types of shock: distributive, obstructive, and cardiogenic. Any diagnosis of shock carries the risk of metabolic acidosis, hypothermia, organ failure, and death. Therefore, it is important that vital signs be assessed after delivery and when there is a postpartal hemorrhage until the blood pressure is higher than 90 mm Hg systolic and the mean arterial pressure is 60 mm Hg or higher (Dagan et al., 2007). Hypothermia can actually impair coagulation. Using a blood or fluid warmer may be life saving. Application of warm blankets is essential after a postpartal hemorrhage.

TRANSFUSIONS
If a transfusion is needed, you may be administering blood and/or blood products (see Exhibit 3.17). The infusion of packed red blood cells should increase the delivery of oxygen to tissues. The primary risk of a blood transfusion is infection. However, the risk of transmission of hepatitis B is 1 in 82,000 units of blood. The risk of HIV transmission is 1 in 4.7 million units. The risk of hepatitis C transmission is 1 in 3.1 million units (Tien, Nascimento Jr., Callum, & Rizoli, 2007). Massive transfusion can cause hypothermia, acidosis, coagulopathy, excess plasma potassium (hyperkalemia), low calcium, and citrate toxicity. Rarely, a mistransfusion occurs (1 in 40,000 units) that can result in death due to a major hemolytic reaction. The hemoglobin level is not used to determine the need for blood because it will not equilibrate with the total circulat-

Exhibit 3.16: Types of Shock

Classes	Signs/Symptoms	Possible Treatments
DISTRIBUTIVE • SEPTIC • ANAPHYLACTIC • Neurogenic*	SEPTIC Temp < 36° C or > 38° HR > 90 bpm RR > 20/min WBCs > 12,000/mm³ or WBCs < 4,000/ mm³ or > 10% bands	• Antibiotics, if sepsis • Crystalloid bolus • Possible dobutamine, dopamine, packed RBCs
	ANAPHYLACTIC • Histamine release • Hypotension • Increased capillary permeability • Angioedema (airway constriction) • Bronchospasm	• Maintain airway (ETT) • IV bolus crystalloid • IV epinephrine
OBSTRUCTIVE CARDIOGENIC	e.g., Pulmonary embolism • Decreased urine output • Altered mentation • Hypotension • Jugular venous distension • Cardiac gallop • Pulmonary edema • Systolic BP < 90 mmHg for > 30 minutes • Oliguria (< 30 mL/hr)	• Thrombectomy • Target the cause
HEMORRHAGIC	• HR > 120 bpm • Systolic BP < 90 mm Hg • Urine < 15 mL/hr • Cold extremities • Cyanotic • May become unconscious	• Crystalloids • Colloids • Dopamine • Blood products • Surgery

*Uncommon in labor and delivery.

ing plasma volume at the time of the transfusion (Tien, Nascimento, Callum, & Rizoli, 2007).

VASOPRESSORS

Drugs such as dopamine or dobutamine may be needed to maintain blood pressure. Usually the woman will be transported to the intensive care unit when these drugs are needed.

CONCLUSIONS

Labor is divided into four stages. The first stage is divided into the latent phase and the active phase. It can also be divided into three parts: early labor, active labor, and transition. During active labor and transition, functional, mechanical, and/or emotional dystocia may slow or stop dilatation and/or de-

scent. Dystocia is the most common reason for a cesarean section.

The second stage of labor has two phases, the latent phase and the active phase. The latent phase of the second stage of labor is a time for laboring down, delayed pushing, and passive descent. Ferguson's reflex may be related to an increased secretion of oxytocin. Women will have a strong urge to push. The active phase of the second stage is a time for pushing and fetal descent. Fundal pressure should not be used during the second stage of labor because it increases the risk of maternal and fetal injuries.

It is important to continue to monitor the fetus throughout the second stage of labor and avoid monitoring the mother's heart rate with the external ultrasound transducer. Maternal

Exhibit 3.17: Blood-product transfusion recommendations	
Platelets	1 pool or 1 unit or as ordered.
Fresh frozen plasma	15 to 20 mL/kg, 4 units at a time to increase blood clotting factors to 30% of normal, 10–15 mL/kg is 3–4 units.
Cryoprecipitate	To replace fibrinogin when less than 1.0 g/L. As ordered. Usually 1 unit/10 kg (8.12 units/dose).

heart rate patterns can mimic fetal heart rate patterns. Nurses have a critical role in preventing the misidentification of the maternal heart rate as the fetal heart rate. At times, a spiral electrode will be needed to help monitor the fetus. The transmission of group B streptococcus to the fetus can occur when a spiral electrode is used. The midwife or physician must weigh the risks and benefits prior to electrode use.

The third and fourth stages of labor are a time when hemorrhage can occur. During the third stage of labor, the placenta is delivered. During the fourth stage of labor, recovery occurs. The goal is to control or stop the bleeding. The first line of treatment for uterine atony is medications. Excessive intravenous fluid can be life threatening. Occasionally, balloon compression will be needed to stop the bleeding. If a woman suffers from hemorrhagic shock, transfusions of blood and blood products may be needed, as well as the administration of vasopressors. Nurses who understand labor, delivery, and their complications, should be able to provide satisfactory care that promotes patient well-being and decreases the risk of harm.

REVIEW QUESTIONS

True/False: Decide if the statements are true or false.

1. Normal labor should last 6 to 12 hours.
2. A birth plan is a form of communication between the patient and her health care providers.
3. In the case of mechanical dystocia, a higher dose of oxytocin will be beneficial.
4. A benefit of delayed pushing or laboring down when an epidural is in place may be fewer midforceps procedures.
5. Shoulder dystocia is more common when labor is slow and there is an arrest of 2 or more hours in the active phase of labor.
6. Fundal pressure during the second stage of labor is a safe procedure.
7. A second-degree tear may precede fecal incontinence.
8. Important goals during the fourth stage of labor include maintaining stable vital signs, controlling vaginal bleeding and pain, and supporting maternal–infant interaction.
9. The usual dose of subcutaneous terbutaline is 0.25 micrograms.
10. Fundal massage during the fourth stage of labor is best accomplished using the two-handed technique.

References

Adair, C. E., Kowalsky, L., Quon, H., Ma, D., Stoffman, J., & McGeer, A. (2003). Risk factors for early-onset group B streptococcal disease in neonates: A population-based case-control study. *Canadian Medical Association Journal, 169*(3), 198–203.

Airede, L. R., & Nnadi, D. C. (2008). The use of the condom-catheter for the treatment of postpartum haemorrhage: The Sokoto experience. *Tropical Doctor, 38,* 84–86.

Albers, L. (1999). The duration of labor in healthy women. *Journal of Perinatology 19,* 114–119.

Albers, L., Schiff, M., & Gorwoda, J. (1996). The length of active labor in normal pregnancies. *Obstetrics & Gynecology, 87,* 355–359.

Althabe, F., Buekens, P., Bergel, E., Belizán, J. M., Campbell, M. K., & Moss, N. (2008). A behavioral intervention to improve obstetrical care. *New England Journal of Medicine, 358*(18), 1929–1940.

Alperin, M., Krohn, M., & Parviainen, K. (2008). Episiotomy and increase in the risk of obstetric laceration in a subsequent vaginal delivery. *Obstetrics & Gynecology, 111*(6), 1274–1278.

American College of Obstetricians and Gynecologists. (2003). Dystocia and the augmentation of labor. *ACOG Practice Bulletin No. 45.* Washington, DC: Author.

Arrabal, P. P., & Nagey, D. A. (1996). Is manual palpation of uterine contractions accurate? *American Journal of Obstetrics and Gynecology, 174,* 217–219.

Association of Women's Health, Obstetric and Neonatal Nurses. (2000). Evidence-based clinical practice guideline. *Nursing management of the second stage of labor.* Washington, DC: Author.

Bakker, P. C. A. M., & van Geijn, H. P. (2008). Uterine activity: Implications for the condition of the fetus. *Journal of Perinatal Medicine, 36,* 30–37.

Bao-Ping, Z., Grigorescu, V., Le, T., Lin, M., Copeland, G., & Barone, M. (2006). Labor dystocia and its association with interpregnancy interval. *American Journal of Obstetrics and Gynecology, 195,* 121–128.

Baruah, M., & Cohn, G. M. (2008). Efficacy of rectal misoprostol as second-line therapy for the treatment of primary postpartum hemorrhage. *Journal of Reproductive Medicine, 53*(3), 203–206.

Bloom, S. L., Casey, B. M., Schaffer, J. I., McIntire, D. D., & Leveno, K. J. (2006). A randomized trial of coached versus uncoached maternal pushing during the second stage of labor. *American Journal of Obstetrics and Gynecology, 194*(1), 10–13.

Brancato, R. M., Church, S., & Stone, P. W. (2008). A meta-analysis of passive descent versus immediate pushing in nulliparous women with epidural analgesia in the second stage of labor. *Journal of Obstetric, Gynecologic, and Neonatal Nursing, 37*(1), 4–12.

Buhimschi, C. S., Buhimschi, I. A., Malinow, A. M., Kopelman, J. N., & Weiner, C. P. (2002). The effect of fundal pressure manoeuvre on intrauterine pressure in the second stage of labor. *British Journal of Obstetrics and Gynaecology, 57*(11), 727–728.

Buhimschi, C., Buhimschi, I., Malinow, A., & Weiner, C. (2001). Second stage of labor performance in obese women. [Abstract]. *American Journal of Obstetrics and Gynecology, 185*(6), S209.

Burtelow, M., Riley, E., Druzin, M., Fontaine, M., Viele, M., & Goodnough, L. T. (2007). How we treat: Management of life-threatening primary postpartum hemorrhage with a standardized massive transfusion protocol. *Transfusion, 47*(9), 1564–1572.

Caruna, E. (2008). Review summaries: Moore, E. R., Anderson G. C., & Bergman N. (2007). Early skin to skin contact for mothers and their healthy newborn infants. *Journal of Advanced Nursing, 62*(4), 439–440.

Cavus, E., Maybohm, P., Dörges, V., Stadlbauer, K.-H., Wenzel, V., & Weiss, H. (2008). Regional and local brain oxygenation during hemorrhagic shock: A prospective experimental study of the effects of small-volume resuscitation with norepinephrine, *Journal of Trauma, 64*(3), 641–649.

Cesario, S. (2004). Reevaluation of Friedman's labor curve: A pilot study. *Journal of Obstetric, Gynecologic, and Neonatal Nursing, 33*(6), 713–722.

Chanimov, M., Gershfeld, S., Cohen, M. L., Sherman, D., & Bahar, M. (2006). Fluid preload before spinal anaesthesia in caesarean section: The effect on neonatal acid-base status. *European Journal of Anaesthesiology, 23*, 676–679.

Cohen, W. R., & Friedman, E. A. (1983). *Management of labor*. Baltimore: University Park Press.

Dagan, I., Gabay, M., & Barnea, O. (2007, August 23–26). Fluid resuscitation: Computer simulation and animal experiments. *Proceedings of the 29th Annual International Conference of the IEEE EMBS Cité* (pp. 2992–2995). Lyon, France.

Danilenko-Dixon, D., Tefft, L., Cohen, R. A., Haydon, B., & Carpenter, M. (1996). Positional effects on maternal cardiac output during labor with epidural analgesia. [Transactions of the Sixteenth Annual Meeting of the Society of Perinatal Obstetricians]. *American Journal of Obstetrics and Gynecology, 175*(4), 867–872.

Davies, G. A. L., Tessler, J. L., Woodman, M. C., Lipson, A., & Hahn, P. M. (2005). Maternal hemodynamics after oxytocin bolus compared with infusion in the third stage of labor: A randomized controlled trial. *Obstetrics & Gynecology, 105*, 294–299.

Donnelly, V., Fynes, M., Campbell, D., Johnson, H., O'Connell, P. R., & O'Herlihy, C. (1998). Obstetric events leading to anal sphincter damage. *Obstetrics & Gynecology, 92*(6), 995–961.

Ferguson, J. K. W. (1941). A study of the motility of intact uterus at term. *Surgery, Gynecology, and Obstetrics, 73*, 359–366.

Frankel, D. A. Z., Acosta, J. A., Anjaria, D. J., Porcides, R. D., Wolf, P. L., & Coimbra, R. (2007). Physiologic response to hemorrhagic shock depends on rate and means of hemorrhage. *Journal of Surgical Research, 143*, 276–280.

Fraser, D. M., & Cooper, M. A. (2003). *Myles textbook for midwives*. Edinburgh: Churchill Livingstone.

Fraser, W., Marcoux, S., Krauss, I., Douglas, J., Goulet, C., & Boulvain, M. for the Pushing Early or Pushing Late with Epidural (PEOPLE) Study Group. (2000). Multicenter randomized controlled trial of delayed pushing for nulliparous women in the second stage of labor with continuous epidural analgesia. *American Journal of Obstetrics and Gynecology. 182*(5), 1165–1172.

Friedman, E. (1978). *Labor: Clnical evaluation and management* (2nd ed.). New York: Appleton-Century-Crofts.

Geller, S. E., Adams, M. G., & Miller, S. (2007). A continuum of care model for postpartum hemorrhage. *International Journal of Fertility, 52*(2–3), 97–105.

Gennaro, S., Mayberry, L., & Kafulafula, U. (2007). The evidence supporting nursing management of labor. *Journal of Obstetric, Gynecologic, and Neonatal Nursing, 36*(6), 598–604.

Gill, P., Sobeck, J., Jarjoura, D., Hillier, S., & Benedetti, T. (1997). Mortality from early neonatal group B streptococcal sepsis: Influence of obstetric factors. *Journal of Maternal-Fetal Medicine, 6*(1), 35–39.

Gilson, G. J., Kramer, R. L., Barada, C., Izquierdo, L. A., & Curet, L. B. (1998). Does labetalol predispose to pulmonary edema in severe pregnancy-induced hypertensive disease? *Journal of Maternal-Fetal Medicine, 7*, 142–147.

Greenberg, M. B., Cheng, Y. W., Hopkins, L. M., Stotland, N. E., Bryant, A. S., & Caughey, A. B. (2006). *American Journal of Obstetrics and Gynecology, 195*, 743–748.

Greves, C., Curtin, W., Florescue, H., Metlay, L., & Katzman, P. (2007). The effect of histologic chorioamnionitis on risk factors for intrapartum fever in the term parturient. [Abstract]. *American Journal of Obstetrics and Gynecology, 197*, S69.

Gurewitsch, E., Fong, J., Diament, P., Lesser, M., McClintock, R., & Chervenak, F. (1999). The effect of obstetric interventions on labor curves of nullipara, multipara and grandmultipara. [Abstract]. *American Journal of Obstetrics and Gynecology, 180*(1, Part 2), S128.

Gutierrez, G., Reines, H. D., & Wulf-Gutierrez, M. E. (2004). Clinical review: Hemorrhagic shock. *Critical Care, 8*(5), 373–381.

Haas, T., Fries, D., Holz, C., Innerhofer, P., Streif, W., & Klingler, A. (2008). Less impairment of hemostasis and reduced blood loss in pigs after resuscitation from hemorrhagic shock using the small-volume concept with hypertonic saline/hydroxyethyl starch as compared to administration of 4% gelatin or 6% hydroxyethyl starch solution. *Anesthesia & Analgesia, 106*(4), 1078–1086.

Halpern, S. H., Leighton, B. L., Ohlsson, A., Barrett, J. R., & Rice, A. (1998). Effect of epidural vs. parenteral opioid analgesia on the progress of labor: A meta-analysis. *Journal of the American Medical Association, 280*(24), 105–110.

Hansen, S. L., Clark, S. L., & Foster, J. C. (2002). Active pushing versus passive fetal descent in the second stage of labor: A randomized controlled trial. *Obstetrics & Gynecology, 99*(1), 29–34.

Holmes, P., Oppenheimer, L., Walker, M., & Wen S. W. (2001). [Abstract #0372]. Cervical dilation at first assessment in labour as a predictor of obstetric outcome. *American Journal of Obstetrics and Gynecology, 184*(1), S114.

Impey, L. W. M., Greenwood, C. E. L., Black. R. S., Yeh, P. S.-Y., Sheil, O., & Doyle, P. (2008). The relationship between intrapartum maternal fever and neonatal acidosis as risk factors for neonatal encephalopathy. *American Journal of Obstetrics and Gynecology, 198*, 49.e1–e6.

Jarrar, D., Wang, P., Cioffi, W., Bland, K., & Chaudry, I. H. (2000). Critical role of oxygen radicals in the initiation of hepatic depression after trauma hemorrhage. *Journal of Trauma, 49*(5), 879–885.

Kheirabadi, B. S., Crissey, J. M., Deguzman, R., Perez, M. R., Cox, A. B., & Dubick, M. A. (2008). Effects of synthetic versus natural colloid resuscitation on inducing dilutional coagulopathy and increasing hemorrhage in rabbits. *Journal of Trauma, 64*(5), 1218–1229.

Kirkpatrick, A. W., Ball, C. G., D'Amours, S. K., & Zygun, D. (2008). Acute resuscitation of the unstable adult trauma patient: Bedside diagnosis and therapy. *Canadian Journal of Surgery, 51*(1), 57–69.

Langenbach, C. (2006). Misoprostol in preventing postpartum hemorrhage: A meta-analysis. *International Journal of Gynecology and Obstetrics, 92*, 10–18.

Lausman, A. Y., Ellis, C. A. J., Beecroft, J. R., Simons, M., & Shapiro, J. L. (2008). A rare etiology of delayed postpartum hemorrhage. *Canadian Journal of Obstetrics and Gynaecology, 30*(3), 239–243.

Lee, C.-C., Chang, I.-J., Yen, Z.-S., Hsu, C.-Y., Chen, S.-Y., & Su, C.-P. (2006). Delayed fluid resuscitation in hemorrhagic shock induces proinflammatory cytokine response. *Annals of Emergency Medicine, 49*(1), 37–44.

Leung, A.S., Leung, E. K., & Paul, R. H. (1993). Uterine rupture after previous cesarean delivery: Maternal and fetal consequences. *American Journal of Obstetrics & Gynecology, 169*(4), 945–950.

Low, J. A., Victory, R., & Derrick, E. J. (1999). Predictive value of electronic fetal monitoring for intrapartum fetal asphyxia with metabolic acidosis. *Obstetrics and Gynecology, 93*, 285–291.

Lu, Y.-Q., Cai, X.-J., Gu, L.-H., Wang, Q., Huang, W.-D., & Bao, D.-G. (2007). Experimental study of controlled fluid resuscitation in the treatment of severe and uncontrolled hemorrhagic shock. *Journal of Trauma, 63*(4), 798–804

Mahlmeister, L. (1999). Professional accountability and legal liability for the team leader and charge nurse. *Journal of Obstetric, Gynecologic, and Neonatal Nursing, 28*(3), 300–309.

Martin, E. J. (2002). *Intrapartum management modules: A perinatal education program.* Philadelphia: Lippincott Williams & Wilkins.

Merhi, Z. O., & Awonuga, A. O. (2005). The role of uterine fundal pressure in the management of the second stage of labor: A reappraisal. *Obstetrical & Gynecological Survey, 60*(9), 599–603.

Mikolajczyk, R. T., Zhang, J., Troendle, J., & Chan, L. (2008). Risk factors for birth canal lacerations in primiparous women. *American Journal of Perinatology, 25*(5), 259–264.

Minato, J.E. (2000). Is it time to push? Examining rest in second-stage labor. *Lifelines, 4* (6), 20–25.

Murray, M. (2004). Maternal or fetal heart rate? Avoiding intrapartum misidentification. *Journal of Obstetric, Gynecologic, and Neonatal Nursing, 33*(1), 93–104.

Ness, A., Goldberg, J., & Berghella, V. (2005). Abnormalities of the first and second stages of labor. *Obstetrics and Gynecology Clinics of North America, 32*, 201–220.

Parer, J. T., King, T., Flanders, S., Fox, M., & Kilpatrick, S. J. (2006). Fetal academic and electronic fetal heart rate patterns: Is there evidence of an association? *Journal of Maternal, Fetal, and Neonatal Medicine, 19*(5), 289–294.

Patriarco, M. S., Viechnicki, B. M., Hutchinson, T. A., Klasko, S. K., & Yeh, S-Y. (1987). A study of intrauterine fetal resuscitation with terbutaline. *American Journal of Obstetrics and Gynecology, 157*(2), 384–387.

Philipsen, N., & Haynes, D. (2005). The similarities between birth plans and living wills. *Journal of Perinatal Education, 14*(4), 46–48.

Physicians' desk reference (2001). Oradell, NJ: Medical Economics Company, Inc.

Pitkin, R. M. (2003). Primigravid labor: A graphicostatistical analysis. *Obstetrics & Gynecology, 101*(2), 216.

Porter, M., van Teijlington, E., Yip, L. C. Y., & Bhattacharya, S. (2007). Satisfaction with cesarean section: Qualitative analysis of open-ended questions in a large postal survey. *Birth, 34*(2), 148–154.

Reid, F., Lobo, D. N., Williams, R. N., Rowlands, B. J., & Allison, S. P. (2003). (Ab)normal saline and physiological Hartmann's solution: A randomized double-blind crossover study. *Clinical Science, 104*, 17–24.

Roberts, J. (2002). The "push" for evidence: Management of the second stage. *Journal of Midwifery & Women's Health, 47*(1), 2–15.

Roberts, J. E. (2007). A new understanding of the second stage of labor: Implications for nursing care. *Journal of Obstetric, Gynecologic, and Neonatal Nursing, 32*(6), 794–801.

Rouse, D. J., Owen, J., Savage, K. G., & Hauth, J. C. (2001). Active phase labor arrest: Revisiting the 2-hour minimum. *Obstetrics & Gynecology, 98*(4), 550–554.

Schaffer J., Bloom, S., Casey, B., McIntire, D., Nihira, M., & Leveno, K. (2005). A randomized trial of the effects of coached vs. uncoached maternal pushing during the second stage of labor on postpartum pelvic floor structure and function. *American Journal of Obstetrics and Gynecology, 192,* 1692–1696

Schlicher, N. R. (in press). Balloon compression as treatment for refractory vaginal hemorrhage. *Annals of Emergency Medicine.*

Sharma, S. K., Gajraj, N. M., & Sidawi, J. E. (1997). Prevention of hypotension during spinal anesthesia: A comparison of intravascular administration of hetastarch versus lactated Ringer's solution. *Anesthesia & Analgesia, 84,* 111–114.

Shults, C., Sailhamer, E. A., Lik Y., Liu, B., Tabbara, M., & Butt, M. U. (2008). *Surviving blood loss without fluid resuscitation, 64*(3), 629–640

Simkin, P. (2007). Birth plans: After 25 years, women still want to be heard. *Birth, 34*(1), 49–51.

Simkin, P., & Ancheta, R. (2005). *The labor progress handbook.* (2nd ed.). Oxford, England: Blackwell Publishing.

Simpson, K.R., & James, D.C. (2005). Effects of immediate versus delayed pushing during second stage labor on fetal well-being: A randomized clinical trial. *Nursing Research, 54*(3), 149–157.

Simpson, K. R., & Knox, G. E. (2001). Fundal pressure during the second stage of labor: Clinical perspectives and risk management issues. *American Journal of Maternal/Child Nursing, 26*(2), 64–71.

Spaniol, J. R., Knight, A. R., Zebley, J. L., Anderson, D., & Pierce, J. (2007). Fluid resuscitation therapy for hemorrhagic shock. *Journal of Trauma Nursing, 14*(3), 152–160.

Spratto, G. R., & Woods, A. L. (2001). *PDR nurse's drug handbook.* Montvale, NJ: Medical Economics Company.

Studd, J. (1975). Identification of high-risk labours [Letter to the editor]. *British Medical Journal,* 702.

Tien, H., Nascimento Jr., B., Callum, J., & Rizoli, S. (2007). An approach to transfusion and hemorrhage in trauma: Current perspectives on restrictive transfusion strategies. *Canadian Journal of Surgery, 50*(3), 202–209.

Tranmer, J. E., Hodnett, E. D., Hannah, M. E., & Stevens B. J. (2005). *Journal of Obstetric, Gynecologic, and Neonatal Nursing,* 34(3), 219–328.

Vahratian, A., Zhang, J., Troendle, J. F., & Savitz, D. A., & Siega-Riz, A.M. (2004). Maternal prepregnancy overweight and obesity and the pattern of labor progression in term nulliparous women. *Obstetrics & Gynecology, 104*(5), 943–951.

Verheijen, E., Raven, J. H., & Hofmeyr, G. J. (2008). Fundal pressure for shortening the second stage of labour (Protocol). *Cochrane Database of Systematic Reviews.* Issue 3. Art. No.: CD006067.doi: 10.1002/14651858.CD006067.

Westgate, J. A., Wibbens, B., Bennet, L., Wassink, G., Parer, J. T., & Gunn, A. J. (2007). The intrapartum deceleration in center stage: A physiologic approach to the interpretation of fetal heart rate changes in labor. *American Journal of Obstetrics and Gynecology, 197,* 236.e1–236.e11.

Williams, K. P., & Galerneau, F. (2003). Intrapartum fetal heart rate patterns in the prediction of neonatal acidemia. *American Journal of Obstetrics and Gynecology, 188*(3), 820–823.

Wise, A., & Clark, V. (2008). Strategies to manage major obstetric haemorrhage. *Current Opinion in Anaesthesiology, 21*(3), 281–287.

Yang, P., Zhao, Z., & Reece, A. (2008). Activation of oxidative stress signaling that is implicated in apoptosis with a mouse model of diabetic embryopathy. *American Journal of Obstetrics and Gynecology, 198,* 130.e1–130.e7.

Zakaria, E. R., Campbell, J. E., Peyton, J. C., & Garrison, R. N. (2007). Post-resuscitation tissue neutrophil infiltration is time-dependent and organ-specific. *Journal of Surgical Research, 143*(1), 119–125.

Zhang, J., Troendle, J. F., & Yancey, M. K. (2002). Reassessing the labor curve in nulliparous women. *American Journal of Obstetrics and Gynecology, 187*(4), 824–828.

4

Pain Management

Those who do not feel pain seldom think that it is felt.

—Samuel Jackson

PAIN DURING LABOR AND BIRTH

Pain causes suffering and stress. Catecholamines are released from the adrenal medulla and are related to decreased stomach emptying, nausea, vomiting, and increased blood pressure. Acute pain also triggers the adrenal cortex to release glucocorticoids. As a result of stress, acute pain increases muscle tension, blood pressure, pulse, and respirations. Blood glucose increases and blood coagulation may increase. Unrelieved pain may heighten the response to subsequent pain. Emotions related to pain may include anxiety, fear, anger, or hopelessness (Schaffer & Yucha, 2004).

Labor pain is due to contractions, distention of the lower uterine segment, pulling on pelvic ligaments, dilation of the cervix, and stretching of the vagina and pelvic floor (Lowe, 2002; Smith, Collins, Cyna, & Crowther, 2007). Referred labor pain may be felt in the abdominal wall, lower back, iliac crests, buttocks, and thighs. Uterine dysfunction can occur as a result of unrelieved pain (Lowe, 1996; Lowe, 2002; Roberts, 1983). Pain causes fatigue (Roberts, 1983). Nurses have a vital role in reducing pain, diminishing distress, decreasing anxiety, and helping women take control of their childbirth experience.

Pain is related to maternal tachycardia (especially during pushing in the second stage of labor), increased oxygen consumption, lactic acid (lactate) production, hyperventilation with a risk of respiratory alkalosis, and increased skeletal muscle tension.

Some women choose to endure labor pain without anesthesia. After the delivery, they may feel that they mastered the experience and did the safest thing for the baby (Stotland &

Stotland, 2005). Women who attend childbirth preparation classes may report less pain than women who are unprepared for childbirth (Lowe, 1996). This may be related to knowledge of what to expect, as well as decreased fear and anxiety. In some women, unrelieved labor pain and a sense of a loss of self-control during delivery may predispose them to posttraumatic stress disorder. Women who have unrelieved pain during labor may have a longer labor than women who received labor anesthesia or nitrous oxide and acupuncture during labor (Hiltunen, Raudaskoski, Ebeling, & Moilanen, 2004).

SEVEN DIMENSIONS OF PAIN

There are seven dimensions of pain: physical, sensory, behavioral, sociocultural, cognitive, affective, and spiritual (Silkman, 2008). The physical dimension is related to the transmission of noxious stimuli from the muscles, bones, nerves, and organs. The sensory dimension is related to the location, quality, and intensity of the pain. The behavioral dimension is related to the verbal and nonverbal expression of pain.

The sociocultural dimension of pain is related to the perception of and response to pain as a result of the patient's social and cultural background. Culture is the way of life of a group of people with shared concepts and learned patterns of behavior that are handed down from one generation to the next. A person's culture affects both the perception and expression of pain. For example, Chinese women may value silence and feel they will dishonor themselves and their families by loud expressions of pain. Moslem women may vocalize their pain and pray during labor. Jewish and Italian patients may vocalize more than Irish patients (Weber, 1996).

The cognitive dimension of pain is related to one's thoughts, beliefs, attitudes, intentions, and motivations with regard to pain. For some women, the pain of labor is accepted as a natural phenomenon that should be experienced with little intervention. Others believe that little or no pain should be tolerated.

The affective dimension of pain is related to the emotions surrounding pain and the woman's outlook on the pain. The spiritual dimension refers to the meaning and purpose one attributes to the pain, to herself, to others, and to the divine. All of these dimensions have an impact on how a woman in labor experiences labor and birth.

THE NURSE'S ROLE

As an intrapartal nurse, you will assess, treat, and reassess your patient to evaluate the effectiveness of your actions in reducing her perception of pain (Manworren, 2006). Assessment includes looking for physical signs of pain. It is unwise to assume all abdominal pain is related to labor. Assessment should include the intensity, timing, and location of the pain, as well as the type of pain, such as, stabbing, dull ache, cramping, or constant.

The woman's face should appear relaxed when she is pain free. If the pain intensifies, she may lower her brow, close her eyes, or grimace. Look at her arms. Are they bent and relaxed or are they tense? Is she grasping the side rail or the sheet? Does she have clenched fists or tightly curled toes? Are her shoulders hunched? Listen for the sounds that indicate pain. Is she groaning, moaning, or chanting (Lowe, 1996)? Is she crying? If she is grunting or using foul or explicit language, she may be close to delivery.

Self-report is the best way to assess pain. Therefore it is important to listen carefully to the patient's complaints (D'Arcy, 2008). The choice of medication should be based on that self-report, plus her activity level, fetal and maternal status, prior response to analgesics, and known allergies. A pain scale may help her assign a number to the intensity of the pain (see Figure 4.1). Validate your assessments by asking the woman about her pain. Ask her how she feels and where it hurts. Of course, if she does not speak English, obtain a translator or use a translator service. If she cannot come up with a number to rate her pain, or she picks a number that seems inconsistent with her vocalizations, reevaluate her. If the physical findings of pain seem inconsistent with her rating, or she constantly rates her pain at a high level even after analgesics or anesthetics, she will need to be reevaluated by the midwife or physician. It is possible that the source of pain is related to something other than labor.

Determine the location of the pain source(s). For example, backache is present in approximately half of all pregnant women (Davis, 1996). Assess for the presence of epigastric pain, the presence or absence of a headache, and other signs of preeclampsia. Some headaches are simply related to being pregnant or even caffeine withdrawal. If she points to the location of the pain in her uterus, there could be a placental

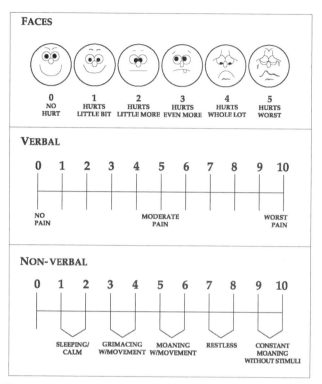

Figure 4.1: Pain rating scales.

abruption. If she has a history of a cesarean section and says she felt something pop or the baby move toward the ceiling, her uterus has probably ruptured.

Assess pain with and without contractions. Determine when the pain began, and what makes it worse. If the pain occurs during and between contractions, she may be in labor or she may have another cause of pain such as appendicitis or gallbladder disease. Notify the midwife and/or physician when pain is unrelated to contractions and when the patient needs analgesia or anesthesia.

You should always assess pain in the clinical context. What is the degree of dilatation? Has her expression of pain changed since admission? For example, if she is only dilated 1 centimeter but she is moaning constantly, and even screaming and thrashing in the bed, think placental abruption. On the other hand, if she is grimacing slightly during 30-second contractions that are 3 to 4 minutes apart, has not slept in 24 hours, is 3-centimeters dilated and it is her first baby, then her pain is appropriate for the situation.

Next, assess the location of the pain. If it is in her lower back and she has coupling of her contractions, is the fetus in an occiput posterior position? Has she been given an epidural and has she had a prior cesarean section? If so, jaw, neck, or shoulder pain can be referred pain from a uterine rupture. Is there pain over her kidneys? Perhaps she has pyelonephritis. Pain in the groin is common as labor advances.

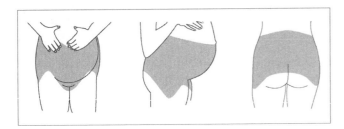

Figure 4.2: Sites of pain during the first stage of labor.

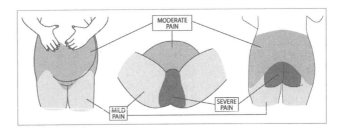

Figure 4.3: Sites of pain during the second stage of labor (10 cm until the birth of the baby).

Educate your patient about the nonpharmacologic and pharmacologic pain management techniques you have at your institution. When pain relief measures are provided, evaluate their effectiveness in helping her cope with pain. Reduce her anxiety. Evaluate the maternal and fetal response when medications are administered.

Documentation example: Patient denies any contractions at this time. Pain 0/10.

Documentation example: Patient becoming more uncomfortable with contractions. Breathing through them. Pain rated as 2 to 3/10.

Documentation example: Patient requests medication for pain. Rates pain as 4/10. Stadol 1 mg given slow IVP.

Documentation example: Patient states Stadol has helped take the edge off of the contractions but "I still feel them." Pain rated as 2/10.

Documentation example: Patient complains of feeling increased pressure. Epidural continues at 10 mL/hr. 9/100%/0. Patient and husband informed of SVE findings.

Documentation example: Patient crying. Complains of increased pain with contractions. Rates pain 10/10. Contractions every 2 to 3 minutes × 50–70 seconds palpate moderate. Options for analgesia and anesthesia discussed. 10 mg Nubain given IVP slowly.

Documentation example: Patient sleeping on right side. Husband is at bedside.

PAIN LOCATIONS DURING LABOR

The normal sites of pain during the first and second stages of labor are illustrated in Figures 4.2 and 4.3. The spinal dermatomes related to these areas are T10 to L1. Note that T10 is near the umbilicus. The goal of neuraxial analgesia/anesthesia during labor is to block the pain at those levels.

Pain during the second stage is located in areas of S2 to S4, which are affected by the pudendal nerves and somatic pain nerves (see Figure 4.3).

PAIN MANAGEMENT: NONPHARMACOLOGIC MEASURES

Nonpharmacologic pain management techniques may help reduce the perception of pain and are usually safe (Stotland & Stotland, 2005). They are also known as complementary and alternative therapies for pain management. They work to change the mind–body interactions or the affective (not sensory) component of pain perception.

Acupressure

Acupressure is the application of pressure on the hands, feet, and ears at points used in acupuncture. This therapy has not been proven to be effective in reducing labor pain. Reflexologists believe that there are points on the feet that correspond to organs or structures of the body and that gentle manipulation or pressing on certain parts of the foot may be helpful to anesthetize other parts of the body (Smith et al., 2007). A person trained in the technique should apply pressure during contractions.

Acupuncture

Acupuncture requires the insertion of delicate, thin needles into the hands, feet, and ears to reduce labor pain. It appears that acupuncture blocks pain signals from reaching the spinal cord and brain, or that it stimulates endorphin release, which acts like natural opioids. Acupuncture and hypnosis are the most effective alternative methods in decreasing the perception of labor pain (Smith et al., 2007). One study in Sweden of 128 pregnant women found that 4 to 8 sterile water injections over the area where the woman felt pain were more effective in reducing pain and increasing relaxation than acupuncture with 2-hour effect. The acupuncture group, on the other hand, received needles in 4 to 7 points that remained in place for 40 minutes and were manually stimulated every 10 minutes by a midwife (Mårtensson, Stener-Victorin, & Wallin, 2008).

Aromatherapy

Essential oils from plants do not change blood pressure or heart rate, but may improve mood and anxiety levels. Their mechanism of action is unclear (Smith et al., 2007). Lavender is often used because it is believed to decrease tension and anxiety.

Audio Analgesia

Listening to "white noise," the sounds of the ocean or other relaxing sounds offer no benefit during labor. Smith and colleagues found that they are ineffective in reducing the perception of pain (Smith et al., 2007).

Controlled Breathing

Controlled, slow breathing during a contraction is a learned behavior that requires practice and a focal point. Women who attend childbirth preparation classes learn to use this technique. Relaxation may not decrease the pain, but it may help keep blood pressure within a normal range, decrease oxygen consumption, decrease muscle tension, and improve blood flow and oxygen delivery (Kwekkeboom & Gretarsdottir, 2006).

Cool Compresses

Women in labor may complain of being warm, and therefore it is soothing to apply a cool cloth to the forehead during labor. Washing the inner arms or face is also refreshing, although cold cloths or compresses are rarely effective in reducing the sensation of labor pain. When a washcloth filled with ice was rubbed over the web space between the index finger and thumb (Hoku point), women reported less pain (Waters & Raisler, 2003). However, cold applications may damage the skin, or cause hives, blisters, itching, and even vasoconstriction or blanching. Some women avoid cold food and drink, and even cold compresses, based on their cultural beliefs (Simkin & Bolding, 2004). Therefore, permission should be obtained prior to the use of cold cloths in labor.

Warm Compresses

Washcloths soaked in water, or wet, warm towel rolls may be used to apply heat, especially to the perineum when a woman is pushing. The warmth seems to help women focus on the location where they should direct their pushing efforts. However, it is not helpful in reducing labor pain. In addition, the wet towel can be used to clean off those "little signs of progress" that are expressed from the bowels during pushing.

You should use caution before using warm compresses heated in a microwave. Consult your hospital's guidelines regarding the use of microwave heat packs.

Hydrotherapy

Immersion in a bath or pool of warm water during labor may reduce the need for analgesia and anesthesia during the first stage of labor (Cluett, Nikodem, McCandlish, & Burns, 2008). If a woman takes a warm tub bath, her body temperature may rise. Therefore, it is a good idea to assess her temperature before and after the bath. Hydrotherapy may be associated with better uterine perfusion, less painful contractions, shorter labors, a decreased need for oxytocin augmentation, fewer perineal tears and episiotomies, a reduction in blood pressure, and increased maternal satisfaction. However, the woman who desires water immersion/hydrotherapy must also expect and understand its benefits, and desire nonpharmacologic management of labor pain.

Hydrotherapy is not a good choice when there is a need for continuous fetal monitoring, vaginal bleeding of undetermined cause, or imminent birth.

Hypnotherapy

Hypnosis may suppress nerve activity between sensory nerves in the brain (sensory cortex) and lower centers related to emotions (limbic system). Hypnosis may inhibit the emotional interpretation of sensations related to pain and promote relaxation, reduce stress and anxiety, and decrease pain perception. Hypnosis also reduces the need for medications for pain relief, including epidural anesthesia. A certified clinical hypnotherapist practitioner is needed to provide this intervention. It is an educational communication process that allows the subconscious and conscious minds to have the same message. Hypnosis and acupuncture are the most effective complementary therapies for pain management during labor. However, acupressure, aromatherapy, audio analgesia, and massage are not as effective in reducing labor pain (Smith et al., 2007).

Injections for Severe, Continuous Low Back Pain

Subcutaneous and intradermal injections of sterile water or sterile normal saline have been used to reduce the perception of back pain. The injection(s) appear to work because the painful stimulus caused by the injection(s) act as a counter-irritant that reduces the perception of pain elsewhere in the body. This decreased perception response induced by a counterirritant has been called "diffuse noxious inhibitory control" (Bahasadri, Ahmadi-Abhari, Dehghani-Nik, & Habibi, 2006).

One or more injections appear to reduce the perception of low-back pain. For example, in Iran, a subcutaneous injection of 0.5 mL of sterile water or saline was administered to 100 women in labor to the most painful point in their lower back. A 1-mL syringe was used with a fine, 30-gauge needle. Both sterile water and saline injections decreased the women's perception of labor pain (Bahasadri et al., 2006). In Canada, four injections (0.5 mL of sterile water) were given subcutaneously and resulted in pain reduction for at least 45 minutes (Reynolds, 2000). When sterile, preservative-free water is used, the injections are called water-block injections.

Intradermal and subcutaneous injections usually require an order from a physician or midwife. They are usually given before an epidural is needed and there are no side effects. Generally, this technique is not used more than twice as pain increases to the point of needing pharmacologic measures or delivery occurs. The effect may last 1 to 2 hours (Mårtensson, Stener-Victorin, & Wallin, 2008). Massage, the application of pressure to the lower back during contractions, and heat may

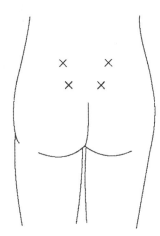

Figure 4.4: Possible sites for intradermal or subcutaneous injections. One injection may be enough to reduce severe back pain. If one injection is used, the injection of 0.5 mL should be at the most painful point in the lower back.

act to reduce pain and are less invasive (see Figure 4.4). Prior to the injection, be sure your patient is not latex hypersensitive. If she is, remove the rubber stopper from the vial of preservative-free sterile water prior to drawing up the fluid.

The location and characteristics of the woman's pain should be assessed and recorded before and after the procedure. Low-back pain is common when the fetus is occiput posterior and in women who had back pain throughout their pregnancies (Reynolds, 2000) Sterile water is more commonly injected than sterile normal saline, although both appear to reduce back pain.

Your patient should verbally consent to the procedure. She should be told there will be intense stinging, burning, and pain that will subside in 20 to 30 seconds (Simkin & Bolding, 2004). She should also be told that within a few minutes pain should be relieved in her lower back (Mårtensson, McSwiggin, & Mercer, 2008). Document who informed her about the procedure, how she would feel, and her change in pain perception.

Massage

Women may experience extreme pain in the lower back, especially when the fetus is in the occiput posterior position. Sacral pressure and shoulder and back kneading may help relax the woman's muscles. Massage may relieve pain by inhibiting pain signals or by improving blood flow and oxygenation to tissues (Smith et al., 2007).

To reduce back pain, a woman in labor should find her position of comfort. Often it is standing or even on "all fours." A warm compress to the lower back may be helpful. Because of the risk of burns, it is best to use a device such as a heating pad. Avoid creating a heating pad in the microwave because it has been associated with third-degree burns to the lower

back. It is best to apply counterpressure with the palm of your hand and push into the lower back during contractions. By applying strong counterpressure, you support her lower back during contractions.

Transcutaneous Electrical Nerve Stimulation

Another nonpharmacological means of labor pain relief is the application of transcutaneous electrical nerve stimulation (TENS) to acupuncture points using a TENS unit. A TENS unit is a portable, battery-powered unit with electrode pads that are placed on the skin. The electrical intensity is between 10 and 18 milliamperes, based on body weight. It causes a tingling sensation. During the first and second stages of labor, a TENS unit applied for 30 minutes decreases the perception of pain (Chao et al., 2007).

PAIN MANAGEMENT: PHARMACOLOGIC MEASURES

Between 1995 and 2003, 21% of 276 sentinel events related to medication error involved the administration of opioids, and 98% of the patients died (Manworren, 2006). Therefore, when administering drugs, it is a critical nursing duty to choose the right patient, right route, right drug, right dose, and right time. Prior to administration of any medication, verify the patient's allergies and the provider's order(s). Assess vital signs. Assess cervical dilatation. Withhold analgesics if she is ready to deliver and notify the midwife or physician that you have done so and your reasons.

Analgesics increase the risk of respiratory depression in the mother, which may decrease maternal and fetal oxygenation. Since narcotics reach the fetus, they also can cause neonatal respiratory depression. Therefore, it is important to be sure it is safe to administer a narcotic to your patient. Prior to analgesic administration, assess and document the fetal heart rate and uterine activity. Any drug that suppresses the central nervous system should not be administered if the fetus has a nonreassuring or abnormal pattern because it may increase the risk of fetal decompensation. Assess your patient's knowledge about the drug you will be administering. Provide information in simple language, especially when your patient is in pain, because her ability to listen is limited. Let her know that she may become sleepy, that you will pull up the side rails, that her call light is within reach, and that you will look in on her frequently. Ask your patient to empty her bladder prior to administration of narcotics or an epidural.

ANALGESIA FOR LABOR PAIN RELIEF: TOPICAL, ENTERAL, AND PARENTERAL ROUTES

Analgesic drugs can be administered by the staff nurse in labor and delivery by three routes: topical, enteral, and parenteral. Topical medications are applied directly where its action is desired but are not used during labor for pain relief. The enteral route is used when the desired drug effect is systemic, not local. Drugs are administered via the digestive tract or per os (PO). PO medications, such as acetaminophen (Tylenol) may be given during labor to reduce the pain associated with headache. PO medications are not given to reduce the pain of contractions. The parenteral route is also used when the desired drug effect is systemic. Parenteral medications use a route other than the digestive tract, such as a subcutaneous (SQ), intramuscular (IM), or intravenous (IV) injection. The IV route is now the most commonly used route for the administration of narcotics during labor.

IV push medications, however, are dangerous. When these medications are administered too rapidly, speed shock will occur (Nicholas & Agius, 2005). Speed shock is the result of the rapid introduction of a foreign substance, usually a medication, into the circulation. Patients may experience flushing, severe headache, and chest pain. In extreme cases, circulatory and cardiac disturbances, including cardiac arrest, can occur. To avoid this complication, medications for IV push administration should always be diluted to an appropriate concentration and administered over 5 minutes. Speed shock can cause hypotension, which can then cause injury to both the mother and her baby.

OPIOIDS ARE NARCOTICS

Opioids are narcotic drugs that depress the central nervous system and act directly on nerve synapses to relieve pain. Opioids may be natural (derived from opium), semisynthetic (partially derived from opium), or synthetic. Natural and synthetic opioids are commonly found in the labor and delivery setting.

Opioids work by binding to pain receptors in the brain and spinal cord. These receptors are known as mu receptors and kappa receptors. Opioids that bind with mu receptors are called mu agonists. Mu agonists produce euphoria. Opioids that bind with kappa receptors are called kappa agonists. Kappa agonists produce dysphoria.

OPIOIDS CROSS THE FETAL BLOOD–BRAIN BARRIER

All opioids given by any route readily cross the fetal blood–brain barrier (Courtney, 2007). After opioid administration, fetal central nervous system depression will occur. Baseline variability will decrease and there may be a benign sinusoidal (pseudosinuosidal) pattern (see Figure 4.5). A benign sinusoidal pattern has regular undulations in the baseline but is preceded and followed by accelerations and fetal movement.

After opioid administration, fetal heart rate accelerations will decrease in number and size until the drug dissipates over the next hour. Prior to narcotic administration, you should confirm that your patient is not allergic to the drug. Assess and record the maternal blood pressure, pulse, respirations, and uterine activity, as well as the fetal heart rate pattern.

Do not administer a narcotic if the fetal heart rate pattern is abnormal or nonreassuring. An already oxygen-deprived fetus who receives a narcotic may decompensate. Instead, act to improve fetal oxygenation and notify the midwife or physician of the fetal heart rate pattern and your intrauterine resuscitation actions.

NATURAL NARCOTICS (MU AGONISTS)

A mu agonist is a drug that binds with the mu opioid receptors in the brain and spinal cord. Naturally occurring narcotics derived from opium are mu agonists. Codeine and oxycodone are two mu agonists that are administered via the enteral route. Diacetylmorphine (heroin) and hydromorphone (Dilaudid) are also mu agonists.

Parenteral mu agonists administered to women in labor may include such medications as fentanyl, meperidine or pethidine, and morphine. The name morphine is a derivative of the name Morpheus, the Greek god of dreams. Morphine is the most potent mu agonist.

The side effects of mu agonists include respiratory depression, nausea, sleepiness, fatigue, dizziness, and mental clouding. Since mu agonists often cause nausea and vomiting, you should have an emesis basin close to the patient. Women treated with mu agonists may also complain of dry mouth or itching, or they may have urinary retention.

Breathing slows as a result of opioid administration. Therefore, you should assess your patient's blood pressure, pulse, and respiratory rate before and after narcotic administration. Also assess and record characteristics of her pain and her pain perception before and after narcotic administration.

One adverse reaction to opioid administration is respiratory depression. If the respiratory rate is depressed, carbon dioxide will be retained. Retention of carbon dioxide is called either hypercapnia or hypercarbia. Hypercapnia increases the risk of respiratory acidosis (Bricker & Lavender, 2002). If respiratory depression is severe, bradypnea with a respiratory rate of 8 breaths per minute or less will occur. Bradypnea precedes metabolic acidosis and is life threatening. Naloxone (Narcan) will be needed.

Since pulse oximetry is a poor monitor for ventilation, you must carefully assess the respiratory rate before and after analgesic administration. Report a respiratory rate of 10 or fewer breaths per minute to the midwife or physician. Maternal desaturation, that is, an SpO_2 of less than 90%, should also be reported. If she has a slow respiratory rate, elevate the head of the bed. Administer oxygen by applying a tight-fitting face mask. Oxygen should flow at 10 L/minute. Encourage the patient to take deep breaths. Even if her SpO_2 increases to 100%, she could still be hypoventilating! Closely monitor and record the respiratory rate and SpO_2 before and after you administer a narcotic antagonist.

SYNTHETIC NARCOTICS (KAPPA AGONISTS)

Synthetic narcotics are kappa agonists that produce dysphoria. Examples of kappa agonists administered during labor are nalbuphine hydrochloride (Nubain) and butorphanol (Schlaepfer et al., 1998). Nubain is primarily a kappa agonist

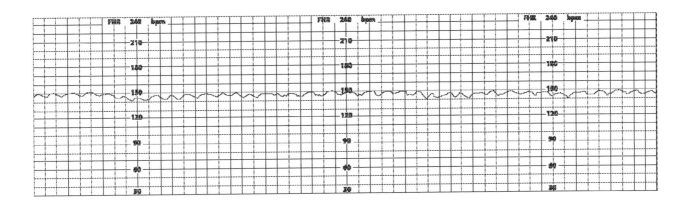

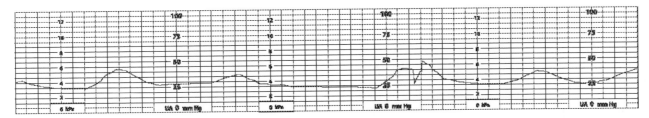

Figure 4.5: Benign sinusoidal pattern following the administration of Nubain 10 mg and promethazine (Phenergan) 25 mg. The fetal heart rate is mostly between 140 and 150 bpm. There were accelerations and no decelerations before narcotic administration. Paper speed is 3 cm/minute.

with a partial mu antagonist action (Nubain, 2003). Butorphanol, sold in the past under the brand name Stadol, has partial mu agonist and antagonist activity, and kappa agonist activity. Synthetic narcotics such as nalbuphine hydrochloride (Nubain) or butorphanol should not be administered to women who are addicted to opiates because these drugs may precipitate opiate withdrawal symptoms.

> **Clinical example of the dysphoria a woman experienced after 10 mg of Nubain**: "I remember thinking it was supposed to help with the pain, but it didn't. It just made me feel like I was in another world. I remember looking at my husband thinking 'What are we here for?' It just made me feel weird, the Nubain did."

LABOR MEDICATIONS AND SELF-DESTRUCTIVE BEHAVIOR

Addiction is a biopsychosocial disease that may be the result of a genetic predisposition or be related to events during pregnancy and labor. Addiction and suicide later in life may be related to what happens during labor and birth. Procedures during childbirth that traumatize the infant may have lasting effects. For example, researchers found that suicides that included hanging, strangulation, jumping from heights, or firearms were more common in men who suffered mechanical birth trauma involving the head or neck. In a number of in-

stances, the mechanical birth trauma occurred as a result of a breech or forceps delivery, or when there were multiple loops of cord around their neck (Jacobson et al., 1987).

In another study, researchers found that when women received 50 to 100 mg of meperidine hydrochloride (Demerol) during labor, especially during the 10 hours prior to delivery, their child was twice as likely to become addicted to drugs than the woman's other children who did not receive the same amount of opiates (Jacobson et al., 1987). Children who were exposed to three or more doses of narcotics or barbiturates in utero during labor were 4.7 times more likely to become an opiate abuser than siblings who were exposed to less medication during the labor of the mother. Medications that seemed to be related to this increase in addiction included meperidine (Demerol) 50 to 100 mg per dose, phenobarbital (100 to 150 mg per dose) and secobarbital (1.5 to 3 grams per dose) (Nyberg, Buka, & Lipsitt, 2000). What this means is that when drugs are given to reduce labor pain or to help a woman rest or sleep, the risk of her infant becoming a drug addict increased four to five times. Even the use of nitrous oxide to reduce labor pain increased the risk of amphetamine addiction in the offspring, especially if the mothers used the gas for more than 4.5 hours during labor (Jacobson, Nyberg, Eklund, Bygdeman, & Rydberg, 1988). Researchers have speculated that the reason for the increase in addictive and self-destructive behavior may be related to the high level of catecholamines in the fetus, which enhanced the imprinting process (Jacobson et al., 1990).

Currently, there are no studies that have examined addiction or other lasting effects on the children of women who received continuous epidural medications such as fentanyl, or agonist–antagonist narcotics such as buprenorphine (Buprenex), butorphanol (Stadol), nalbuphine (Nubain), or dezocine (Dalgan).

MEPERIDINE IS THE SAME DRUG AS PETHIDINE

Meperidine or pethidine are used to treat moderate to severe pain. In the United States and Canada, meperidine is sold as Demerol. However, this drug is also sold in other countries as Algil, Alodan, Centralgin, Dispadol, Dolantin, Isonipecaine, Lidol, Pethanol, Petidin, Dolargan, Dolestine, Dolosal, Dolsin, and Mefedina. The half-life of meperidine is 3 to 6 hours. If it is administered more than 3 hours prior to delivery, it can linger in the neonate for 15 to 23 hours. When meperidine is given within 1 hour of delivery, there are negligible effects on the newborn (Bricker & Lavender, 2002).

FENTANYL (SUBLIMAZE)

Fentanyl was introduced in the 1960s as an intravenous anesthetic called Sublimaze, but has since been found to be useful as an analgesic for labor pain. It is 50 or more times as potent as morphine, but with a shorter analgesic effect (2 hours versus 4 to 6 hours with morphine) (Atkinson et al., 1994). Fentanyl may be ordered for use every hour as needed (PRN) at a dose of 50 to 100 micrograms, slow IV push. It has been called a "fast-in, fast-out" drug because it relieves pain quickly but only lasts a few hours. It is best used late in labor and it seems to help women who need to relax more when they are near 5 centimeters of dilatation. Sometimes after fentanyl is administered, women fall asleep, and then wake up ready to deliver! Side effects include sedation and dizziness. The elimination half-life in neonates is 75 to 440 minutes (Nikkola et al., 1997). Contractions will not diminish when fentanyl is administered (Atkinson et al., 1994). The fetus will receive the drug (Nikkola et al., 1997). Expect variability and the number and size of accelerations to decrease for 1 hour after drug administration (Nikkola, Ekblad, Kero, Alihanka, & Salonen, 1997). Side effects include nausea, vomiting, and sedation. As with any narcotic, fentanyl should not be given when there is a nonreassuring fetal heart rate pattern, a maternal respiratory rate of 8 breaths per minute or less, or when her oxygen saturation is low, that is, less than 95% at sea level. Vital signs should be assessed before, and within 30 minutes after, narcotic administration. To avoid speed shock, take a full 5 minutes to administer the drug IV push. Inject a small amount during each contraction. The ordered dose is usually 50 or 100 micrograms by slow IV push. The protocol may be to administer 1 to 2 mL of fentanyl diluted in 8 mL of normal saline in a syringe, or to inject the drug directly into the port on the IV tubing with the infusion of fluid between each small push of the drug over a 5-minute period.

If fentanyl (75 micrograms) is administered in the epidural, the fetus will have a decrease in variability and fewer accelerations for up to 1 hour (Viscomi, Hood, Melone, & Eisenach, 1990). Sufentanil (Sufenta) is at least five times more potent than fentanyl and is usually administered with epidurals or intrathecals. Remifentanil (Ultiva) is the shortest-acting opioid and is rarely used in labor and delivery. When it is used, it is used for neuraxial analgesia.

NALBUPHINE HYDROCHLORIDE (NUBAIN)

Nubain is a synthetic opioid, kappa-agonist, mu-antagonist analgesic. Milligram per milligram, it produces analgesia equivalent to morphine. It is also chemically related to oxymorphone (agonist) and naloxone (Narcan, a narcotic antagonist). Therefore, it should never be administered to a woman who is addicted to opioid narcotics such as heroin because it may induce withdrawal.

The effects of Nubain occur within 2 to 3 minutes after intravenous administration, and in less than 15 minutes following intramuscular injection. It can produce respiratory depression similar to morphine. It has a 5-hour half-life, with a 3- to 6-hour duration (see Figures 4.6 and 4.7).

There is a high, rapid, and variable transfer of Nubain to the fetus. One of the fetal side effects is severe bradycardia resulting in neurologic damage. Neonates may have respiratory depression and cyanosis (Nubain, 2003). Nubain administration may result in the birth of a neonate with respiratory depression. Therefore, its use is usually early in labor, that is, prior to or at 4 or 5 centimeters of dilatation.

Adverse effects of Nubain include nervousness, depression, restlessness, crying, euphoria, a floating feeling, hostility, unusual dreams, confusion, faintness, hallucinations, dysphoria, a feeling of heaviness, numbness, tingling, and a sense of unreality (Nubain, 2003).

In the past, Nubain contained sodium metabisulfite that caused anaphylactic symptoms and asthmatic episodes in women allergic to sulfites (Nubain, 1990). Today, it contains sodium citrate hydrous, citric acid anhydrous, hydrochloric acid, and sodium chloride. Allergic reactions may include anaphylactic or anaphylactoid reactions with shock, respiratory distress, respiratory arrest, bradycardia, cardiac arrest, hypotension, or laryngeal edema. Other reports include pulmonary edema, agitation, seizures, stridor, bronchospasm, wheezing, swelling, rash, itching, nausea, vomiting, diaphoresis, weakness, and shakiness (Nubain, 2003).

Following the administration of Nubain, the fetal heart rate pattern may have a benign sinusoidal appearance. Severe and prolonged fetal bradycardia has also been reported (Nubain, 2003). Because it can have a strong effect on the fetus, Nubain should be used only when the benefits outweigh the risks. It is metabolized in the liver and excreted by the kidneys. Therefore, your patient should not have impaired renal or liver function.

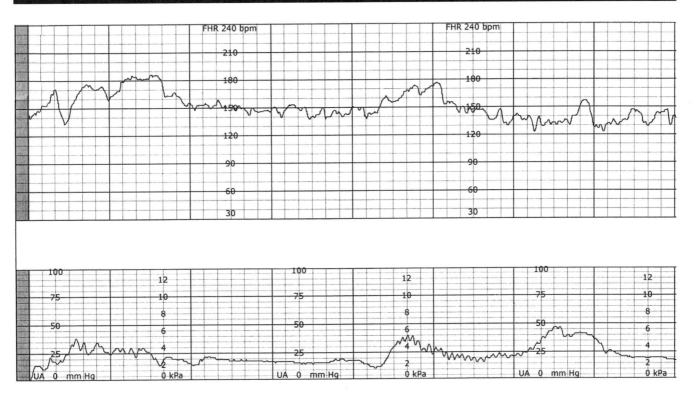

Figure 4.6: Nubain 10 mg was given by slow IV push. Note the accelerations from a baseline in the 140s and 130s. Paper speed is 3 cm/minute.

Documentation example: 142/88–102–22. FHR 145. Patient assisted to bathroom, voided 200 mL amber urine, trace protein. Assisted back to bed and medicated with Nubain 10 mg slow IV push over 5 minutes for 10/10 pain. IV push given during contractions.

Documentation example 1/2 hour later: Patient resting on left side. 124/78–88–20. Pain now 3/10. Baseline 135 bpm, absent (long term) variability with early decelerations.

NITROUS OXIDE

Women may be asked to self-administer analgesic concentrations of inhalation agents such as trichloroethylene, methoxyflurane, or nitrous oxide. Nitrous oxide affects the brain and may induce the release of endogenous opioid peptides that modulate pain stimuli. The gas is not flammable and has no pungent odor. It is minimally toxic and can cause slight depression of the cardiovascular system. It has no effect on contractions. One third of the women who inhale nitrous oxide may experience nausea or vomiting. Adverse effects include dizziness, dry mouth, buzzing in the ears, and a feeling of pins and needles or numbness. One fourth of women who inhale nitrous oxide may have dreams or drowsiness, and as many as 37% may have hazy memories of labor. There is also a risk

of unconsciousness of 0.4% with a 50% nitrous oxide mixture, and of 3% with a 70% nitrous oxide mixture (Rosen, 2002).

Maternal SpO$_2$, vital signs, and the level of consciousness should be assessed and documented before, during, and after the use of nitrous oxide. Instruct your patient in the use of the hand-held device and tell her the pain will not be eliminated, but decreased. Tell her she may feel dizzy or nauseous. If nitrous oxide is used after analgesics have been administered, the risk of unconsciousness increases. Therefore, the use of nitrous oxide may not be reasonable. Inhalation should begin approximately 30 seconds before a contraction or at the moment she feels a contraction. Inhalation of the gas should stop as the contraction wanes. The mask or mouthpiece should be removed between contractions, and she should breathe normally. During the second stage, 2 to 3 inhalations should be taken before each contraction and pushing (Rosen, 2002). Consult your hospital protocol for specific recommendations.

PROMETHAZINE (PHENERGAN)

To prevent nausea and vomiting associated with narcotic administration, promethazine (Phenergan) or another type of antiemetic may be ordered. In the past it was believed that Phenergan given with the narcotic lengthened the duration of analgesia, but this is not true. The addition of Phenergan increases sedation without added pain relief. Phenergan also

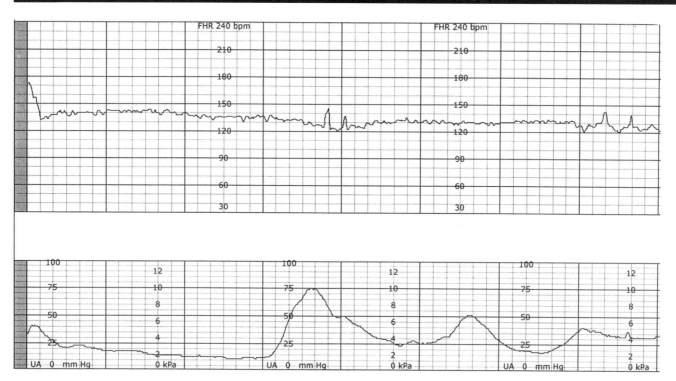

Figure 4.7: Twenty minutes later, note the significant decrease in variability and decreased number of accelerations. Paper speed is 3 cm/minute.

appears to reduce the effectiveness of meperidine (Pethidine) (Bricker & Lavender, 2002).

NEURAXIAL ANALGESIA OR ANESTHESIA

Neuraxial analgesia or anesthesia is achieved when medication is placed around the nerves of the spinal cord and is therefore considered regional analgesia or anesthesia. Medication is delivered to the epidural space in an epidural or spinal-epidural procedure. Medication is delivered to the subarachnoid space during a spinal procedure. Narcotics placed in the subarachnoid space are called intrathecal narcotics (ITN). The epidural space surrounds the dura mater (dura) within the spinal canal and extends to the brain (see Figure 4.8). Fat cells and blood vessels are found in the epidural space.

TO PRELOAD OR NOT TO PRELOAD?

In the past, neuraxial anesthesia was given with a single injection into the caudal space, epidural space, or subarachnoid space (spinal). This was believed to cause a sympathetic blockade to the vessels in the legs resulting in vasodilation and hypotension. To prevent hypotension, clinicians infused a large volume of crystalloid fluid prior to these procedures because they believed increased intravascular volume would prevent hypotension.

Today, neuraxial analgesia and anesthesia medications and the techniques to administer these medications have evolved.

The bolus infusion or preload of crystalloid solution prior to a low-dose epidural does not prevent hypotension and is not needed. For example, when women received one liter of crystalloid prior to the epidural administration of 0.1% or 0.2% bupivacaine (Marcaine) and 50 micrograms of fentanyl there was no difference in the incidence of hypotension compared with women who received no preload (Kinsella, Pirlet, Mills, Tuckey, & Thomas, 2000). A 2000 mL preload of lactated Ringer's solution prior to a spinal and cesarean section may actually decrease vascular tone (Pouta, Karinen, Vuolteenaho, & Laatikainen, 1996).

The infusion of colloids has no effect on blood pressure. However, the administration of 500 mL of a colloid solution increased uterine blood flow prior to a cesarean section and epidural anesthesia (Gogarten et al., 2005).

Possible maternal consequences of receiving a bolus of intravenous fluid are fluid overload, pulmonary edema, and even congestive heart failure in vulnerable patients (Hofmeyr, Cyna, & Middleton, 1996). A fetal consequence of the mother's receiving a bolus of a glucose-containing crystalloid is hyperglycemia and a neonatal consequence is hypoglycemia. Hyperglycemic fetuses produce more insulin and have an increased risk of hypoxemia (Philipps, Rosenkrantz, Porte, & Raye, 1985). Therefore, an interavenous bolus or preload with any glucose-containing solutions should be avoided.

A bolus of intravenous fluid decreases the number of uterine contractions. When women in labor received 500 mL to 1

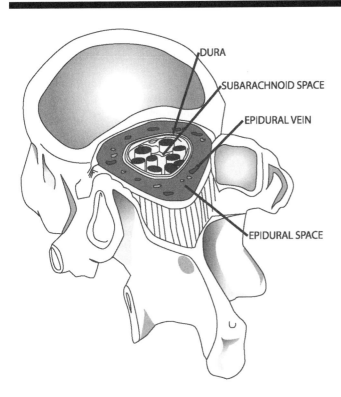

Figure 4.8: Epidural space and subarachnoid spaces where neuraxial analgesia or anesthesia medication may be administered.

DURA

SUBARACHNOID SPACE

EPIDURAL VEIN

EPIDURAL SPACE

liter of either lactated Ringers' solution or normal saline, they had fewer contractions for an average of 20 minutes (Cheek, Samuels, Miller, Tobin, & Gutsche, 1996).

The decrease in uterine activity may be related to a decrease in circulating vasopressin and oxytocin or an increase in circulating atrial natriuretic peptide (ANP), or both. Vasopressin and oxytocin stimulate uterine contractions (Wing et al., 2006). A bolus of intravenous fluid may inhibit the release of vasopressin (antidiuretic hormone) and oxytocin from the posterior pituitary gland (neurohypophysis) (Valenzuela, Cline, & Hayashi, 1983). Rapid distension of the atria in the heart from the infusion of a bolus of fluid stimulates the release of ANP which inhibits uterine smooth-muscle contractions in rats (Bek, Ottesen, & Fahrenkrug, 1988). By inhibiting the release of vasopressin and oxytocin, and the possible increase in circulating ANP, the number of contractions diminishes. Therefore a preload or prehydration with a bolus of 500 mL or more is not helpful prior to the administration of neuraxial analgesia or anesthesia, and it may actually lengthen the duration of labor.

PREPARATIONS FOR THE PROCEDURE

Prior to the insertion of an epidural, the patient must have a functioning intravenous line. Baseline vital signs should be taken and the fetal heart rate and uterine activity should be assessed and documented. The woman should empty her bladder, if possible. She should read the consent. If she has questions, she should wait until the anesthesia provider is present to answer any questions you cannot answer for her. She should sign the consent. A baseline measurement of her oxyhemoglobin concentration (SpO_2) should be obtained and documented.

Usually visitors are asked to leave the room prior to the procedure. In the past, the patient's husband or support person would stand in front of her to help her hunch her shoulders and remain still during the procedure. However, an incident occurred in a hospital in which the husband became dizzy, fell, hit his head on the corner of a sink, became comatose, and died 2 days later. Since that time, many hospitals have changed their policy. The support person may remain in the room, but must be seated during the epidural catheter insertion. Follow your hospital policy regarding who may help the patient remain in the proper position during the procedure.

You should explain to your patient and her support person how the patient will be positioned for the procedure. You may be asked to bring the anesthesia medication to the room. Read the label on the bag prior to its removal from the refrigerator and verify that it is the correct medication. Read the label again when you hand it to the anesthesia provider. The nurse or anesthesia provider should bring the anesthesia cart to the labor room. If you are asked to bring additional narcotics, such as fentanyl, sign it out in the narcotics book and in the computer (if that is your hospital procedure). Read the label before you remove it from the drawer, after you remove it, and prior to handing it to the anesthesia provider. Usually, the anesthesia provider will program the epidural pump and be called to the bedside when needed to adjust the rate or administer another bolus dose.

PAUSE BEFORE THE PROCEDURE

The Joint Commission has recommended a universal protocol to prevent an invasive procedure at the wrong site, the wrong procedure, or the wrong patient. The time-out is a pause for patient safety. Elements of the time out include the correct patient, the correct side and site, an agreement on the procedure to be done, the correct patient position, and the availability of special equipment or special requirements. In the case of the epidural, there is only one site, the back (usually between L2–3 and L3–4). The equipment is usually contained in the epidural cart. You will also need a pulse oximeter and the epidural pump on an IV pole (see Figure 4.9).

Prior to the procedure, the time-out is usually called by the nurse or physician. Saying "time-out" is readily understood by most people, patients, and clinicians. The pause or time out should include the identification of the patient, pertinent information such as allergies, the planned procedure, site and side (if applicable), and implants or special equipment or special requirements. Document the time-out, for example, "Time-out prior to procedure."

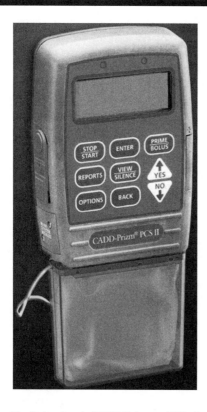

Figure 4.9: Photograph of CADD-Prizm® PCS II ambulatory infusion pump. This pump is usually programmed by anesthesia personnel for the continuous epidural infusion. (Reproduced with permission of Smiths Medical MD, Inc., St. Paul, Minnesota.)

The patient will need to be identified by two methods. For example, you can ask the patient her name and you can confirm her identity by examining her identification band. Of course, she needs to confirm that the information on her identification band is correct and that her name is spelled correctly before the band is placed on her wrist.

The site and the procedure will be verified by two licensed professionals, usually yourself and the anesthesia provider. The site need not be marked if the person doing the procedure has been in continuous attendance with the patient from the time of the decision to do the procedure and consent has been obtained for the procedure. If you leave the room to get equipment or supplies after the time-out is called, the time-out should still be in effect provided the anesthesiologist or nurse anesthetist have not left the room.

Example of a time-out prior to an epidural: Patient identified using 2 identifiers. Site verified, procedure verified by anesthesia provider [name] and nurse [name].

Example of a time-out prior to an epidural: RN: "What is your name and date of birth?" Patient states her name

and birth date. "Doctor, I have confirmed the patient information with her armband. We are doing a labor epidural. [Patient's name] is allergic to penicillin and latex. She has no other chronic health problems. The latex-free cart is in the room. We have the epidural pump and it's unlocked. Her CBC results are on your cart. Platelets are 236,000. Is there anything else I can get for you?"

Anesthesiologist: "Thank you. I do need an extra fentanyl and have you educated the family about leaving the room?"

RN to family: "Please wait in the waiting room. Someone will notify you when the procedure is completed."

MATERNAL OXYGEN SATURATION, PATIENT POSITIONING, AND VITAL SIGNS

You should continue to monitor and document the maternal SpO$_2$. Some anesthesia providers may want the maternal electrocardiogram to be continuously monitored prior to and during the administration of the test dose of the anesthetic. If a separate pulse oximeter device is used (not the one attached to the fetal monitor), turn the volume up so that the anesthesia provider can listen to the pulse rate. This will help him or her identify a possible intravascular administration of the anesthetic drug. If he or she desires a continuous electrocardiogram (ECG), bring a portable ECG monitor into the room prior to the procedure and turn up the volume so that the anesthesia provider can listen to the maternal heart rate. Some fetal monitors are now equipped with leads for the maternal ECG (MECG). In that case, be sure you apply the active electrodes to the maternal chest and attach the MECG before the anesthesia provider arrives at the bedside.

Position your patient according to the anesthesia provider's preference. Most providers seem to like the patient sitting up with her back arched out in the shape of a "C." It is important to inform your patient to remain totally still during the procedure. Bring her shoulders forward and down to assist her into position. It is also helpful to place a pillow in front of her abdomen for her to hold (see Figure 4.10).

Assess and record the maternal blood pressure and pulse before the procedure and after the test dose is administered. Your hospital protocol will define how often to reassess the blood pressure and pulse. The blood pressure and maternal heart rate should be assessed every 2 to 5 minutes, at a minimum, during the first 15 to 30 minutes, every 15 to 30 minutes if there is a continuous infusion of anesthetic medication, and every 5 minutes after any redose or rebolus of anesthetic medication. Once the blood pressure is stable again, resume assessments at 15- to 30-minute intervals. Maternal respirations should be assessed once an hour or more frequently, as needed. Comfort should be assessed at least once an hour. The bladder should be assessed every 30 minutes and, if ordered, an indwelling catheter can be inserted. Labor progress is usually assessed when there are changes in the fetal heart rate that

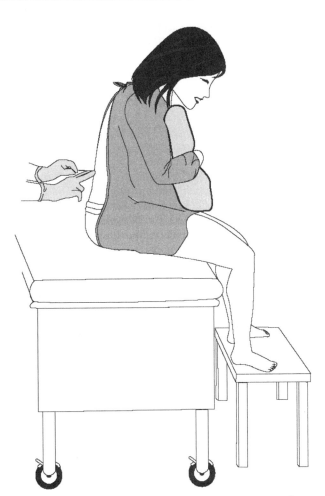

Figure 4.10: This is an example of the sitting position prior to administration of epidural, spinal-epidural, or intrathecal (spinal) analgesia or anesthesia.

tion of the anesthesia provider. The patient may say, "I can't breathe" or "I feel sick." Check her blood pressure immediately. Assess her respiratory rate. Assess the fetal heart rate and uterine activity. Record your findings and any communications (see Exhibit 4.1).

EPIDURAL ANALGESIA/ANESTHESIA

Epidural anesthesia has become the most commonly used method of labor pain relief in the United States (Canton et al., 2002). In the United States, many women enter the birthing suite expecting an epidural, even before they are fully assessed. What these women probably do not know is that the epidural is associated with significant risks to themselves and their child. Unfortunately, if they are in pain and demanding an epidural, it is not a "teachable moment" and the anesthesia provider will need to discuss the risks and benefits of the procedure. However, it is highly unlikely he or she will discuss all the risks of the procedure.

Epidural anesthesia decreases the number of spontaneous vaginal deliveries and increases the risk of a vacuum-assisted delivery. Women who have an epidural often needed oxytocin to augment their labors. Their neonates have more evaluations for sepsis, receive antibiotics more often, and have hyperbilirubinemia more often than neonates of women who do not receive an epidural (Ohana et al., 2007). Epidural anesthesia also increases the risk of fetal malpresentation, neonatal hypotonia, neonates requiring bag and mask ventilation, and neonatal seizures. Neonates of women who have epidurals perform differently from those born to nonmedicated mothers on a comprehensive Neonatal Behavioral Assessment Scale and have poorer muscle tone compared with infants of women who receive opioids during labor (Canton et al., 2002).

CONTRAINDICATIONS AND COMPLICATIONS

Women who have a coagulopathy such as thrombocytopenia purpura, gestational thrombocytopenia, preeclampsia,

suggest progress, that is, variable decelerations when there previously were none, or if the patient says "I feel different" or she feels pressure. Some providers assess the cervix every 2 hours after regional anesthesia has been administered.

SYMPTOMS OF MATERNAL HYPOTENSION

Hypotension has been defined as a 30% or greater reduction from the baseline blood pressure, or a systolic pressure of less than 90 mm Hg. Women whose anxiety drops or pain precipitously decreases with the administration of neuraxial analgesia or anesthesia may experience hypotension and report nausea or shortness of breath. Difficulty breathing, headache, ringing in the ears, sweating, light-headedness, and a systolic blood pressure that drops 10% from the baseline value or preanesthetic level, especially if it falls to near 80 or less, are findings that need to be immediately brought to the atten-

eclampsia, HELLP syndrome, clotting disorders such as von Willebrand Disease, or infection in the lower back where the epidural is inserted are at risk of developing an epidural complication. However, a specific platelet count that predicts complications is not clear (American Society of Anesthesiologists Task Force on Obstetric Anesthesia, 2007). In some hospitals, a complete blood count is not ordered at admission. Therefore, you will not have the ability to report a platelet count to the anesthesia provider prior to the procedure. In that case, report any unusual bleeding that you observed, such as bleeding from the gums, vagina, nose, or ears, or report bleeding at the site when the intravenous line was initiated. Unusual bleeding may be a sign of thrombocytopenia or disseminated intravascular coagulopathy (DIC).

A rare but serious complication of an epidural, spinal-epidural, or spinal is a spontaneous epidural hematoma, which occurs in one person per million (Case & Ramsey, 2005). The hematoma could compress her spinal cord and cause her lifelong paralysis. Several factors (described below) predispose a woman to rupture a preexisting pathological venous system and develop a spontaneous epidural hematoma.

Factors that predispose a woman for a spontaneous epidural hematoma include an abnormally low platelet count, hypertension, a clotting disorder, vasculitis, anticoagulant use, and the Valsalva maneuver. In addition, some herbs can increase bleeding tendencies. Garlic, ginko biloba, and ginseng increase the risk of bleeding, a spontaneous hematoma, and paraplegia. Usually this risk is increased if the patient is also using heparin during her pregnancy (Kuczkowski, 2006).

Women are generally not well informed of the risks to themselves and their infants. Instead, they decide they want an epidural because someone in their family had one or they saw it on a television program. It is the duty of the anesthesia provider to explain the risks and benefits of the procedure. But it is also the nurse's duty to prevent harm. Therefore, the nurse must know prior to the procedure if there are any contraindications for her patient, such as a clotting disorder or an abnormally low platelet count.

PREPARATION FOR THE EPIDURAL

You should review the platelet count and report it to the anesthesia provider. A count near 50,000 significantly increases the risk of hemorrhage and is a contraindication to neuraxial medication administration. Document baseline vital signs, fetal heart rate, and uterine activity. The patient should sign her written consent after her questions have been answered by the anesthesia provider.

You may be asked to bring the anesthesia cart, the intravenous bag of anesthetic or analgesic medication, and the programmable pump to the bedside. To help with positioning your patient, place a chair at the edge of the bed and place a pillow in front of the maternal abdomen. If protocol allows, position the support person in front of your patient. If this is against your hospital's protocol, you may need to stand in front of the patient and gently hold her shoulders to help her

arch her back in a "C" (see Figure 4.10). Some anesthesia providers prefer the patient to be lying on her side. In that case, you should place one pillow in front of her abdomen and a pillow between her legs. Place a chair near your patient's head for her partner or support person to sit during the procedure.

Anesthesia providers will use a technique known as "loss of resistance." After disinfecting and numbing the skin, a needle is inserted (usually between L2–3 and L3–4). The needle will pass through fascia and ligaments and enter the epidural space. Once the anesthesia provider is able to inject air into the space without meeting resistance, he or she will insert a catheter and administer the test dose of an anesthetic agent. The test dose is often lidocaine 1.5% with a dilute concentration of epinephrine. If the catheter tip is in a vein, the epinephrine will cause the patient to feel palpitations and become tachycardic and hypotensive. She may become dizzy, have blurred vision, tinnitus (ringing in the ears), and a metallic taste in her mouth, or even lose consciousness. Rarely, seizures may occur, or respiratory or cardiac arrest. Because of these potential adverse reactions, it is extremely important that the blood pressure, pulse, and SpO_2 be assessed as soon as the test dose is administered and frequently thereafter. Abnormal findings should be reported to the anesthesia provider immediately.

THE TEST DOSE

A test dose of medication is injected to confirm proper catheter placement. Following the test dose, you should assess and record the maternal blood pressure, pulse, respirations, and fetal heart rate approximately every 2 minutes for at least 15 minutes or longer until it is stable. Once the blood pressure is stable, it is usually reassessed every 15 to 30 minutes, depending on the preference of the anesthesia provider or the hospital protocol. If the test dose entered a blood vessel, your patient will report one or more of the following: numbness in the lips, tongue, and/or teeth; a metallic taste in the mouth ("like sucking on a penny"); ringing in the ears; drowsiness; apprehension (with epinephrine solutions); or tachycardia (with epinephrine solutions). If this occurs, the anesthesia provider will stop the injection. Be ready to deliver oxygen at 10 liters per minute with a tight-fitting mask and be prepared to treat seizures or a cardiac arrest. This is a rare occurrence, but being prepared with each epidural is critical. Make sure you have the crash cart nearby.

If the test dose enters the subarachnoid space instead of the epidural space, the patient may report an inability to move her legs or feet or have sudden and complete pain relief. Take her blood pressure immediately because the prompt relief of pain can be accompanied by a significant drop in blood pressure. Be prepared to administer ephedrine as ordered. Usually, if this occurs, the anesthesia provider is still at the bedside and can take action. Rarely, the anesthetic will travel to a high level and impact breathing. Sometimes, the anesthesia provider will have to ventilate the woman if she develops a "high" spinal and stops breathing on her own.

Following the test dose, a continuous infusion of an anesthetic (with or without an added narcotic) such as bupivacaine, ropivacaine, or charoaccaine will be administered via an infusion device. Fentanyl appears to speed up the onset of action and is often added to the anesthetic solution. When these drugs are administered, the patient may also feel a warm tingling sensation down her legs when the initial epidural medication is administered. This is a normal sensation in response to the anesthetic and analgesic. After the epidural catheter is taped, place the patient in a full lateral or supine position, with right or left uterine displacement (using pillows to shift the uterus off the vena cava and aorta), and elevate the head of the bed slightly, that is, 30 to 40 degrees. Assist your patient in changing her position at least once an hour or more often to avoid excessive pressure to one body area.

Once the epidural is in place and the neuraxial analgesia and/or anesthesia is effective, you should not need to administer narcotics to the patient. If she is hurting more than you think she should, perhaps her uterus ruptured or there is another cause of pain. Notify the anesthesia provider if you cannot determine the origin of her pain. Also ask the midwife or physician to evaluate her pain.

If your hospital policy requires you to assess the level of analgesia and anesthesia, you can determine the dermatome by touching the skin with a cool alcohol prep pad and asking your patient if she feels anything when you touch her. Use of a sterile needle for this procedure may be done, but an alcohol swab is less invasive. In some hospitals, you may be asked to determine the anesthesia level by dermatomes (see Figure 4.11). The umbilicus is near T10 and the nipple line is near T4.

After neuraxial analgesia or anesthesia has been administered, it may be more difficult to determine labor progress because of the loss of verbal and nonverbal cues. Therefore, it is imperative that you know the findings of the last vaginal examination. If this is her first baby and the fetus is not engaged in the pelvis, that is, −1, −2, or −3 station, the risk of a cesarean section increases if there is an epidural (Traynor, Dooley, Seyb, Wong, & Shadron, 2000). If she is multiparous or has a history of precipitous labor, observe her behavior and the fetal heart rate pattern closely for subtle changes that suggest she is close to delivery. The onset of variable decelerations or the presence of bloody streaks in the amniotic fluid may indicate that she is nearing 10 centimeters dilatation. It is wise to not let more than 2 hours pass without looking at the perineum or performing a vaginal examination. A vaginal examination is a good idea, especially if there is a history of rapid labors or the fetus is small and oxytocin is infusing. Since vaginal examinations after the rupture of membranes increase the risk of an ascending infection and chorioamnionitis, you will need to think about the reason for the examination and weigh its risks and potential benefits (see Exhibit 4.2).

WHO SHOULD PROGRAM THE EPIDURAL PUMP?

Only an anesthesiologist or certified registered nurse anesthetist (CRNA) should initiate or program a continuous infusion

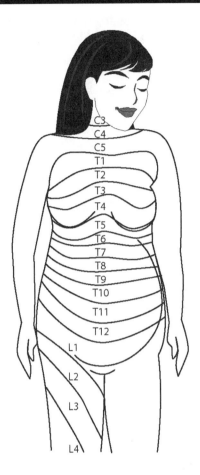

Figure 4.11: Dermatomes.

pump. Only the anesthesiologist or CRNA should add medications to a continuous epidural infusion bag or administer a bolus of epidural medication.

WHO SHOULD CLEAR AIR BUBBLES FROM THE EPIDURAL PUMP TUBING?

If air enters the tubing, the pump will produce an alarm signal. The anesthesia provider should be notified of air in the tubing. He or she may choose to advance the air or may disconnect the tubing between the bag and the epidural catheter to allow the air to escape. Occasionally, a staff nurse will be trained by the anesthesia provider to remove air from the tubing. Consult your hospital policies, procedures, and protocols to know what is accepted at your facility.

SHOULD A STAFF NURSE INCREASE OR DECREASE THE INFUSION RATE ON THE EPIDURAL PUMP?

This is a controversial question. Can a nurse be trained to do this when an order is obtained from an anesthesiologist or CRNA? The Association of Women's Health, Obstetric, and

Exhibit 4.2: Guidelines for nursing care related to epidural anesthesia and analgesia.

1. Assess and record vital signs prior to the procedure.
2. Assess dilatation, effacement, and station close to the time of the procedure.
3. Place the pulse oximeter on the woman's finger (not on the same side as the blood pressure cuff because when it inflates, it will cause the alarm to go off).
4. Notify the anesthesia provider if the SpO₂ remains less than 90 mm Hg or there is a 10% drop in the blood pressure or both.
5. Assess and record the maternal SpO₂ per protocol or at least every 15 minutes.
6. After the test dose is administered, assess and record the blood pressure and pulse every 2 to 3 minutes until stable.
7. Assess and record the blood pressure and pulse every 15 minutes thereafter or as ordered. Assess and record the respirations every 15 to 30 minutes or more often as needed. Assess and record the temperature every 2 hours if the membranes are ruptured and every 4 hours if the membranes are intact. Report elevations to the obstetric provider. If there is an elevation, assess the temperature hourly or more often.
8. If there are fewer than 12 respirations per minute, stop the epidural infusion, notify the anesthesia provider STAT, and if ordered, administer Narcan 0.1 mg slow IV push.
9. Once the epidural catheter is removed (wear a disposable glove), confirm that the catheter tip is intact, document that the tip was intact, wash and dry the site, apply a band-aid, and dispose of the catheter in the biohazard bag.
10. Calculate (from the pump) the remaining medication and record the amount of the medication waste in the anesthesia medication book (or per unit protocol).

Neonatal Nurses (2007) in the United States has taken the position that only a qualified, credentialed, licensed anesthesia care provider should increase or decrease the rate of a continuous analgesia or anesthesia infusion. Consult your hospital policies, procedures, and protocols to find out what is accepted at your facility.

The pump should remain in a locked box during use. The pump should be programmed in mL. The nursing role in some hospitals is to obtain the bag of anesthetic and sign it out and provide it to the anesthesiologist or CRNA prior to initiation of the procedure. Inadvertent administration of magnesium sulfate through the epidural catheter has occurred (Goodman, Haas, & Kantor, 2006). It is critical that you read the medication label on the bag as you remove it from the medication refrigera-

tor and read it again before handing it to the anesthesia provider.

Once the continuous epidural infusion is set up by the anesthesia provider and is working, you should not have to give any intravenous or intramuscular narcotics. In fact, it is expected that you will discontinue all previous narcotics orders. If the patient is not getting adequate pain relief, especially by 30 to 40 minutes after the epidural was inserted, notify the anesthesia provider.

Documentation example related to epidural anesthesia: "4/100%/–1, requested epidural. Consent signed for epidural. Time-out prior to procedure. Dr. Nopain present during time-out. Test dose given at 1000."

WHO SHOULD PUSH THE PCEA BUTTON?

Epidural pumps usually have an attached "button" that can be pushed to administer a bolus dose of analgesia/anesthesia. When the button is used by the patient, the pump becomes a patient-controlled epidural analgesia or anesthesia (PCEA) device. PCEA gives women in labor the opportunity to manage their own pain (Marshall & Baker, 2006; Sia, Lim, & Ocampo, 2007; Stienstra, 2000) and offers women in labor the psychological benefit of being in control. Another benefit of PCEA with intermittent boluses is a more uniform epidural "spread" and pain relief (Sia et al., 2006). Anesthesia providers benefit when patients use PCEA because there is less intervention and thus a reduced workload (Chen et al., 2006; Smiley & Stephenson, 2007).

The first study of PCEA use in labor was in 1988. The epidural anesthesia was 0.125% bupivacaine at 12 mL/hour and the patient could deliver doses of 4 mL no faster than every 20 minutes when she pushed the PCEA button. Researchers believe that the benefit of using a PCEA device is psychological because 30% of the women observed reported immediate pain relief when they pushed the PCEA button (Smiley & Stephenson, 2007). The use of PCEA did not delay cervical dilatation compared with dilatation in women who had a continuous spinal-epidural without a PCEA (Sezer & Gunaydin, 2007). PCEA use had no effect on maternal or neonatal outcomes (Vallejo, Ramesh, Phelps, & Sah, 2007).

If a PCEA device will be used, the patient needs to provide her informed consent and she should be the only person pressing the button. The anesthesia provider will discuss when and how to use the PCEA button. After the anesthesia provider leaves the room, ask your patient and her family to use the call light if you are out of the room when the PCEA button is pushed. Explain that you need to assess her pain, her labor progress, and her vital signs any time she uses the PCEA button.

If the PCEA button is pushed, significant hypotension (defined in this study as a systolic reduction of 25% or more) can occur within the next 10 minutes if the epidural catheter was misplaced and is in the subdural space (Sia, Lim, & Ocampo, 2007). The challenge for the nurse is to be at the bedside when the PCEA button is pushed, or soon thereafter, so that maternal vital signs can be monitored every 5 minutes for the next 30 minutes.

If your patient pushes the PCEA button, in addition to assessing and recording her vital signs, you should assess and record the fetal heart rate pattern and uterine activity. Could she be close to delivery? Perhaps you should don a glove and check her cervix and the fetal station. What are the characteristics of the pain she was feeling when she pushed the button? Record her description of the pain or pressure that motivated her to press the PCEA button and evaluate a change, if any, in her pain or pressure.

THE RISKS OF A PATIENT-CONTROLLED EPIDURAL ANESTHESIA DEVICE VERSUS A PATIENT-CONTROLLED ANALGESIA DEVICE

A PCEA device is different from a patient-controlled analgesia (PCA) device. A PCA device infuses narcotics into a vein. A PCEA device infuses narcotics or anesthetics or both into the epidural space.

A PCA device can cause serious injury or death, especially if it is misused. Adverse reactions include nausea, sedation, and respiratory depression. Sedation precedes opioid-induced respiratory depression (Pasero, & McCaffery, 2005). Untreated respiratory depression from use of the PCA device can result in death. In 2004, the Food and Drug Administration of the United States reported 22 deaths and 106 adverse drug events associated with PCA devices (Weinger, 2008). Also in 2004, The Joint Commission issued a sentinel-event alert on unauthorized PCA administration that was reported to them over a 5-year period. There were 460 reports of PCA-related errors that resulted in patient death or serious injury. Fifteen patients died or were harmed as a direct result of family members or clinical staff pressing the PCA button, even though patients, family, visitors, and the health care providers knew that the PCA was authorized only for patient use. The Institute for Safe Medication Practices has also issued similar precautions about PCA devices (Pasero & McCaffery, 2005).

At the time of this writing, no adverse effects were identified in the literature related to use of PCEA. The Association of Women's Health, Obstetric, and Neonatal Nurses (AWHONN) has not taken a position related to the use of PCEA by a patient. In 2006, Carvalho, Wang, and Cohen wrote that only 25% of California hospitals used PCEA for analgesia in labor. Reasons for not using PCEA were cost, clinician preference, safety concerns, and the inconvenience of change.

DOES AN EPIDURAL INCREASE THE DURATION OF LABOR?

The answer is that an epidural may be related to a longer labor, but researchers have never considered the preload of crystalloid and its impact on decreasing the number of contractions. The presence of an epidural in women who are near term (37 weeks or more) seemed to prolong labor an average of 1 hour and dilatation was slower (1.6 cm/hr versus 1.4 cm/hr without the epidural) (Alexander, Sharma, McIntire, & Leveno, 2002; Sharma et al., 1997). Nulliparous women who received an epidural early in labor reached 10-cm dilatation sooner (median time 295 minutes) than nulliparous women who only received opioids (median time 385 minutes) (Wong et al., 2005).

Furthermore, women who had an epidural had a longer second stage of labor and more procedures, such as the use of rotational forceps, than women who did not have an epidural (Alexander, Sharma, McIntire, & Leveno, 2002; Fraser et al., 2000). However, epidural anesthesia given early in labor does not seem to increase a woman's chance of having a cesarean section. Researchers confirmed that women who had an "early" epidural had an 18% cesarean section rate and women who received parenteral opioids had a 21% cesarean section rate (Wong et al., 2005).

If a woman has received neuraxial analgesia or anesthesia, it is important to keep her bladder as empty as possible so that there are no unnecessary obstructions for descent and delivery. Therefore, it is important to assess her bladder at least every 30 minutes and to catheterize her (as ordered) if the bladder fills full. After you catheterize the patient, record the color and amount of her urine. Perhaps it will be "bright yellow" or "amber" or "blood-tinged." If there is blood in the urine, there probably has been bladder trauma. Consider the possibility that a large fetus was pushing on her bladder. Notify the obstetrician or certified nurse midwife if there is blood in the urine.

DOES AN EPIDURAL INCREASE THE RISK OF OPERATIVE VAGINAL DELIVERY OR CESAREAN SECTION?

The answer is "yes" to the first question, and "possibly" to the second. Epidural analgesia was associated with an increased use of forceps and vacuum extraction, but not cesarean sections (Anim-Somuah, Smyth, & Howell, 2005; Klein, 2006). However, some physicians still believe the epidural, spinal, and combined spinal-epidurals do increase the risk of cesarean delivery (American College of Obstetricians and Gynecologists, 2002). Epidural analgesia with low-dose oxytocin augmentation increased the risk of fetal malposition, operative vaginal delivery, perineal trauma, and cesarean section, especially in nulliparous woman (Kotaska, Klein, & Liston, 2006). If there was a persistent occiput posterior position, a malposition, there were more operative deliveries and fewer normal vaginal births (Fitzpatrick, McQuillan, & Herlihy, 2000). Women with twins had an increased risk of a cesarean section if they also had an epidural (Ben-Aroya et al., 2001). Should a cesarean be needed, the epidural can be redosed avoiding the use of general anesthesia (Chestnut, 1997). If the patient has a scheduled cesarean section and she is not in labor, an epidural injection with 2% lidocaine without epinephrine should have no adverse effect on the fetus (Marquette, Mechas, Charest, & Rey, 1994).

DOES AN EPIDURAL INCREASE THE RISK OF MATERNAL FEVER?

Yes, fever (100.4° F or 38° C) is associated with the duration of the epidural and the use of an anesthetic (versus a narcotic). However, fever may also be related to chorioamnionitis. Both possibilities should be considered any time a woman in labor who has had an epidural develops a fever. Fever occurred in 14% of women who had an epidural with ropivacaine for at least 6 hours, but in only 2% of women who received remifentanil in the epidural (Evron et al., 2008). In another study, fever occurred in 14.5 to 33% of nulliparous women who had an epidural. The average rise in temperature after 8 hours was 1.3° F (Goetzl et al., 2007). The reason women who have had an epidural have an elevated temperature is not clear. It has been proposed that there may be a perturbation of thermoregulation in the brain (Goetzl et al., 2004). On the other hand, it was also found that epidurals prolong labor, and that fever during labor was associated with longer labor, a longer time since the rupture of the membranes, and the use of epidural analgesia (Reilly & Oppenheimer, 2005). Longer labors mean more vaginal examinations, and repeated vaginal examinations increase the risk of chorioamnionitis. Nulliparous women in labor who received an epidural had higher average tympanic temperatures within 1 hour after the onset of epidural anesthesia (Goetzl et al., 2007).

SHOULD YOU DISCONTINUE THE EPIDURAL INFUSION DURING THE SECOND STAGE?

Discontinuing an epidural infusion is not a good idea because it does not lead to better outcomes and it is associated with inadequate maternal pain relief (Torvaldsen, Roberts, Bell, & Raynes-Greenow, 2004). If you are asked to do so, discuss this plan with the provider. With teaching, encouragement, and the use of warm compresses on the perineum later in the second stage, women will be able to push their babies out, even with the epidural infusing up to the time of birth.

ONGOING ASSESSMENTS

Usually maternal vital signs, the fetal heart rate pattern, and uterine activity are documented every 15 minutes once an epidural is in place. The dermatome level of the anesthesia block may also be documented, as well as the woman's self-reported pain score. Assess pain at least once an hour or more often. You should also monitor the patient's temperature once an hour and report an elevation, especially a fever, to the midwife or physician.

> **Documentation example**: Epidural tubing in place. Site clear. Transparent dressing intact, clean, and dry. Left tilt with head of bed elevated 30 degrees. Reports pain 2/10 with low abdominal pressure. Dermatome level T10.

The IV should remain intact until the epidural has worn off and your patient has normal movement and sensation.

If you work in a labor-delivery-recovery-postpartum (LDRP) setting, assess the site of insertion every 12 hours for pain, redness, swelling, and drainage, or all of the above. You should report an elevation in the patient's temperature, and any pain, redness, swelling, or drainage, as soon as it is observed.

Anesthesia providers should be informed of a respiratory rate less than 10 to 12 breaths per minute, or as ordered. The obstetric provider should be informed of abnormal vital signs as well as the fetal heart rate pattern. The anesthesia provider should be informed of an increasing level of anesthesia (based on the dermatomes), sedation, or a maternal hemoglobin oxygen saturation (SpO$_2$) less than 90%. Finally, they need to know if the woman has inadequate pain relief; leaking, redness or tenderness at the insertion site; changes in the fetal heart rate; or, maternal tachycardia, bradycardia, or hypertension. Other worrisome findings that should be reported to an anesthesia provider include dizziness, tinnitus, a metallic taste in the mouth, loss of consciousness or seizures, stiff neck, headache, nausea, vomiting, itching, redness, or disruption of the tape, dressing, or tubing. When the epidural tubing becomes disconnected from the filter where it is connected and taped near her shoulder, do not attempt to reconnect the tubing. Call the anesthesia provider immediately. He or she may decide to replace the epidural catheter.

REMOVAL OF THE EPIDURAL CATHETER

After delivery, if there are no future procedures planned, and if the patient does not have any coagulation abnormalities, you will have to remove the epidural catheter. Do not remove the epidural catheter, however, if your patient will have a tubal ligation during the postpartum period. Nurses must complete a training program before being allowed to remove epidural catheters, and many institutions require competency validation.

To remove the catheter, raise the head of the bed and ask your patient to lean forward. Remove the tape. Ask the patient to arch her back. Slowly remove the catheter. Do not continue removing the epidural catheter if she has pain when you begin to remove it. Stop and call the anesthesia provider. Do not try to remove the epidural catheter if you feel resistance. Stop and call the anesthesia provider. Once the catheter is removed, you must confirm that the tip is intact. Document the time of removal and note "tip intact." Ask the patient if she would like to see the catheter. If she says "yes," show the catheter to the patient. If you suspect any breakage of the epidural catheter, alert the anesthesia provider immediately. Save the catheter for inspection.

INTRATHECAL NARCOTICS

The subarachnoid space is also called the "intrathecal" or "subdural" space. The area outside the dura (that lines the spinal cord) is called the epidural space. Although epidural medication does not enter the dura or the subdural space, intrathecal medication does enter that space.

Intrathecal anesthesia prior to cesarean section is called a "spinal block." A spinal block may be achieved with the administration of bupivacaine (Marcaine) injected through the dura into the spinal fluid. Changes in maternal blood pressure are dependent on the dose of the anesthetic agent. The stronger and higher the dose of the drug, the lower you can expect the maternal blood pressure to fall. Therefore, you should monitor maternal vital signs before and after the injection of intrathecal medication (see Exhibit 4.3). For cesarean section, Marcaine and sufentanil (Sufenta) may be administered (Van de Velde, Van Schoubroeck, Jani, Teunkens, Missant, & Deprest, 2006).

During labor, a low-dose spinal or intrathecal, not a spinal block, is created with a low dose of morphine, fentanyl, or sufentanil. Morphine (Duramorph) may be administered. Duramorph is a preservative-free morphine from Elkins-Sinn, Inc., Cherry Hill, New Jersey. A prerequisite for its use is that the patient be in active labor with no fetal compromise. In addition, she must not be allergic to the drug that will be injected into the subdural space.

Pain relief should last 1.5 to 3.5 hours after the administration of intrathecal Duramorph. Duramorph is a mu agonist. Some hospitals require a dilatation of 5 or more centimeters prior to intrathecal injection. However, when intrathecal morphine is administered late in labor, it may not lessen the pain. Expect no decrease in the number of contractions. The goal is to reach 10 centimeters before it wears off. Your patient should still be able to move her legs and feel the urge to push. She will need a pudendal block or local anesthetic if an episiotomy is required.

Position your patient as you would for an epidural. Expect the duration of pain relief to be at least 1 to 2 hours. One side effect may be headache, depending on the size of the needle that is used. Mu-receptor activation produces intense analgesia, but can also cause respiratory depression and even fetal bradycardia (Friedlander, Fox, Cain, Dominguez, & Smiley, 1997). Therefore, it is critical that maternal SpO_2, vital signs, and the fetal heart rate be assessed and recorded before and after an intrathecal injection, especially in the 30 minutes after the procedure. Hypotension and fetal bradycardia can occur with a frequency similar to that observed after an epidural. Any abnormality should be reported immediately to the anesthesia provider. The fetal heart rate should be stable, and contractions should continue and strengthen. Your patient should remain mobile in the bed with no decrease in her second-stage pushing efforts (Manning, 1996).

Side effects of intrathecal narcotics include itching, nausea, vomiting, and urinary retention for up to 12 hours after the intrathecal injection. Some believe the itching is a reflection of pain. You should assess the patient's back and the injection site every 1 to 2 hours for pain, redness, swelling, and drainage, and you should notify the anesthesia provider of abnormalities. Assess the patient's bladder every 30 minutes by palpation. Place your hand above the pubic bone and push down. If you feel an enlarged soft object, like a sponge, she probably has a full bladder. Catheterize her as ordered or PRN. Assess labor progress (dilatation, effacement, and station) at least every 2 hours or more frequently. She should still feel the urge to push and be able to work with the contractions during the second stage.

A change in the fetal heart rate pattern, such as a variable deceleration, may herald the onset of the second stage of labor. Therefore, be attentive to the patient's reports of pain and other changes that signal birth is imminent.

Intrathecal Duramorph use may result in delayed respiratory depression, peaking at 7 to 9 hours, but lasting for 12 hours, after the intrathecal injection (Manning, 1996). Therefore, it is very important that you report the use of Duramorph to the recovery and postpartum nurse. They will also need to watch her for symptoms of a spinal headache, which occurs when there is a loss of cerebral spinal fluid through the puncture site.

Documentation example: Patient sitting at edge of bed and anesthesia provider is here to administer intrathecal.

Documentation example: Prolonged deceleration to 80 bpm × 140 seconds after intrathecal. Oxygen on by face mask at 10 L/min, patient to left side. SVE done. 6/80%/0. Scalp stimulation after FHR returned to baseline. Acceleration noted and baseline now at 120 to 125 bpm. Dr. Gottucee notified.

Documentation example: FHR at 120–130 bpm with acceleration to 145 bpm × 15 seconds. Oxygen removed. Patient instructed to let RN know if there is an increase in pain, pressure, or feeling the need to have a bowel movement. Patient confirms understanding. Pain was 9/10 preblock, now no pain with last contraction.

COMBINED SPINAL–EPIDURAL ANESTHESIA OR ANALGESIA

Combined spinal–epidural anesthesia (CSE) is achieved when the anesthesia provider injects a narcotic and an anesthetic into the epidural and subdural spaces. The anesthetic may be 2.5 mg of bupivacaine (Marcaine) with 25 micrograms of fentanyl (Viitanen, Viitanen, & Heikkilä, 2005). This is accomplished by first inserting the epidural needle into the epidural space and then inserting a longer spinal needle through the epidural needle. Once they puncture the dura mater, medication will be injected and the spinal needle will be removed. Then the epidural catheter is inserted into the epidural space. The goal of the procedure is to provide a fast-onset, reliable block (with the administration of medications into the spinal fluid), and continuous epidural anesthesia (Lewis & Calthorpe, 2005).

The administration of 10 mg of intrathecal sufentanil followed by epidural bupivacaine, with or without fentanyl or sufentanil, is an example of combined spinal–epidural anesthesia. This has been called the needle-through-needle technique

Exhibit 4.3: Guidelines for nursing care related to an intrathecal injection.

1. Assist the patient to the bathroom to urinate.
2. Have her sit on the side of the bed with her back flexed (forming a "C") or lie down on her side in a lateral decubitus position (as preferred by the anesthesia provider) (see Figure 4.10).
3. The anesthesia provider will perform a lumbar puncture and inject the medication.
4. Apply the pulse oximeter (it should remain on continuously for 8 hours after fentanyl or sufentanil is injected and for 24 hours after Duramorph (morphine) is injected (Manning, 1996).
5. Assess and record vital signs every 5 minutes x 4.
6. Report a drop in blood pressure, especially before the systolic reaches 80 mm Hg to prevent fetal bradycardia and to allow time to treat hypotension with ephedrine.
7. Monitor vital signs every 15 minutes thereafter or per anesthesia orders.
8. As continuously as possible, monitor the fetal heart rate and uterine activity.
9. Assess and record pain per protocol and PRN.
10. Assess and record side effects, such as pruritus, nausea, and vomiting.
11. Notify provider of side effects and provide medication as ordered. For example, metoclopramine hydrochloride (Reglan, A. H. Robins Company, Richmond, VA) may be given for nausea and vomiting.
12. Monitor the bladder by palpation. Continue to record intake and output.
13. Catheterize PRN (or as ordered).
14. Continue to assess maternal SpO_2 and respirations and provide Narcan as ordered (0.2 mg) slow IV if the respiratory rate drops below 10/minute or oxygen saturation drops below 89% or as ordered by the anesthesia provider.
15. Provide oxygen by a tight-fitting face mask at 10 liters per minute PRN (Manning, 1996).

tion. In another study, women who received a spinal–epidural had a similar complication rate as women who received a continuous epidural. These complications included a spinal headache or failed epidural analgesia (Norris, Fogel, & Conway-Long, 2001). After the CSE, anesthesia providers instructed women to use a patient-controlled analgesic device. Twenty-nine women had a 5-minute lockout (where no medication would be delivered by the pump) and 31 women had a 15-minute lockout. The 5-minute lockout was the most efficient and was found to be safe (Stratmann et al., 2005).

Prior to the spinal-epidural, you should perform a time-out. The care of the patient should be similar to the care you provide with an epidural. After the epidural or the spinal-epidural with the woman in a sitting position, she is then placed supine with left uterine displacement. A blanket roll or a pillow can be used to tilt her. Blood pressure should be monitored every 2 minutes for at least 10 minutes, and then every 5 minutes for 20 minutes. Subsequently, the patient may be monitored every 30 minutes until delivery, or as ordered by the anesthesia provider (Nageotte, Larson, Rumney, Sidhu, & Hollenbach, 1997). The benefit of a CSE censurs a low-dose epidural is faster onset. The disadvantage is that there is increased pruritus (Simmons, Cyna, Dennis, & Hughes, 2007).

CONCLUSIONS

Pain is the fifth vital sign and it has seven distinct dimensions: physical, sensory, behavioral, sociocultural, cognitive, affective, and spiritual. Women in labor need pain relief. Nonpharmacologic measures to assist women in perceiving less pain include acupressure, acupuncture, aromatherapy, audio analgesia, controlled breathing, cool compresses, warm compresses, hydrotherapy, hypnotherapy, intradermal or subcutaneous injections in the lower back, massage, and transcutaneous electrical nerve stimulation. Pharmacologic measures include the use of parenteral opioids, which may be mu or kappa agonists. In addition, neuraxial analgesia and anesthesia may be administered via an epidural catheter, a spinal–epidural, or in the intrathecal space. Nurses have a critical role in assessing a woman's pain, communicating with the obstetric and anesthesia providers, and administering pain therapy. Nurses also must evaluate the woman's response to therapeutic measures and evaluate the maternal and fetal response after the administration of analgesics and anesthetics.

REVIEW QUESTIONS

True/False: Decide if the statements are true or false.

1. Pain has two dimensions: the physical sensation and the emotional response to it.
2. Hypnosis is one of the most effective nonpharmacologic treatments to reduce labor pain.
3. Subcutaneous injections of sterile water to treat severe back pain during labor cause burning and stinging for 1 to 2 minutes.
4. Parenteral opioid administration is the most common method of pain relief in the United States.

(Norris, Fogel, & Conway-Long, 2001). The spinal–epidural has resulted in fetal bradycardia and emergent cesarean delivery for a nonreassuring fetal heart rate pattern. Compared with the babies of women who received meperidine (Demerol) 50 mg on demand for a maximum of 200 mg in 4 hours, there were similar neonatal outcomes (Gambling et al., 1998). Dr. Nageotte and his colleagues (1997) at Women's Hospital in the Long Beach Memorial Medical Center in California found that nulliparous women in spontaneous labor who received a continuous lumbar epidural or a combination spinal and epidural had similar rates of a cesarean section, dystocia, maternal and fetal complications, and reduced patient satisfac-

5. It is safe to remove the epidural catheter when the platelet count is 50,000.
6. An intrathecal injection is the administration of drugs into the epidural space.
7. Maternal respirations usually increase after an intrathecal injection.
8. Side effects of intrathecal narcotics such as itching, nausea, vomiting, and urinary retention may last for 24 hours after the intrathecal injection.

9. An adverse effect of intrathecal narcotics is fetal bradycardia.
10. The complication rate after a spinal–epidural is similar to the complication rate after a continuous epidural.

References

Alexander, J. M., Sharma, S. K., McIntire, D. D., & Leveno, K. J. (2002). Epidural analgesia lengthens the Friedman active phase of labor. *Obstetrics & Gynecology, 100*, 46–50.

American College of Obstetricians and Gynecologists. (2002). Analgesia and cesarean delivery rates. *ACOG Committee Opinion Number 339.* Washington, DC: Author.

American Society of Anesthesiologists Task Force on Obstetric Anesthesia. (2007). Practice guidelines for obstetric anesthesia: An updated report by the American Society of Anesthesiologists Task Force on Obstetric Anesthesia. *Anesthesiology, 106*(4), 843–863.

Anim-Somuah, M., Smyth, R., & Howell, C. (2005). Epidural versus non-epidural or no analgesia in labour. *Cochrane Database of Systematic Reviews,* Issue 4. Art No.: CD000331. doi:10.1002/14651858.CDE000331.pub2.

Association of Women's Health, Obstetric, and Neonatal Nursing. (2007). *Role of the registered nurse (RN) in the care of the pregnant woman receiving analgesia/anesthesia by catheter techniques (epidural, intrathecal, spinal, PCEA catheters).* Washington, DC: Author.

Atkinson, B. D., Truitt, L. J., Rayburn, W. F., Turnbull, G. L., Christensen, H. D., & Wlodaver, A. (1994). Double-blind comparison of intravenous butorphanol (stadol) and fentanyl (sublimaze) for analgesia during labor. [Transactions of the fourteenth annual meeting of the Society of Perinatal Obstetricians]. *American Journal of Obstetrics and Gynecology, 171*(4), 993–998.

Bahasadri, S., Ahmadi-Abhari, S., Dehghani-Nik, M., & Habibi, G. R. (2006). Subcutaneous sterile water injection for labour pain: A randomized controlled study. *Australian and New Zealand Journal of Obstetrics and Gynaecology, 46*, 102–106.

Bek, T., Ottesen, B., & Fahrenkrug J. (1988). The effect of gallanin, CGRP and ANP on spontaneous smooth muscle activity of rat uterus. *Peptides, 9*, 497–500.

Ben-Aroya, Z., Bar-David, J., Hallak, M., Zolotnik, L., Friger, M., & Katz, M. (2001). Epidural analgesia in twin gestation is associated with adverse obstetrical outcome. [Abstract]. *American Journal of Obstetrics and Gynecology, 184*(1), S164.

Bricker, L., & Lavender, T. (2002). Parental opioids for pain relief: A systematic review. *American Journal of Obstetrics and Gynecology, 186*(5), 94–109.

Carvalho, B., Wang, P., & Cohen, S. E. (2006). A survey of labor patient-controlled epidural anesthesia in California hospitals. *International Journal of Obstetric Anesthesia, 15*(3), 217–222.

Canton, D., Corry, M. P., Frigoletto, F. D., Hopkins, D. P., Lieberman, E., & Mayberry, L. (2002). The nature and management of labor pain: Executive summary. *American Journal of Obstetrics and Gynecology, 186*(2 Suppl.), S1–S15.

Case, A. S., & Ramsey, P. S. (2005). Spontaneous epidural hematoma of the spine in pregnancy. *American Journal of Obstetrics and Gynecology, 193*, 875–877.

Chao, A.-S., Chao, A., Wang, T.-H., Chang, Y.-C., Peng, H.-H., & Chang, S.-D. (2007). Pain relief by applying transcutaneous electrical nerve stimulation (TENS) on acupuncture points during the first stage of labor: A randomized double-blind placebo-controlled trial. *Pain, 127*, 214–220.

Cheek, T. G., Samuels, P., Miller, F., Tobin, M., & Gutsche, B. B. (1996). Normal saline fluid load decreases uterine activity in active labour. *British Journal of Anaesthesia, 77*(5), 632–635.

Chen, S. H., Liou, S. C., Hung, C. T., Shih, M. H., Chen, C., & Tsai, S. C. (2006). Comparison of patient-controlled epidural analgesia and continuous epidural infusion for labor analgesia. [Abstract]. *Chang Gung Medical Journal, 29*(6), 576–582.

Chestnut, D. H. (1997). Epidural analgesia and the incidence of cesarean section: Time for another close look. *Anesthesiology, 87*, 472–476.

Cluett, E. R., Nikodem, V. C., McCandlish, R. E., & Burns, E. E. (2008). Immersion in water in pregnancy, labour and birth (Review). *Cochrane Library,* Issue 2.

Courtney, K. (2007). Maternal anesthesia: What are the effects on neonates? *Nursing for Women's Health, 11*(5), 499–502.

D'Arcy, Y. (2008). Be an expert in pain assessment. *2008 Pathways Directory, Nursing Spectrum & NurseWeek,* 10–15.

Davis, D. C. (1996). The discomforts of pregnancy. *Journal of Obstetric, Gynecologic, and Neonatal Nursing, 25*(1), 73–80.

Evron, S., Ezri, T., Protianov, M., Muzikant, G., Sadan, O., & Herman, A. (2008). The effects of remifentanil or acetaminophen with epidural ropivacaine on body temperature during labor. *Journal of Anesthesia, 22*(2), 105–111.

Fitzpatrick, M., McQuillan, K., & O'Herlihy, C. (2000). Influence of occipito-posterior position on delivery outcome. [Abstract]. *American Journal of Obstetrics and Gynecology, 182*(1, Part 2), S134.

Fraser, W. D., Marcoux, S., Krauss, I., Douglas, J. K., Goulet, C., & Boulvain, M. (2000). Multicenter, randomized, controlled trial of delayed pushing for nulliparous women in the second stage of labor with continuous epidural analgesia. *American Journal of Obstetrics and Gynecology, 182*(5), 1165–1172.

Friedlander, J. D., Fox, H. E., Cain, C. F., Dominguez, C. L., & Smiley, R. M. (1997). Fetal bradycardia and uterine hyperactivity following subarachnoid administration of fentanyl during labor. Case report. *Regional Anesthesia, 22*(4), 378–381.

Gambling, D. R., Sharma, S. K., Ramin, S. M., Lucas, M. J., Leveno, K. J., Wiley, J. & Sidawi, J. E. (1998). A randomized study of combined spinal-epidural analgesia versus intravenous meperidine during labor: Impact on cesarean delivery rate. *Anesthesiology, 89*, 1336–1344.

Goetzl, L., Rivers, J., Evans, T., Citron, D. R., Richardson, B. E., & Lieberman, E. (2004). Prophylactic acetaminophen does not prevent epidural fever in nulliparous women: A double-blind placebo-controlled trial. *Journal of Perinatology, 24*, 471–475.

Goetzl, L., Rivers, J., Zighelboim, I., Wali, A., Badell, M., & Suresh, M. S. (2007). Intrapartum epidural analgesia and maternal temperature regulation. *Obstetrics & Gynecology, 109*, 687–690.

Gogarten, W., Struemper, D., Gramke, H. F., Van Aken, H., Buerkle, H., & Durieux, M. (2005). Assessment of volume preload on uteroplacental blood flow during epidural anaesthesia for caesarean section. *European Journal of Anaesthesiology, 22*, 359–362.

Goodman, E. J., Haas, A. J., & Kantor, G. S. (2006). Inadvertent administration of magnesium sulfate through the epidural catheter: Report and analysis of a drug error. *International Journal of Obstetric Anesthesiology, 15*(1), 63–67.

Hiltunen, P., Raudaskoski, T., Ebeling, H., & Moilanen, I. (2004). Does pain relief during delivery decrease the risk of postnatal depression? *Acta Obstetricia et Gynecologica Scandinavica, 83*, 257–261.

Hofmeyr, G. J., Cyna, A. M., & Middleton, P. (1996). Prophylactic intravenous preloading for regional analgesia in labour. *Cochrane Database of Systematic Reviews*, Issue 2. Art. No.: CD000175. doi:10.1002/14651858. CD000175.pub2.

Jacobson, B., Eklund, G., Hamberger, L., Linnarsson, D., Sedvall, G., & Valverius, M. (1987). Perinatal origin of adult self-destructive behavior. *Acta Psychiatricia candinavica, 75*, 364–371.

Jacobson, B., Nyberg, K., Eklund, G., Bygdeman, M., & Rydberg, U. (1988). Obstetric pain medication and eventual adult amphetamine addiction in offspring. *Acta Obstetricia et Gynecologica Scandinavica, 67*, 677–682.

Jacobson, B., Nyberg, K., Gronbladh, L., Eklund, G., Bygdeman, M., & Rydberg, U. (1990). Opiate addiction in adult offspring through possible imprinting after obstetric treatment. *British Medical Journal, 301*, 1067–1070.

Kinsella, S. M., Pirlet, M., Mills, M. S., Tuckey, J. P., & Thomas, T. A. (2000). Randomized study of intravenous fluid preload before epidural analgesia during labour. *British Journal of Anaesthesia, 85*(2), 311–333.

Klein, M. C. (2006). Does epidural analgesia increase rate of cesarean section? *Canadian Family Physician, 52*(4), 419–421.

Kotaska, A. J., Klein, M. C., & Liston, R. M. (2006). Epidural analgesia associated with low-dose oxytocin augmentation increases cesarean births: A critical look at the external validity of randomized trials. *American Journal of Obstetrics and ynecology, 194*, 809–814.

Kuczkowski, K. M. (2006). Labor analgesia for the parturient with herbal medicine use: What does an obstetrician need to know? *Archives in Gynecology and Obstetrics, 274*, 233–239.

Kwekkeboom, K. L., & Gretarsdottir, E. (2006). Systematic review of relaxation interventions for pain. *Journal of Nursing Scholarship, 38*(3), 269–277.

Lewis, M., & Calthorpe, N. (2005). Combined spinal epidural analgesia in labour. *Fetal and Maternal Medicine Review, 16*(1), 29–50.

Lowe, N. K. (1996). The pain and discomfort of labor and birth. *Journal of Obstetric, Gynecologic, and Neonatal Nursing, 25*(1), 82–92.

Lowe, N. K. (2002). The nature of labor pain. *American Journal of Obstetrics and Gynecology, 186*(2 Suppl), S16–S24.

Manning, J. (1996). Intrathecal narcotics: New approach for labor analgesia. *Journal of Obstetric, Gynecologic, and Neonatal Nursing, 25*(3), 221–224.

Manworren, R. (2006). A call to action to protect range orders. *American Journal of Nursing, 106*(7), 65–68.

Marquette, G. P., Mechas, T., Charest, J., & Rey, E. (1994). Epidural anaesthesia for elective caesarean section does not influence fetal umbilical artery blood flow indices. *Canadian Journal of Anaesthesia, 41*(11), 1053–1056.

Marshall, K. M., & Baker, J. (2006). Are patients in labor satisfied with PCEA? *Nursing 2006, 36*(6), 18–19.

Mårtensson, L., McSwiggin, M., & Mercer, J. S. (2008). US midwives' knowledge and use of sterile water injections in labor pain. *Journal of Midwifery & Women's Health, 53*, 115–122.

Mårtensson, L., Stener-Victorin, E., & Wallin, G. (2008). Acupuncture versus subcutaneous injections of sterile water as treatment for labour pain. *Acta Obstetricia et Gynecologica, 87*, 171–177.

Nageotte, M. P., Larson, D., Rumney, P. J., Sidhu, M., & Hollenbach, K. (1997). Epidural analgesia compared with combined spinal-epidural analgesia during labor in nulliparous women. *New England Journal of Medicine, 337*(24), 1715–1719.

Nicholas, P. K., & Agius, C. R. (2005). Toward safer IV medication administration. *American Journal of Nursing, 105*(3), (Suppl), 25–30.

Nikkola, E. M., Ekblad, U. U., Kero, P. O., Alihanka, J. J., & Salonen, M. A. (1997). Intravenous fentanyl PCA during labour. *Canadian Journal of Anesthesia, 44*, 1248–1255.

Norris, M. C., Fogel, S. T., & Conway-Long, C. (2001). Combined spinal-epidural versus epidural labor analgesia. *Anesthesiology, 95*(4), 913–920.

Nubain. (1990). Du Pont Pharmaceuticals. Newark, Delaware.

Nubain. (2003). Endo Pharmaceuticals Inc. Chadds Ford, PA.

Nyberg, K., Buka, S. L., & Lipsitt, L. P. (2000). Perinatal medication as a potential risk factor for adult drug abuse in a North American cohort. *Epidemiology, 11*, 715–716.

Ohana, H. P., Levy, A., Rozen, A., Shapira, Y., Greenberg, L., & Sheiner, E. (2007). The influence of epidural analgesia on mode of delivery in nulliparous women. [Abstract]. *American Journal of Obstetrics and Gynecology, 197*, S103.

Pasero, C., & McCaffery, M. (2005). Authorized and unauthorized use of PCA pumps: Clarifying the use of patient-controlled analgesia, in light of recent alerts. *American Journal of Nursing, 105*(7), 30–32.

Philipps, A. F., Rosenkrantz, T. S., Porte, P. J., & Raye, J. R. (1985). The effects of chronic fetal hyperglycemia on substrate uptake by the ovine fetus and conceptus. *Pediatric Research, 19*(7), 659–666.

Pouta, A. M., Karinen, J., Vuolteenaho, O. J., & Laatikainen, T. J. (1996). Effect of intravenous fluid preload on vasoactive peptide secretion during caesarean section under spinal anesthesia. *Anaesthesia, 51*(2), 128–132.

Reilly, D. R., & Oppenheimer, L. W. (2005). Fever in term labour. *Canadian Journal of Obstetrics and Gynaecology, 27*(3), 218–223.

Reynolds, J. L. (2000). Sterile water injections relieve back pain of labor. *Birth, 27*(1), 58–60.

Roberts J. (1983). Factors influencing distress from pain during labor. *American Journal of Maternal Child Nursing, 8*, 62–66.

Rosen, M. A. (2002). Nitrous oxide for relief of labor pain: A systematic review. *American Journal of Obstetrics and Gynecology, 186*(5), S110–S126.

Schaffer, S. D., & Yucha, C. B. (2004). Relaxation & pain management. *American Journal of Nursing, 104*(8), 75–82.

Schlaepfer, T. E., Strain, E. C., Greenberg, B. D., Preston, K. L., Lancaster, E., & Bigelow, G. E. (1998). Site of opioid action in the human brain: Mu and kappa agonists' subjective and cerebral blood flow effects. *American Journal of Psychiatry, 155*(4), 470–473.

Sezer, O. A., & Gunaydin, B. (2007). Efficacy of patient-controlled epidural analgesia after initiation with epidural or combined spinal-epidural analgesia. *International Journal of Obstetric Anesthesia, 16*(3), 226–230.

Sharma, S. K., Sidawi, J. E., Ramin, S. M., Lucas, M. J., Leveno, K. J., & Cunningham, F. G. (1997). Cesarean delivery: A randomized trial of epidural versus patient-controlled meperidine analgesia during labor. *Anesthesiology, 87*(3), 487–494.

Sia, A. T., Lim, Y., Ocampo, C. (2007). A comparison of a basal infusion with automated mandatory boluses in parturient-controlled epidural analgesia during labor. *Anesthesia and Analgesia, 104*(3), 673–678.

Silkman, C. (2008). Assessing the seven dimensions of pain. *American Nurse Today*, 13–16.

Simkin, P., & Bolding, A. (2004). Update on nonpharmacologic approaches to relieve labor pain and prevent suffering. *Journal of Midwifery & Women's Health, 49*, 489–504.

Simmons, S. W., Cyna, A. M., Dennis, A. T., & Hughes, D. (2007). Combined spinal-epidural versus epidural analgesia in labour. *Cochrane Database of Systematic Reviews*. Issue 3. Art. No.: CD003401. doi: 10.1002/14651858. CD003401. pub2.

Smiley, R., & Stephenson, L. (2007). Patient-controlled epidural analgesia in labor. *International Anesthesiology Clinics, 45*(1), 83–98.

Smith, C. A., Collins, C. T., Cyna, A. M., & Crowther, C. A. (2007). Complementary and alternative therapies for pain management in labour. (Review). *The Cochrane Library*. Issue 4. Art. No.: CD003521. doi: 10.1002/14651858. CD003521. pub2.

Stienstra, R. (2000). Patient-controlled epidural analgesia or continuous infusion: Advantages and disadvantage of different modes of delivering epidural analgesia for labour. *Current Opinion in Anaesthesiology, 13*(3), 253–256.

Stotland, N. E., & Stotland, N. L. (2005). Simpson, Semmelweis, and transformational change. [Letter to the editor]. *Obstetrics & Gynecology, 106*(5, Part 1), 1107.

Stratmann, G., Gambling, D. R., Moeller-Bertram, T., Stackpole, J., Pue, A. F., & Berkowitz, J. (2005). A randomized comparison of a five-minute versus fifteen-minute lockout interval for PCEA during labor. *International Journal of Obstetric Anesthesia, 14*, 200–207.

Torvaldsen, S., Roberts, C. L., Bell, J. C., & Raynes-Greenow, C. H. (2004). Discontinuation of epidural analgesia late in labour for reducing the adverse delivery outcomes associated with epidural analgesia. *Cochrane Database of Systematic Reviews*, Issue 4. Art. No.: CED004457. doi: 10.1002/14651858. CD004457.pub2.

Traynor, J. D., Dooley, S. L., Seyb, S., Wong, C. A., & Shadron, A. (2000). Is the management of epidural analgesia associated with an increased risk of cesarean delivery? *American Journal of Obstetrics and Gynecology, 182*(5), 1058–1062.

Valenzuela, G., Cline, S., & Hayashi, R. H. (1983). Follow-up of hydration and sedation in the pretherapy of premature labor. *American Journal of Obstetrics and Gynecology, 147*, 396–398.

Vallejo, M. C., Ramesh, V., Phelps, A. L., & Sah, N. (2007). Epidural labor analgesia: Continuous infusion versus patient-controlled epidural analgesia with background infusion versus without a background infusion. *Journal of Pain, 8*(12), 970– 975.

Van de Velde, M., Van Schoubroeck, D., Jani, J., Teunkens, A., Missant, C., & Deprest, J. (2006). Combined spinal-epidural anesthesia for cesarean delivery: Dose-dependent effects of hyperbaric bupivacaine on maternal hemodynamics. *Anesthesia and Analgesia, 103*(1), 187–190.

Viitanen, H., Viitanen, M., & Heikkilä, M. (2005). Single-shot spinal block for labour analgesia in multiparous parturients. *Acta Anaesthesiologica Scandinavica, 49,* 1023–1029.

Viscomi, C. M., Hood, D. D., Melone, P. J., & Eisenach, J. C. (1990). Fetal heart rate variability after epidural fentanyl during labor. *Anesthesia and Analgesia, 71,* 679–683.

Waters, B., & Raisler, J. (2003). Ice massage for the reduction of labor pain. *Journal of Midwifery and Women's Health, 48,* 317–321.

Weber, S. E. (1996). Cultural aspects of pain in childbearing women. *Journal of Obstetric, Gynecologic, and Neonatal Nursing, 25*(1), 67–72.

Weinger, M. B. (2008). Dangers of postoperative opioids: APSF workshop and white paper address prevention of postoperative respiratory complications. Retrieved July 3, 2008. Available at http://www.apsf.org/resource_center/newsletter/2007/winter/01_opi oids.htm.

Wing, D. A., Goharkhay, N., Felix, J. C., Rostamkhani, M., Naidu, Y. M., & Kovacs, B. W. (2006). Expression of the oxytocin and V1a vasopressin receptors in human myometrium in differing physiologic states and following misoprostol administration. *Gynecologic and Obstetric Investigation, 62,* 181–185.

Wong, C. A., Scavone, B. M., Peaceman, A. M., McCarthy, R. J., Sullivan, J. T., & Diaz, N. T. (2005). The risk of cesarean delivery with neuraxial analgesia given early versus late in labor. *New England Journal of Medicine, 352,*655–665.

Positions for Labor and Birth

This chapter illustrates various positions a woman can assume during labor with some of the advantages and disadvantages of these positions. Today, nurses no longer have to insist that their patients remain flat or semiflat in the bed. Nurses should encourage women to change position frequently to facilitate labor and birth.

UPRIGHT POSITIONS

Women who walk during labor report an increased level of comfort and satisfaction. Many women prefer to walk during labor and indicate they would do so again in a future labor (see Figure 5.1). Walking does not speed up the first stage of labor (Roberts, Algert, & Olive, 2004). It is a safe position, however, for both women and their fetuses (Winslow, Crenshaw, & Jacobson, 2000).

A woman giving birth in an upright position increases her risk of a second-degree laceration. If the woman moves down into a supported squatting position, this may reduce the weight on her legs and feet without adding pressure to her pelvis (Keen, Di Franco, & Amis, 2004).

At times, a woman may wish to lean on the bed (see Figure 5.2). You should elevate the bed height so that she is not straining her back. This position and other upright positions are not harmful to either the mother or the fetus and they do not delay the progression of labor (Gupta & Nikodem, 2000).

Women who are positioned on their sides during labor have less pain, and more oxygen is delivered to their fetus than women who labor on their backs (see Figure 5.3). This position promotes more normal fetal heart rate patterns, more effective uterine contractions, a shorter second stage of labor, and a reduced need for pain medication. A side-lying position

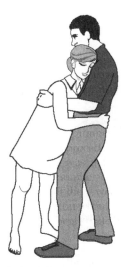

Figure 5.1: Walking during labor.

may also help to slow a rapidly progressing labor and birth (Keen et al., 2004).

Upright positions do not appear to reduce the duration of the first stage of labor (Souza, Miquelutti, Cecatti, & Makuch, 2006). Certain upright positions such as kneeling, however, may interfere with provider tasks such as amniotomy and fetal monitoring. The benefits of an upright position include better circulation to the uterus and therefore better oxygen delivery to the fetus (see Figures 5.6, 5.7, and 5.8).

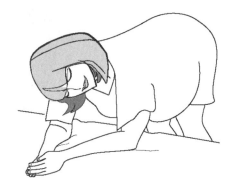

Figure 5.2: Upright and resting on bed.

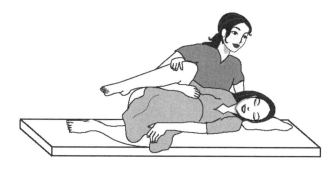

Figure 5.5: Pushing in a lateral position.

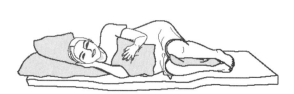

Figure 5.3: Side-lying positions increase blood flow to the uterus.

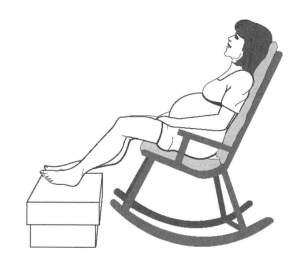

Figure 5.6: Upright position in rocking chair.

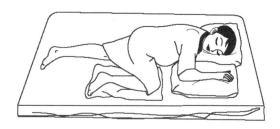

Figure 5.4: Lateral positioning during the second stage with passive descent (laboring down) can reduce the incidence of a difficult delivery (Roberts & Hanson, 2007).

Upright positions are usually well accepted by laboring patients and have no negative effect on fetal or neonatal well-being, the duration of the first and second stages of labor, the cesarean section rate, or other obstetric interventions (Miquelutti, Cecatti, & Makuch, 2006).

HYDROTHERAPY

Hydrotherapy increases maternal comfort (see Figure 5.9) and may improve uterine contractility (Stark, Rudell, & Haus, 2008). It promotes local vasodilatation and muscle relaxation, decreases muscle pain, reduces anxiety, and decreases production of stress-related hormones. It appears to increase oxytocin and endorphin production, which increases contractions and

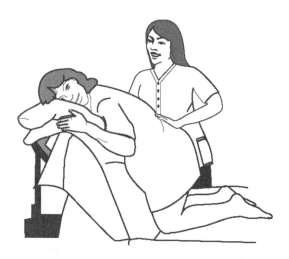

Figure 5.7: Upright kneeling position.

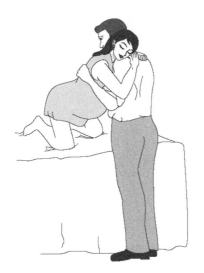

Figure 5.8: Kneeling with support.

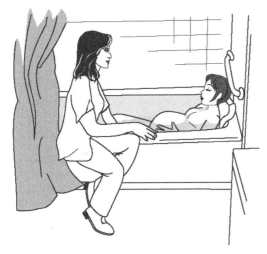

Figure 5.9: Hydrotherapy (warm-water immersion) promotes both relaxation and pain relief (Hofmeyr, 2005).

dilatation. Warm-water immersion also reduces blood pressure and edema (Florence & Palmer, 2003; Simkin, & O'Hara, 2002). It seems to temporarily reduce labor pain, especially when the water temperature does not exceed the maternal body temperature (Eappen & Robbins, 2002).

Labor progress may be shortened when nulliparous women soak in a tub filled with warm water (Cluett, Pickering, Getliffe, & St. George Saunders, 2004). Hydrotherapy appears to be most effective once the woman is in active labor, as entering the warm water at less than a 5-cm dilatation seemed to diminish the strength and frequency of contractions (Mackey, 2001; Simkin & O'Hara, 2002). Some hospitals do not have hydro-

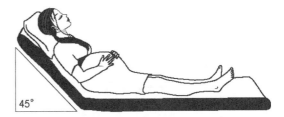

Figure 5.10: Semi-Fowler's position.

therapy tubs and therefore water immersion is not an option (Brown, Douglas, & Flood, 2001).

Fowler's position is a semi-upright position with the head of the bed raised 80 to 90 degrees. Fowler's position is used less often during labor than a semi-Fowler's position with the head of the bed raised 45 to 60 degrees (see Figure 5.10). This variation of an upright position appears to improve maternal comfort and decrease the need for analgesics. It is a safe option for maternal activity during the first stage of labor (Souza et al., 2006). The side rails may be lowered until she is given an analgesic. A nonsupine position such as the semi-Fowler's position may decrease the number of operative vaginal deliveries and cesarean sections (Romano & Lothian, 2008).

Women who have not received an epidural and who remain in an upright position during the second stage of labor should have fewer abnormal fetal heart rate patterns, fewer reports of severe pain, and a slightly decreased duration of the second stage. They also decrease their chances of an episiotomy or operative vaginal delivery. Women who push while they are in an upright position have an increased risk of second-degree perineal tears (Roberts & Hanson, 2007).

An upright position, especially with uterine displacement to the left or right side, should reduce the duration of labor in women who have received an epidural. This position should also increase the number of spontaneous vaginal births, while decreasing the incidence of operative vaginal deliveries and cesarean sections (Roberts, Algert, Cameron, & Torvaldsen, 2005).

During the second stage of labor, elevating the head of the bed 30 degrees (see Figure 5.11) decreases the bladder capacity (Roberts & Hanson, 2007). Therefore, if this position is used the woman should empty her bladder before she begins to push. The semirecumbent position for childbirth is also related to a higher episiotomy rate (Shorten, Donsante, & Shorten, 2002).

The kneeling position (see Figures 5.12 and 5.13) is often helpful in reducing persistent back pain. With patience, even a woman who has received an epidural can be assisted in assuming this position. It is usually well accepted by laboring women, and there is no evidence of harm when this position is used. Use of this position for fetal rotation to an occiput anterior position, or to reduce operative vaginal deliveries may be helpful (Stremler et al., 2005).

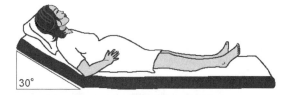

Figure 5.11: Semirecumbent position with the head of bed elevated 30 degrees. This position is lower than the semi-Fowler's position.

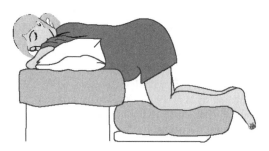

Figure 5.12: Maternal kneeling position or hands-and-knees position may correct a transverse or posterior fetal position (Hofmeyr, 2005).

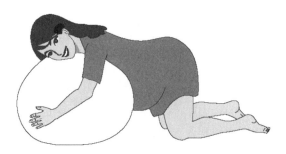

Figure 5.13: Kneeling using the labor ball. It may be helpful to put a pillow under her knees. Sitting on the birthing (labor) ball will displace maternal weight (Eappen & Robbins, 2002).

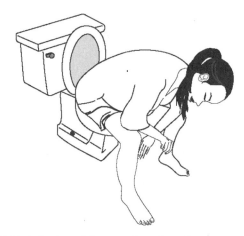

Figure 5.14: Laboring while seated on the toilet.

Some women prefer to labor or push while they are seated on the toilet (see Figure 5.14). If she is pushing, stay with her and observe her perineum. We do not want the baby to fall in! Before delivery, encourage her to return to bed. If you have a birthing chair, she can sit in it for delivery after she leaves the toilet. These specially designed chairs have been associated with a greater blood loss at delivery than when women deliver in other upright or lateral positions (Gupta & Nikodem, 2000). Use of a birthing chair is also associated with more second-degree perineal tears and no significant difference in the length of the second stage of labor (Gupta, Hofmeyr, & Smith, 2004).

The squatting position (see Figure 5.15) widens the pelvic diameter, thus allowing the baby to descend (Romano & Lo-

thian, 2008). This position requires muscular fitness and stamina to maintain a deep squat (Gupta et al., 2004). In some cultures, women assume the squatting position when they are eating or waiting. For example, in Bahrain, women and their children were observed by the primary author to be waiting in a squatting position at the bus stop. Japanese women often squat when they are eating. However, most North American women rarely squat and have not developed their leg muscles. If women are not able to support their weight in a squatting position, they may be supported with a squatting bar or with the help of support persons. The squatting position seems to cause fatigue more than other positions (Keen et al., 2004). The squatting position is also associated with the highest rate of third-degree tears (that require sutures), and the least favorable perineal outcomes (Gupta et al., 2004; Shorten et al., 2002).

The knee–chest position moves the fetus away from the cervix and towards the maternal diaphragm (see Figure 5.16). Therefore, it is the position of choice when the umbilical cord has prolapsed. However, this position should be avoided if there is a suspicion of uterine rupture, especially in a woman who has been induced with prostaglandins after a prior cesarean section. Women who have had a prior cesarean section and who are being induced with prostaglandins tend to rupture their uterus at the site of the prior cesarean scar more often than other locations (Buhimschi, Buhimschi, Patel, Malinow, & Weiner, 2005). If these women are placed in a knee–chest position, the weight of the fetus may extend the rupture and the fetus may be expelled from the uterus.

In the past, it was believed that the knee–chest position was related to an increased risk of an air embolism, but this belief is false. The knee–chest position is not related to any form of embolism. For a pregnant woman to suffer from an air embolism, air must be blown into the vagina in a sufficient quantity to cause an air lock in the heart, pulmonary trunk, or arteries (Collins, Davis, & Lantz, 1994; Hill & Jones, 1993; Kaiser, 1994; Marc, Chadly, & Durigon, 1990). This generally

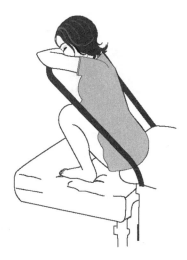

Figure 5.15: The squatting position.

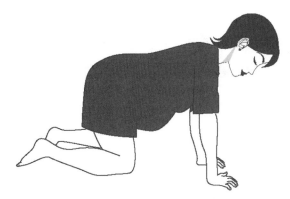

Figure 5.17: Hands-and-knees position, also known as the "all fours" position.

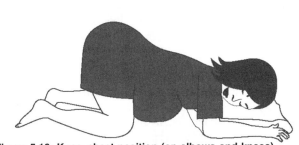

Figure 5.16: Knee–chest position (on elbows and knees).

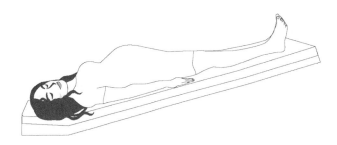

Figure 5.18: The Trendelenburg position.

happens when a sexual partner forcefully blows air into the vagina, and it enters the woman's venous system through damaged veins or open venous sinuses in the wall of the uterus (Truhlar et al., 2007; Varon, Laufer, & Sternbach, 1991).

If women are not pregnant and air is blown forcefully into the vagina, it will travel through the uterus, through the fallopian tubes, and into the abdomen. They will feel lower abdominal pain and chest pain radiating to their shoulders. Air blown forcefully into the vagina is called oral–genital insufflation (Christiansen, Danzl, & McGee, 1980). Therefore, nurses should always discourage women from engaging in activities that introduce a substantial quantity of air under pressure into the vagina.

The hands-and-knees position (see Figure 5.17) may be helpful to rotate a fetus from a posterior position to an anterior position (Kariminia, Chamberlain, Keogh, & Shea, 2004; Simkin & Ancheta, 2000). It may also help disimpact the anterior fetal shoulder when shoulder dystocia is encountered (Gherman et al., 2006). When this position is used to treat shoulder dystocia, it is called "the Gaskin maneuver."

The hands-and-knees position may decrease pressure on the maternal sacrum when a fetus is in the occiput posterior position. Women who have received an epidural will need assistance to turn and reposition themselves on their hands and knees. Some women will find the hands-and-knees position uncomfortable. A woman can be made more comfortable in this position by raising the head of the bed to support her head, or by placing several pillows below her head so she can lower her head and rest between contractions.

The Trendelenburg position is named after Friedrich Trendelenburg, a German genitourinary surgeon who taught the use of this position in his 1873 text (see Figure 5.18). Dr. Willie Meyer, a New York surgeon and a student of Dr. Trendelenburg, described this position in an 1885 article. Now, more than 100 years later, it has been found that this position does not improve vascular resuscitation and is, therefore, an ineffective treatment for hemorrhage (Martin, 1995). Although it has been used in the past to treat hypotension, shock, or both, a review of the results of five research studies found that this position only briefly improves hemodynamic status and may be followed by hemodynamic deterioration with compromised right ventricular ejection fraction. Shammas and Clark (2007) therefore suggest that the Trendelenburg position be avoided as a treatment for acute hypotension or shock until definitive research with larger sample sizes is conducted.

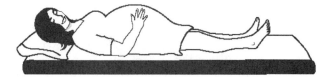

Figure 5.19: Supine position.

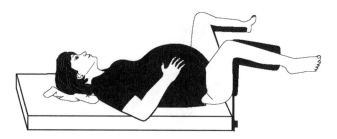

Figure 5.21: Dorsal lithotomy position.

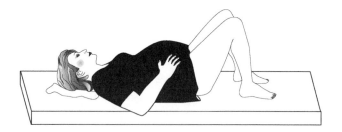

Figure 5.20: Dorsal recumbent position.

In the Trendelenburg position, the head is lower than the body and the diaphragm is forced up toward the woman's face. The weight of the uterus, amniotic fluid, placenta, and fetus will compress her great vessels, further compromising blood flow and oxygen delivery to the uterus. Therefore, this position should not be used as an intervention or position during labor because it is potentially harmful to the mother and her baby. It may be used occasionally when the fetus is preterm, the woman is not in labor, and the membranes are bulging into the vagina. In that case, her head may be lowered slightly. Encourage her to rest on her side. This position, with a slightly lowered head, is called a "modified Trendelenburg position."

AVOID THE SUPINE POSITION

The supine position (see Figure 5.19) is discouraged because the weight of the uterus, fetus, amniotic fluid, and placenta may compress the vena cava and aorta. This position has been associated with maternal orthostatic hypotension.

The dorsal recumbent position, like the supine position, diminishes blood flow to the uterus and oxygen delivery to the fetus (see Figure 5.20). Therefore, the uterus should be tilted with a pillow or towel roll to the right or left side if she will be in this position more than a few minutes. This position, however, is often the position of choice when the cervix is examined.

The dorsal lithotomy position (see Figure 5.21) is often helpful to deliver a large fetus. Encourage your patient to "push straight ahead." This position should be used close to the time of delivery. Prolonged use of this position during the second stage is discouraged as it can diminish blood flow to the uterus and oxygen delivery to the fetus.

In the 18th century, the horizontal or supine position was common during the first stage of labor to facilitate care and the performance of obstetric maneuvers and procedures. In this position, however, the weight of the uterus, amniotic fluid, placenta, and fetus compresses the maternal aorta. Therefore, the supine position is undesirable as it precedes decreased blood flow to the uterus and decreased oxygen delivery to the fetus (Souza et al., 2006). When the maternal position is changed in response to a nonreassuring fetal heart rate pattern, this position should be avoided (De Jong & Lagro-Janssen, 2004).

Labor or delivery in the supine position may make monitoring of the fetal heart rate by electronic means or auscultation easier, but it poses risks for the woman and her baby (Gupta et al., 2004). The needs of the caregiver must be weighed against the need to maximize maternal cardiac output to the uterus and fetal oxygenation. Giving birth in the supine position is related to more maternal complaints of pain, abnormal fetal heart rate patterns, more operative vaginal deliveries, and perineal tears. There is, however, a decrease in maternal blood loss (Gupta et al., 2004).

ENCOURAGE AN UPRIGHT POSITION FOR BIRTH

During the second stage of labor, the benefits of an upright position (see Figures 5.22 and 5.23) include a slight decrease in the length of the second stage of labor, maternal reports of less severe pain, fewer assisted deliveries, and, in some cases, fewer second-degree perineal tears (Gilder, Mayberry, Gennaro, & Clemmens, 2002). An upright position for delivery may increase the overall risk of perineal tears and postpartum hemorrhage (a blood loss of 500 mL or more), even though the duration of the second stage of labor decreases with fewer assisted deliveries, fewer episiotomies, and fewer maternal reports of severe pain (Gupta & Nikodem, 2000; Gupta et al., 2004). In addition, there were fewer abnormal fetal heart rate patterns (Gupta et al., 2004).

McROBERTS' MANEUVER FOR SHOULDER DYSTOCIA OR WHEN A LARGE BABY IS ANTICIPATED

William A. McRoberts Jr. popularized the use of this maneuver (see Figure 5.24) when he was at the University of Texas at

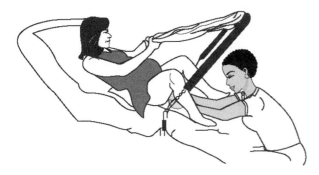

Figure 5.22: Upright position for birth.

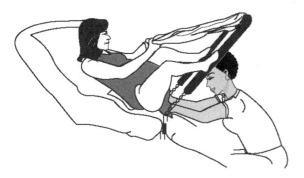

Figure 5.23: Upright position for birth with feet resting on squat bar.

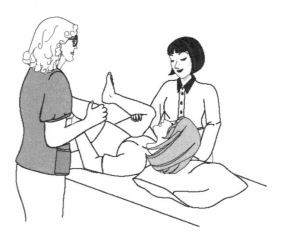

Figure 5.24: McRoberts' maneuver with the woman lying flat (dorsal recumbent position), the knees pulled up to the abdomen, and the hips abducted.

Houston. The legs are removed from the stirrups (if they are used) and sharply flexed. The McRoberts' maneuver is a useful and safe intervention after shoulder dystocia is diagnosed (Poggi et al., 2004). It is usually the first maneuver that is done when shoulder dystocia is recognized (Gherman et al., 1997). A woman can also be placed in this position when the birth of a large fetus is anticipated. The McRoberts' maneuver increases maternal pushing efficiency and strengthens intrauterine pressure (Buhimschi et al., 2005). Another benefit of the McRoberts' maneuver is that it reduces fetal extraction forces and brachial plexus stretching without significantly increasing the degree of symphyseal separation (Gherman, Tramont, Muffley, & Goodwin, 2000; Piper & McDonald, 1994).

> **Documentation example:** Head delivered at 10:00 a.m. Shoulder dystocia encountered. McRoberts' maneuver by this nurse, assisted by charge nurse, L. Rubin. Suprapubic pressure applied by CNM I. Willhelp. Delivery of baby at 10:03 a.m.

The risk of maternal injury increases with the maneuver because of compression of the lateral femoral cutaneous nerve. Injury or entrapment of this nerve is also known as meralgia

paresthetica, derived from the Greek word *meros*, meaning "thigh," and *algo*, meaning "pain." It is a syndrome characterized by numbness and pain in the lateral and anterolateral thigh. Entrapment of this nerve usually occurs at the inguinal ligament. Extreme thigh abduction and external rotation may even result in femoral nerve injury (Wong et al., 2003). Prolonged or aggressive use of the McRoberts' maneuver may also result in a pelvic ligament stretch injury (Gherman et al., 2006). Therefore, you must be very cautious when you use this maneuver.

If your patient reports a feeling of burning, tingling, or numbness in her thigh, and these symptoms increase with standing, walking, or extension of her hip, she may have an injury to her lateral femoral cutaneous nerve. Symptoms usually are on one side, but may be on both sides. Report signs of possible nerve injury to the physician.

CONCLUSIONS

The optimal maternal position for labor and birth is the one chosen by the mother, the one that supports maternal and fetal well-being, and the one that enables the nurse to best care for the patient. As a labor and delivery nurse, you will work to find this somewhat elusive "best position" for your patient. You must understand both physiology and the risks and benefits of different positions during labor and birth. You will also learn to adjust your patient care behaviors to allow her to be comfortable in the position of her choosing. Bath sheets, pillows, wash cloths, and towels will also assist you in providing support, cleanliness, and comfort to your patient.

REVIEW QUESTIONS

True/False: Decide if the statements are true or false.

1. An upright position is a safe option for maternal activity during the first stage of labor.

2. There are fewer abnormal FHR patterns reported in the maternal upright position versus the supine position.
3. Many laboring patients prefer to ambulate and would choose to do so again in a future labor.
4. A side-lying position increases both blood flow to the uterus and oxygen delivery to the fetus, and may be associated with less maternal pain.
5. Lateral positioning during passive fetal descent may reduce the incidence of a difficult delivery, but may increase costs to the hospital.

6. Laboring women report increased maternal comfort and relaxation when they are allowed to bathe or soak in a tub of warm water.
7. Bathing or soaking in a tub may be restricted due to institutional policy.
8. Most laboring women can assume a squatting position for long periods of time without becoming fatigued.
9. The knee–chest position should be avoided if one believes the uterus has ruptured.
10. The McRoberts' maneuver in a supine position is a safe and appropriate external maneuver often used to correct shoulder dystocia.

References

Brown, S. T., Douglas, C., & Flood, L. P. (2001). Women's evaluation of intrapartum nonpharmacological pain relief methods used during labor. *Journal of Perinatal Education, 10*(3), 1–8.

Buhimschi, C. S., Buhimschi, I. A., Patel, S., Malinow, A. M., & Weiner, C. P. (2005). Rupture of the uterine scar during term labour: Contractility or biochemistry? *British Journal of Obstetrics and Gynaecology, 112*, 38–42.

Christiansen, W. C., Danzl, D. F., & McGee, H. J. (1980). Pneumoperitoneum following vaginal insufflation and coitus. *Annals of Emergency Medicine, 9*(9), 480–482.

Cluett, E. R., Pickering, R. M., Getliffe, K., & St. George Saunders, N. J. (2004). Randomised controlled trial of labouring in water compared with standard of augmentation for management of dystocia in first stage of labour. *British Medical Journal*, doi:10.1136/bmj.37963.606412.EE.

Collins, K. A., Davis, G. J., & Lantz, P. E. (1994). An unusual case of maternal-fetal death due to vaginal insufflation of cocaine. *American Journal of Forensic Medical Pathology, 15*(4), 335–339.

De Jong, A., & Lagro-Janssen, A. L. M. (2004). Birthing positions. A qualitative study into the view of women about various birthing positions. *Journal of Psychosomatic Obstetrics & Gynecology, 25*, 47–55.

Eappen, S., & Robbins, D. (2002). Nonpharmacological means of pain relief for labor and delivery. *International Anesthesiology, 40*(4), 103–114.

Florence, D. J., & Palmer, D. G. (2003). Therapeutic choices for the discomforts of labor. *Journal of Perinatal and Fetal and Neonatal Nursing, 17*, 249.

Gherman, R. B., Chauhan, S., Ouzounian, J. G., Lerner, H., Gonik, B., & Goodwin, T. M. (2006). Shoulder dystocia: The unpreventable obstetric emergency with empiric management guidelines. *American Journal of Obstetrics and Gynecology, 195*, 657–672.

Gherman, R. B., Goodwin, T. M, Souter, I., Neumann, K., Ouzounian, J. G., & Paul, R. H. (1997). The McRoberts' manuever for the alleviation of shoulder dystocia: How successful is it? *American Journal of Obstetrics and Gynecology, 176*(3), 656–661.

Gherman, R. B., Tramont, J., Muffley, P., & Goodwin, T. M. (2000). Analysis of McRoberts' maneuver by x-ray pelvimetry. *Obstetrics & Gynecology, 95*(1), 43–47.

Gilder, K., Mayberry, L. J., Gennaro, S., & Clemmens, D. (2002). Maternal positioning in labor with epidural analgesia. *American Womens Health, Obstetric, and Neonatal Nursing Lifelines, 6*(1), 41–45.

Gupta, J., & Nikodem, V. (2000). Woman's position during second stage of labor. *Cochrane Database of Systematic Review*, 2000, Issue 1. Art. No.: CD002006.

Gupta, J. K., Hofmeyr, G. J., & Smith, R. (2004). Position in the second stage of labour for women without epidural anaesthesia. *Cochrane Database of Systematic Reviews*, Issue 1. Art. No.: CD002006.doi:10.1002/14561858.CD002006.pub2.

Hill, B. F., & Jones, J. S. (1993). Venous air embolism following orogenital sex during pregnancy. *American Journal of Emergency Medicine, 11*(2), 155–157.

Hofmeyr, G. (2005). Evidence-based intrapartum care. *Best Practice & Research Clinical Obstetrics & Gynecology, 19*(1), 103–115.

Kaiser, R. T. (1994). Air embolism death of a pregnant woman secondary to orogenital sex. *Academy of Emergency Medicine, 1*(6), 555–558.

Kariminia, A., Chamberlain, M., Keogh, J., & Shea, A. (2004). Randomized controlled trial of effect of hands and knees posturing on incidence of occiput posterior position at birth. *British Medical Journal*, doi:10.1136/bmj.37942.594456.44.

Keen, R., Di Franco, J., & Amis, D. (2004). Care practices that promote normal birth #5: Non-supine (e.g., upright or side-lying) positions for birth. *Journal of Perinatal Education, 13*(2), 30–32.

Mackey, M. (2001). Use of water in labor and birth. *Clinical Obstetrics and Gynecology, 44*(4), 733–748.

Marc, B., Chadly, A., & Durigon, M. (1990). Fatal air embolism during female autoerotic practice. *International Journal of Legal Medicine, 104*(1), 59–61.

Martin, J. T. (1995). The Trendelenburg position: A review of current slants about head down tilt. *Journal of the American Association of Nurse Anesthetists, 63*(1), 29–36.

Miquelutti, M., Cecatti, J., & Makuch, M. (2007). Upright position during the first stage of labor: A randomised controlled trial. *Acta Obstetricia et Gynecologica, 86*, 553–558.

Piper, D. M., & McDonald, P. (1994). Management of anticipated and actual shoulder dystocia: Interpreting the literature. *Journal of Nurse Midwifery, 39*(6), 387–388.

Poggi, S. H., Allen, R. H., Patel, C. R., Ghidini, A., Pezzullo, J. C., & Spong, C. Y. (2004). Randomized trial of McRoberts' versus lithotomy positioning to decrease the force that is applied to the fetus during delivery. *American Journal of Obstetrics & Gynecology, 191*, 874–878.

Roberts, C., Algert, C., Cameron, C., & Torvaldsen, S. (2005). A meta-analysis of upright positions in the second stage to reduce instrumental deliveries in women with epidural analgesia. *Acta Obstetricia et Gynecologica, 84*, 794–798.

Roberts, C. L., Algert, C. S., & Olive, E. (2004). Impact of first-stage ambulation on mode of delivery among women with epidural analgesia. *Australian and New Zealand Journal of Obstetrics and Gynecology, 44*(6), 489–494.

Roberts, J., & Hanson, L. (2007). Best practices in second stage labor care: Maternal bearing down and positioning. *Journal of Midwifery & Women's Health, 52*(3), 238–245.

Romano, A., & Lothian, J. (2008). Promoting, protecting, and supporting normal birth: A look at the evidence. *Journal of Obstetric, Gynecologic, and Neonatal Nursing, 37*, 94–105.

Sahai-Srivastava, S., & Amezcua, L. (2006). Compressive neuropathies complicating normal childbirth: Case report and literature review. *Birth, 34*(2), 173–175.

Shammas, A., & Clark, A. P. (2007). Trendelenburg positioning to treat acute hypotension: Helpful or harmful? *Clinical Nurse Specialist, 21*(4), 181–187.

Shorten, A., Donsante, J., & Shorten, B. (2002). Birth position, accoucheur, and perinatal outcomes: Informing women about choices for vaginal birth. *Birth, 29*(1), 18–27.

Simkin, P., & Ancheta, R. (2000). *The labor progress handbook.* Malden, MA: Blackwell Science.

Simkin, P. P., & O'Hara, M. (2002). Nonpharmacologic relief of pain during labor: Systematic reviews of five methods. *American Journal of Obstetrics and Gynecology, 186*, S131–S159.

Souza J., Miquelutti, M., Cecatti, J., & Makuch, M. (2006). Maternal position during the first stage of labor: A systematic review. *Reproductive Health, 3*(10), 1–10.

Stark, M., Rudell B., & Haus, G. (2008). Observing position and movements in hydrotherapy: A pilot study. *Journal of Obstectric, Gynecologic, and Neonatal Nursing, 37*, 116–122.

Stremler, R., Hodness, E., Petryshen, P., Stevens, B., Weston, J., & Willan, A. (2005). Randomized controlled trial of hands-and-knees positioning for occipitoposterior position in labor. *Birth, 32*(4), 243–251.

Truhlar, A., Cerny, V., Dostal, P., Solar, M., Parizkova, R., Hruba, I., & Zabka, L. (2007). Out-of-hospital cardiac arrest from air embolism during sexual intercourse: Case report and review of the literature. *Resuscitation, 73*(3), 475–484.

Varon, J., Laufer, M. D., & Sternbach, G. L. (1991). Recurrent pneumoperitoneum following vaginal insufflation. *American Journal of Emergency Medicine, 9*(5), 448–448.

Winslow, E. H., Crensaw, J., & Jacobson, A. F. (2000). Managing labor: Does walking help or hurt? *American Journal of Nursing, 100*(3), 52–54.

Wong, C., Scavone, B., Dugan, S., Smith, J., Prather H., & Ganchiff, J. (2003). Incidence of postpartum lumbosacral spine and lower extremity nerve injuries. *Obstetrics & Gynecology, 101*(2), 279–288.

6

Passenger, Placenta, and Cord

Think as you work, for in the final analysis your worth to your company comes not only in solving problems but in anticipating them.

—Herbert H. Ross

BIRTH OF THE PASSENGER: FROM FETUS TO NEONATE

Birth occurs when the fetus exits the uterus and becomes a neonate. The fetus travels through the maternal pelvis to be delivered vaginally. The size and type of the pelvis can impede or facilitate descent. There are four basic pelvic types. The type of pelvis is based on its shape, which is determined by the midwife or physician during prenatal care. The four pelvic types are: gynecoid, android, anthropoid, and platypoid (see Figure 6.1).

A gynecoid pelvis is what you hope to find recorded in the prenatal record because it usually has the greatest capacity with the largest diameter between the right and left side of the pelvis. An android pelvis is more triangular in shape with a narrow arch below the pubic bone (subpubic arch). Large babies have a difficult time passing through an android pelvis.

An anthropoid pelvis has an oval shape similar to a gynecoid pelvis, except that the largest diameter of the pelvis is between the pubic bone and the maternal spine. Women with an anthropoid pelvis may have babies that stay at a high station through most of the labor and then rotate, descend, and deliver.

A platypoid pelvis is flattened at the inlet and has a prominent sacrum and prominent ischial spines. This pelvis is wide but narrow between the pubic bone and maternal spine. Large fetuses might not fit though this pelvis. Fetuses also have a hard time rotating in a platypoid pelvis. Often they cannot move to an occiput anterior position. Therefore, they may stay in an occiput transverse position if they cannot rotate.

FETAL SIZE AFFECTS OUTCOMES

Fetal size is related to labor progress and operative delivery. Nulliparous women with large babies have longer first and second stages of labor, receive more oxytocin to augment labor, have more forceps deliveries, and have more cesarean sections (Turner et al., 1990). Big babies (more than 4,000 grams) also have a higher injury rate (Kolderup, Laros, & Musci, 1997). Shoulder dystocia, cesarean sections, and postpartum hemorrhage are more common when the fetus is large.

If the neonate weighs 3,591 grams (7 pounds 15 ounces) or more, there are more cesarean sections (Witter, Caulfield, & Stoltzfus, 1995). Large babies have an increased risk of injury. When a fetus weighs more than 4,000 grams (8 pounds 13 ounces), there is an increased risk of fractures, nerve injury, intracranial hemorrhage, soft-tissue lacerations (for example, from forceps), and minor scalp lacerations.

If you suspect a large fetus, you must be vigilant in monitoring labor progress and the fetal heart rate. Communicate any abnormalities of the fetal heart rate, uterine activity, dilatation, or descent to the midwife or physician. Also inform your charge nurse or supervisor of your concerns about the passenger, placenta, or cord.

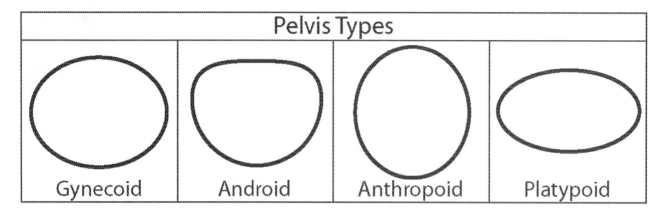

Figure 6.1: Pelvis types based on their shape. The top of the image is the back of the pelvis. A gynecoid pelvis is the most common female pelvis type.

FETAL SIZE AND WEIGHT

The size of the fetal head and the weight of the fetus affect descent. There are many factors that influence fetal size and weight. For example, male fetuses generally have larger heads than female fetuses of similar weight (Eogan, Geary, O'Connell, & Keane, 2003). Babies of women who live at sea level weigh more than babies of women who live at high altitudes. Birth weight was reduced an average of 100 grams (3.5 ounces) per 1,000 meters (3,300 feet) of elevation (Jensen & Moore, 1997; Moore, 2003).

Maternal weight influences fetal weight. Obese mothers have heavier fetuses than mothers who are not obese. Obesity also increases a woman's risk of hypertension, diabetes, the need to induce labor, cesarean section, and wound infection (Bastek, Elovitz, Pare, & Srinivas, 2007; Kieffer, 2000; Lu et al., 2001). Ethnicity may be related to the risk of diabetes, for example, Kieffer et al., (1999) found that diabetes was common in Hispanic women of childbearing age. Learn about the population of women you serve. What is their risk of diabetes?

Uncontrolled diabetes is related to excessive fetal weight (Nahum, 2006). If you have a patient who is obese, it is especially important that an estimated fetal weight be determined. If your patient is obese and has diabetes, it is even more important to estimate the fetal weight.

Women who smoke cigarettes during pregnancy have smaller babies than women who do not smoke. Women who have sickle cell disease and low hemoglobin have an increased risk of having a low-birth-weight neonate (Nahum, 2006).

Paternal height, but not weight, influences fetal weight. Babies of tall fathers were heavier than babies of short fathers (Morrison, Williams, Najman, & Andersen, 1991; To, Cheung, & Knok, 1998). If the father is tall and the mother is short, the baby weighs less than if the mother is also tall (Morrison, Williams, Najman, & Andersen, 1991). Parents who were both born with low birth weight had an increased risk of having a baby with low birth weight. However, the weight of the baby is not related to the father's birth weight unless the father had low birth weight. In that case, there is an increased risk of his infant also being born with low birth weight (Magnus, Gjessing, Skrondal, & Skjaerven, 2001).

Parity and maternal age affect fetal weight. However, the relationship between parity, age, and fetal weight is complex because as women age and have more babies, they also have a greater risk of developing diabetes mellitus. Diabetes is related to bigger babies. As parity increases, the body mass index increases. Big women make big babies. On the other hand, older women have babies who weigh less than babies of younger women (Aliyu et al., 2005). When an older woman with high parity is your patient, you will need to estimate the fetal weight and read the prenatal record to determine the pelvis type in order to anticipate problems with descent and delivery of the fetus. If a young, nulliparous woman is your patient, you should still estimate fetal weight and determine the pelvic type because her baby might also be too big for her pelvis.

ESTIMATE FETAL WEIGHT

Fetal weight can be estimated by a recent ultrasound, by palpation, or by measuring the symphysis-to-fundus height (symphysis–fundal height measurement) (see Figure 6.2). Your ability to approximate the actual fetal weight improves with practice. Use both hands to palpate the abdomen and to push through maternal tissue to feel the baby. You can do this during Leopold's maneuvers or independently of Leopold's maneuvers.

Think: Is the baby small, large, or very large? How much do I think this baby weighs? At the time of delivery, compare the actual weight with your estimate. How close were those weights? Try to determine if you have a pattern of underestimation or overestimation, and then modify your future estimates of fetal weight. With time and experience, your accuracy should increase.

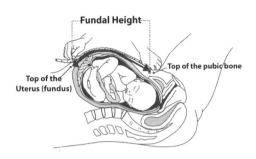

Figure 6.2: Fundal height, measured in centimeters, is the distance from the top of the pubic bone (symphysis pubis) to the top of the uterus (fundus).

The symphysis-to-fundus distance is related to the estimated fetal weight (EFW) (see Figure 6.2). The symphysis–fundal distance is also known as the fundal height. Fundal height is the distance from the top of the pubic bone to the top of the fundus of the uterus and it is measured in centimeters.

Mongelli and Gardosi (2004) proposed a formula for predicting fetal weight from the fundal height (see Figure 6.3). They found a strong relationship between fundal height and fetal weight.

DOCUMENT THE ESTIMATED FETAL WEIGHT (EFW)

After you have palpated the fetus, measured the fundal height, and estimated the fetal weight, document your estimate in the medical records. If the midwife or physician documented the EFW close to the time of admission, or if there was an ultrasound that documented the EFW close to the time of admission, some hospitals consider that a reasonable time frame for an EFW, and the nurse is not required to record an EFW. Consult your hospital's policies, procedures, and protocol.

By documenting the EFW you demonstrate your awareness of the fetal size. The EFW might be documented as "baby is very large" or "mother reports this baby is much larger than her last baby" or "estimated fetal weight is 8 1/2 lbs." You should also document the mother's height.

Documentation example: Leopold's maneuvers done. EFW 8 1/2 lbs. Mom 5′ tall. SVE 4/80%/–3. Discussed findings with CNM Aleers. CNM discussed plan of care with patient.

A fetus may be too big to safely pass through the pelvis or passageway. The pelvis may not be adequate and gynecoid (based on your review of the prenatal record). Communicate with the midwife or physician and inform them about your concerns. Discuss the plan of care. It may need to change.

One sign that indicates the fetus may be having difficulty passing through the pelvis is scalp swelling or

caput. When you combine the information from the EFW with the information on her pelvis (from the prenatal record) and your assessment of caput at 0 station with a dilatation of 7 cm, what does this constellation of facts suggest? The answer is that this baby may be too big for the passageway. After recording your assessments, communicate with the obstetric care provider. Discuss your assessments and concerns. Ask the provider to evaluate the fetal fit and descent.

Documentation example: Now 7/100%/caput at 0, station –1 to –2. FHR 140 to 150 with accelerations and variable decelerations for 20 to 30 seconds, dropping to 100 to 110 bpm. CNM Redy notified of SVE results. CNM confirmed SVE results and conferred with Dr. Obsconsult. Physician discussed plan of care with patient and her husband. Patient consented to a cesarean section.

DOCUMENT FETAL WELL-BEING

Fetal well-being means that the fetus is well oxygenated. A well-oxygenated fetus has accelerations in the fetal heart rate pattern (see Figure 6.4). Accelerations are transient increases in the fetal heart rate that rise above the baseline and return to the baseline. Accelerations are not part of a deceleration. Fetal accelerations rule out metabolic acidosis. When the fetal heart rate accelerates 10 or more beats per minute (bpm) above the baseline, and the acceleration lasts 10 or more seconds at its base, the fetus is not acidotic (Skupski, Rosenberg, & Eglinton, 2002). A nonstress test is classified as a reactive test when there are two or more accelerations that rise 15 or more bpm and last 15 or more seconds during a 20-minute period. Accelerations in a reactive nonstress test also rule out metabolic acidosis at the time of the accelerations.

An acceleration with a dip (see second to last acceleration in Figure 6.4) is called a Lambda pattern. Clinicians do not document Lambda patterns. A Lambda pattern is innocuous and thought to be related to a baroreceptor–vagal response to the rise in the fetal blood pressure with the rise in the fetal heart rate (acceleration).

Documentation example: Baseline 135 bpm (may also be recorded at 130 to 140), accelerations to 155 to 160 bpm, no decelerations. Contractions every 2 minutes for 70 seconds, palpating strong, resting tone soft. Oxytocin decreased to 6 mU/minute.

EXPECT FETAL ACCELERATIONS DURING LABOR

Fetal heart rate accelerations during labor are to be expected. Accelerations of the fetal heart rate should occur often during labor. Accelerations should occur no further than 90 minutes apart (Spencer & Johnson, 1986). If you assume the care of a patient who is in labor, determine when the last acceleration occurred. Even if a standard dose of narcotics was adminis-

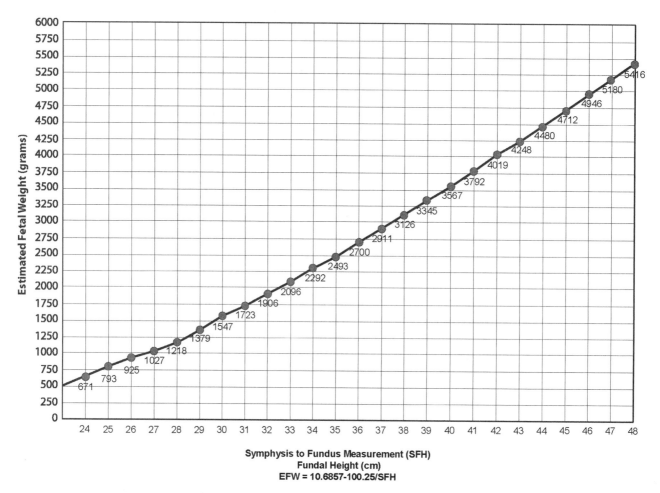

Figure 6.3: Symphysis to fundus measurement (fundal height) in centimeters and corresponding estimated fetal weight in grams. Graph developed with data from Mongelli and Gardosi (2004).

tered, the fetal heart rate should have accelerated within 90 minutes from the time of the narcotic administration.

A low umbilical artery pH (less than 7.2) was found when the admission test strip (first 30 minutes of monitoring) and the test strip at 30 minutes before delivery had a thin baseline (bandwidth of less than 3 beats per minute) or there were less than three cycles per minute (see Figure 6.5). A wider baseline without accelerations can also be related to a low pH. Fetuses with a baseline range of 5 or more bpm, or 5 or more cycles per minute *without accelerations*, also had a low umbilical artery pH (less than 7.2) (Samueloff et al., 1994). Do not administer a uterine stimulant such as oxytocin until fetal well-being is established. If there are no accelerations or there is a nonreactive admission strip, the physician or midwife should perform a bedside evaluation.

MACROSOMIA

Macrosomia means "a large body." A fetus who is macrosomic will have a high birth weight. A neonate whose weight is above the 90th percentile for its gestational age is classified as macrosomic. An EFW of 4,000 or more grams raises the suspicion that the neonate will be macrosomic.

When the neonate weighs 4,000 grams or more (8 lbs 13 ounces or more), it is likely to be large for gestational age. At 4,000 or more grams, there is an increased risk of cephalopelvic disproportion, prolonged labor, operative vaginal delivery, cesarean section, postpartum hemorrhage, shoulder dystocia, brachial plexus palsy (Erb's palsy), and asphyxia. Therefore, it is critical that you be aware of the EFW, that you have determined if labor progress is normal or abnormal, and that you have anticipated and prepared for complications related to birth.

THE FETAL–PELVIC FIT: FLOATING, DIPPING, OR ENGAGED?

You may have heard the saying, "one size fits all." This saying does not apply to the fetus or the pelvis, which vary between

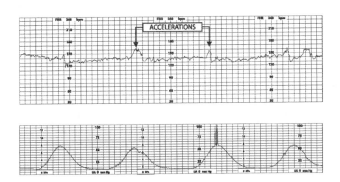

Figure 6.4: Accelerations of the fetal heart rate during labor that rise 10 or more bpm above their base and last 10 or more seconds at their base. Paper speed is 3 cm/minute. The accelerations rule out metabolic acidosis at the time of the test and reflect fetal well-being.

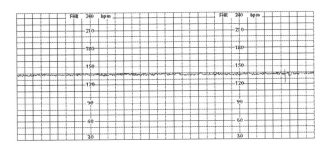

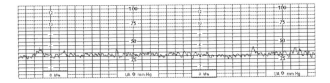

Figure 6.5: Part of a nonreactive admission strip. Paper speed is 3 cm/minute.

patients. Your assessment of the fetal–pelvic fit during the course of labor is crucial to maternal and fetal safety.

A fetus with an EFW of 4,000 grams or more may be floating or dipping in the pelvis when a woman arrives at the hospital for induction (see Figure 6.7). If the fetal head is floating or dipping, and the fetus is 41 or more weeks of gestation, the risk of a cesarean section is 12.4 times greater than the risk of a cesarean section if the fetus is engaged in the pelvis at the time of admission (Shin, Brubaker, & Ackerson, 2004). An unengaged fetal head more likely predicts the need for a cesarean section than the need for an induction. You will need to consider the increased risk for a cesarean section in your patient if she is being induced and the fetus is not at 0 station or lower. Pay attention to dilatation and descent during the

induction. Communicate the EFW, dilatation, and station to the nurse who will assume care during your report.

When the presenting part is entirely out of the pelvis and is freely movable above the pelvic inlet, it is floating. When the presenting part has passed through the plane of the inlet but is not engaged (0 station or lower), it is dipping. When the biparietal diameter has passed through the plane of the pelvic inlet and the tip of the skull is at or below the level of the ischial spines (0 station), the fetus is engaged.

Most primigravid women in the latent phase of spontaneous labor (67%) will have a fetus who is dipping at a −2 or a −1 station. Women with a body mass index of 25 or higher are more likely to present in the latent phase of labor with a fetus who was floating at a −3 station or higher. Fetuses who are floating descend almost 1 cm an hour slower than fetuses who are dipping or engaged. If the fetus is floating in the latent phase of labor, there is an increased incidence of a protracted active phase of labor and an arrest of dilation (Murphy, Shah, & Cohen, 1998).

A high fetal station is associated with fetopelvic disproportion, especially if the woman is nulliparous and has a term or postdates fetus (Murphy, Shah, & Cohen, 1998). Almost 24% of nulliparous women with an unengaged fetus at the onset of labor have an abnormally slow labor. However, only 13.8% of nulliparous women have a slow labor if their fetus is engaged at the onset of the labor (see Figure 6.8 and Exhibit 6.1) (Friedman & Sachtleben, 1965a, b, c).

Forty-three percent of nulliparous women with a floating fetus at the onset of their induction delivered by cesarean section. If the fetus was engaged, only 6.9% of the women had a cesarean section. Multiparous women with a term fetus who were induced were 37% more likely to require a cesarean section than multiparous women in spontaneous labor (Battista, Chung, Lagrew, & Wing, 2007). Induction increases the risk of a cesarean section. If the fetal presenting part is floating at the onset of the induction, this also increases the risk of a cesarean section.

DIPPING OR FLOATING AT 7 CENTIMETERS

If the fetal head is not engaged when a nulliparous woman is dilated 7 cm, there is a significant risk of a prolonged second stage of labor, vaginal delivery is not feasible, and a cesarean section will be needed (Debby et al., 1999). If labor is allowed to continue even though there is an unengaged fetus at 7 cm, it is probable that the fetal head and cord will be significantly compressed as labor progresses. Augmentation with oxytocin at this point may force the fetus deeper into the pelvis, which can increase the risk of fetal oxygen deprivation as the umbilical cord becomes compressed. If you have a nulliparous patient whose fetus is unengaged when she is 7-cm dilated, inform the midwife or physician of your findings and discuss the plan of care.

Clinical example: A nulliparous laboring woman was 5 feet 1/2 inch tall and she weighed 155 pounds, a 28-

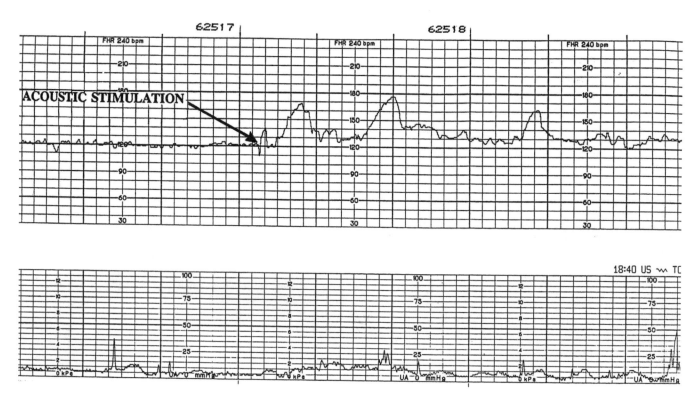

Figure 6.6: An acceleration rules out fetal metabolic acidosis at that time. Paper speed is 3 cm/minute. Note the three accelerations after a 3-second acoustic simulation with a device that emitted 110 dB of sound.

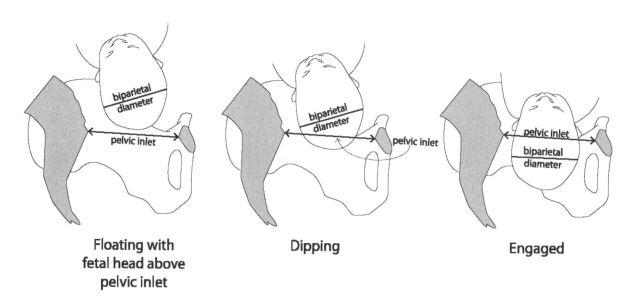

Floating with fetal head above pelvic inlet

Dipping

Engaged

Figure 6.7: Floating, dipping, and engaged fetal head.

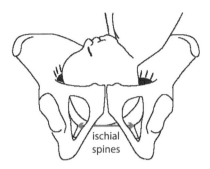

Engaged at
zero station

Figure 6.8: The fetus is engaged when the tip of the skull bone is at the level of the ischial spines.

pound weight gain. The estimated fetal weight was 3,500 grams. At 0700, her cervix was a fingertip dilated, thick, and with a station estimated to be –2. The tip of the skull was not palpated. She was contracting regularly and by 1015 she was 5 cm/100%/–2. By 1200, she had an anterior lip and the station was –1. At 1230, she was 10 cm and the station was –1.

Question: Does she have an increased risk of a cesarean section? Answer: Yes.

VARIABLE DECELERATIONS

If the fetus of a nulliparous woman is not engaged at 7-cm dilatation, you should closely monitor the fetal heart rate and fetal descent. If the baby descends, cord compression is likely. Head compression and cord compression will produce variable decelerations with pushing during contractions (see Figures 6.9 and 6.10).

FETAL HEART RATE DECELERATES AND MATERNAL HEART RATE ACCELERATES DURING PUSHING

Analyze the tracing carefully. Maternal accelerations occur during pushing and contractions while the external ultrasound transducer is over the maternal aorta and the monitor is re-

cording the maternal heart rate (see Figures 6.11 and 6.12). If this occurs, you must differentiate the maternal from the fetal heart rate and reposition the ultrasound over the fetal heart.

To differentiate the maternal heart rate pattern from the fetal heart rate pattern, you need to simultaneously record both the maternal heart rate and the fetal heart rate and compare the two images. To obtain a continuous printout of the maternal heart rate, rest the second ultrasound transducer over her heart or apply the two-lead or three-lead maternal ECG device for the fetal monitor, or place a pulse oximeter for the fetal monitor on her finger or ear lobe. Locate the equipment available at your hospital for simultaneously recording the maternal heart rate with the fetal heart rate. Comparing the two images, rather than just taking the maternal pulse, should help you distinguish between the two.

The sound from the fetal monitor should not be used to confirm that the mother, instead of the fetus, is being recorded. It is a misconception that sounds from the electronic fetal monitor when the mother is recorded are different from those obtained when the fetus is recorded. Sounds you hear are not from the fetus or the mother. They are produced when the computer in the fetal monitor analyzes the ultrasound or spiral electrode input and converts the calculated rate into a sound.

There is no audible difference in decibels (loudness) when the signal source is maternal or fetal. The difference you might hear would be the rate. When a woman is in labor without a fever, she usually has a slower heart rate than the fetus. When she is pushing and in significant pain during labor, particularly during the second stage, it is common for her to have tachycardia and to accelerate during contractions. Her heart rate and the fetal heart rate during the second stage may be at a similar level. The difference is in the image they produce. During the second stage, fetuses may decelerate during contractions but women accelerate during contractions. That is why it is important to watch the changes in the recorded heart rate pattern between and during contractions. If you remove the tocotransducer, you must palpate contractions and watch the change in the heart rate tracing. If the fetal monitor paper is saved (in addition to the computer disk), mark the paper with a vertical line at the beginning and end of contractions or use the mark button when the contraction begins and ends. Evaluate your marks and the changes in the heart rate pattern. Does the rate increase or decrease with contractions?

Exhibit 6.1: Outcomes of nulliparous women with a high fetal station.			
Station	Cesarean Sections (%)	Protracted Active Phase Arrest of Dilation	Birthweight > 4,000 gm
–4	*77%		
–3	27%, *43%	40%	13.3%
–2/–1	6.8%, *20% if –2, 6% if –1	15%	4.5%
0	6.9%	17%	3.4%
Note: Based on Murphy, Shah, and Cohen (1998) at term, with spontaneous labor and *Shin, Brubaker, and Ackerson (2004) at 41 or more weeks of gestation, during induction.			

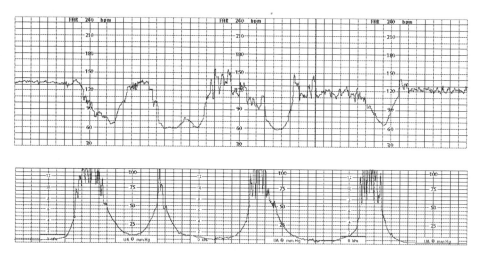

Figure 6.9: Variable decelerations during the second stage of labor. Paper speed is 3 cm/minute.

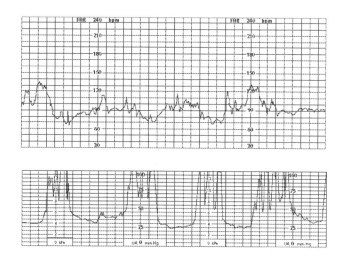

Figure 6.10: Variable decelerations with a falling baseline during the second stage of labor. Paper speed is 3 cm/minute. Note the fetal heart rate decelerates during pushing. There are too many contractions with inadequate rest between them.

The second stage of labor is a time of increased fetal vulnerability. The fetal heart rate is your means of assessing fetal oxygenation (see Figure 6.13). If you cannot determine the fetal status due to the lack of a fetal heart rate or fetal heart rate pattern, act quickly to obtain this information. Discuss the application of a spiral electrode with the obstetric care provider, or ask a skilled nurse to apply the electrode. In some hospitals, nurses do not apply spiral electrodes. In that case, ask your charge nurse or supervisor to help you locate a midwife or physician who can apply the electrode. You should never leave the patient while she is in the second stage of labor.

FETAL EXTRUSION: AN UNPLANNED EXIT

If a fetus cannot leave the uterus through the usual path, it might push through the lower uterine segment and create another exit, a uterine rupture. The most common risk factor for uterine rupture, however, is previous uterine surgery (Walsh & Baxi, 2007). Abnormal labor also increases the risk of uterine rupture (Bujold, Bujold, & Gauthier, 2001). Several studies and case reports document a relationship between the use of oxytocin and uterine rupture in women who have never had a cesarean section as well as in women with a history of a cesarean section (Catanzarite, Cousins, Dowling, & Daneshmand, 2006; McDonagh, Osterweil, & Guise, 2005; Mishra, Morris, & Uprety, 2006; Walsh & Baxi, 2007; Zelop et al., 1999).

A fetal weight of 4,000 or more grams does not appear to increase the chance of uterine rupture, but the technique used to close the uterus at the time of the prior cesarean section is related to the risk of subsequent uterine rupture during labor or delivery (Landon et al., 2006). If the surgeon who performed the prior cesarean used a one-layer closure rather than a two-layer closure of the uterus, there was a significant risk of uterine rupture (Gyamfi, Juhasz, Gyamfi, Blumenfeld, & Stone, 2006). Only 0.6% of women with two-layer closures had subsequent uterine ruptures, but 3.3% with one-layer closures suffered uterine ruptures (Bujold, Bujold, & Gauthier, 2001). Other factors related to uterine rupture, even in an unscarred uterus, include fibroid removal or uterine surgery, trauma, placenta increta, a uterine anomaly, a thin lower segment or weak uterus due to multiparity, and oxytocin use (Wang & Su, 2006). If the patient has an anomalous uterus, or if she has had a prior dilatation and curettage (D & C) and an instrument punctured the uterine wall, she also will have an increased risk of uterine rupture at that site (Wang & Su, 2006).

The time lapse between the cesarean section and the subsequent trial of labor is related to the risk of uterine rupture. If it has been less than 2 years since the patient's last cesarean and

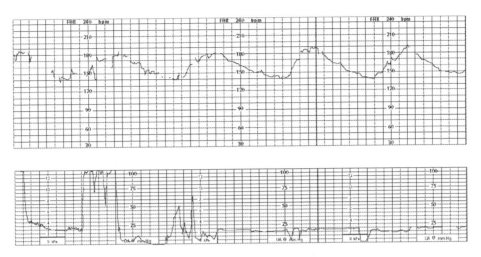

Figure 6.11: Maternal accelerations during the second stage of labor. Paper speed is 3 cm/minute. The tocotransducer stopped recording well. Note the large accelerations with a maternal tachycardic baseline near 140 bpm.

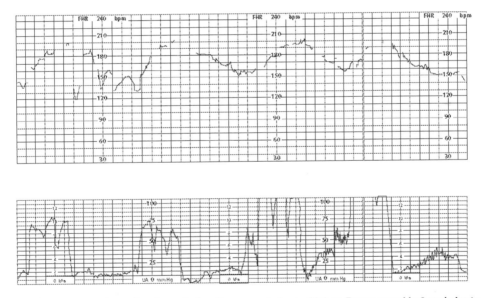

Figure 6.12: Maternal accelerations during the second stage of labor. Paper speed is 3 cm/minute. Note her baseline is tachycardic in the 140s and 150s. Also note her accelerations last for the duration of the contraction or longer.

the current birth, she has an increased risk of uterine rupture (Landon et al., 2006). If she has had a cesarean section but has never had a vaginal delivery, she has an increased risk of uterine rupture. A history of cesarean section and vaginal delivery, however, do not prevent uterine rupture if there is an abnormal labor (Bujold, Bujold, Hamilton, Harel, & Gauthier, 2002).

Labor and delivery nurses must know when their patient had a cesarean section or sections, when she delivered vagi-

nally, and the type of incision and repair that was performed on the uterus. An external abdominal scar from a prior cesarean section does not mean that the uterine incision and the scar are in the same location. For example, she may have a midline scar on her abdomen but a low transverse scar in her uterus. A vertical or midline (classical) uterine incision is a contraindication for labor (Landon et al., 2006).

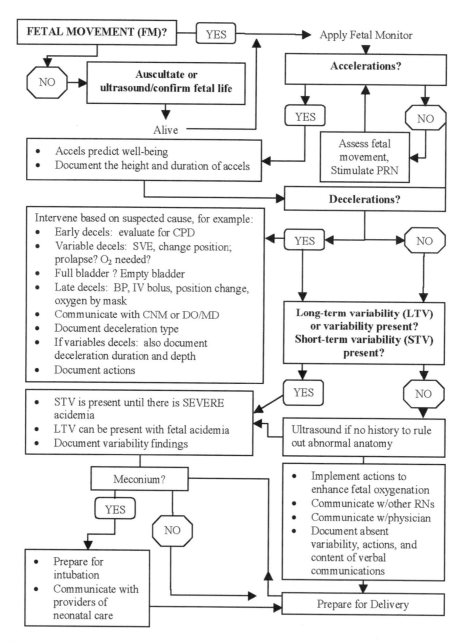

Figure 6.13: Interpretation of FHR patterns, decisions, and actions.

PROSTAGLANDINS AND OXYTOCIN INCREASE THE RISK OF UTERINE RUPTURE

Prostaglandin use is correlated with rupture of a scarred uterus. Uterine rupture occurred in 25 of 1,000 women who received prostaglandins after a previous cesarean section. Rupture occurred in only 8 of 1,000 women who were induced without prostaglandins and in 5 of 1,000 women who were attempting to have a vaginal birth after cesarean (VBAC) but were in spontaneous labor (American College of Obstetricians and Gynecologists, 2002). If prostaglandins are not used to soften an unripe, hard, closed cervix, a significant barrier exists between the fetus and the exit.

Induction and augmentation with oxytocin also increase the risk of uterine rupture (Bujold, Bujold, Hamilton, Harel, & Gauthier, 2002; McDonagh, Osterweil, & Guise, 2005). Rupture of an unscarred uterus occurred in a primigravid woman who was in labor and receiving oxytocin. Her fetus was at $40^1/2$ weeks of gestation, and she was in the second stage of labor when her uterus ruptured. She had four to five contractions every 10 minutes at that time (Catanzarite, Cousins, Dowling, & Daneshmand, 2006). A multigravid woman had a spontaneous uterine rupture after induction with misoprostol and oxytocin (Mazzone & Woolever, 2006). It is clear that the use of oxytocic drugs and fundal pressure during a prolonged second stage of labor increases the risk of uterine rupture (Mishra, Morris, & Uprety, 2006).

Documentation example after prostaglandin E₂ vaginal insert 25 minutes previously: Patient complains of heartburn and shortness of breath. Reports somewhat painful contractions now. Pulse oximeter applied. SpO_2 100% on room air. Physician notified of patient complaints and SpO_2.

Documentation example: Received patient from triage. Patient oriented to room and plan of care for a trial of labor after cesarean discussed by physician. Verbal informed consent given for the oxytocin induction. Patient verbalizes understanding of the plan of care. Husband at bedside. Patient reports irregular contractions at this time. Fetal monitor applied. Abdomen palpates soft between contractions, with mild contractions every 6 to 10 minutes for 50 to 80 seconds. IV started in right hand with 18-gauge catheter and lactated Ringer's solution at 125 mL/hour.

FETAL HEART RATE PATTERNS RELATED TO UTERINE RUPTURE

If your patient has had a previous cesarean section, you must watch for signs of an impending uterine rupture. The fetus will often let you know there is a problem less than 2 hours before the actual uterine rupture. It was found that the fetus had variable decelerations prior to the diagnosis of uterine rupture. After the uterus ruptures and the fetus extrudes (leaves the uterus), the fetus will have bradycardia (see Figure 6.14).

PERSISTENT PAIN IS A SIGN OF UTERINE RUPTURE

The woman whose uterus is rupturing may have persistent abdominal pain with or without abnormally frequent contractions (Pryor et al., 2007).

Epidural anesthesia is related to uterine rupture, but this is not a cause-and-effect relationship (Landon et al., 2006). Instead, the epidural masks the pain associated with the rupture. Women who have received an epidural may have different complaints when their uterus is rupturing. They will complain of jaw, neck, upper-back, or shoulder pain because the pain is referred to a higher level.

Clinical example: The patient was multiparous, 5 feet tall, a gestational diabetic with an estimated fetal weight of 4,000 grams. She was 30 years old, weighed 190 pounds, a gain of 42 pounds, and she had a history of one prior cesarean section for cephalopelvic disproportion. She was admitted for induction at 38 weeks due to rising blood pressure and "impending macrosomia." Her cervix was closed and thick. She had a birth plan that included an epidural at 4-cm dilataton. In addition, her last delivery was 23 months ago.

Her physician has ordered you to follow a protocol for low-dose oxytocin. Is initiating the oxytocin infusion appropriate with this constellation of facts? Yes, as long as you are totally aware of her risk factors for uterine rupture. Report any abnormalities of labor, pain, uterine activity, and the fetal heart rate. Have an operating room, operating room crew, neonatal team, and surgeon immediately available. Your role is to recognize, vocalize, and mobilize. You also have a right to hold the oxytocin until a clear plan of care is developed, you have confirmed that the patient has received information about the risks and benefits of the induction procedure, and she has given verbal consent or has signed a written consent for the induction.

RECOGNIZE, VOCALIZE, MOBILIZE

Women who are attempting a VBAC may vomit with such force that a uterine rupture occurs. The cause of uterine rupture after a woman vomits is not clear. The increase in intraabdominal pressure during vomiting may be related to the uterine rupture. However, a more likely cause is the increase in uterine contractions as a result of the vomiting reflex. Vomiting precedes the release of antidiuretic hormone (vasopressin) (Shelton, Kinney, & Robertson, 1976). The surge of vasopressin causes a dramatic increase in the number, duration, or strength of contractions (Chan, Wo, & Manning, 1996). Other stimulants for vasopressin release are hypotension and hypovolemia (Baylis, 1989).

After your patient has vomited, you should immediately assess the fetal heart rate pattern, uterine activity, blood pressure, pulse, and the presence of any vaginal bleeding or clots. Obviously, if you feel a fetal body part under her skin, there may be a uterine rupture. Communicate abnormal findings to the obstetric provider without delay. You should always know where the surgeon is when you have a patient in labor who is attempting a vaginal birth after cesarean (VBAC).

There may be very little or no bleeding when the uterus ruptures, or there may be active bleeding if there is a uterine rupture and a concurrent placental abruption. Pull the emergency cord, call for help, and communicate your need to call the obstetrician or surgeon. The charge nurse or supervisor should be informed so that the operating crew can be mobilized for the emergency cesarean section.

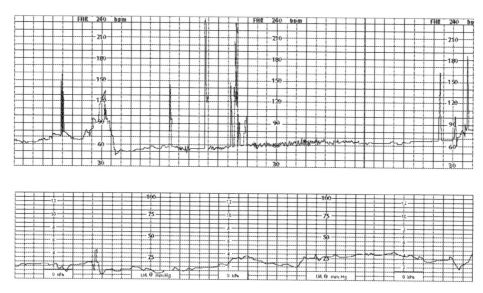

Figure 6.14: Fetal heart rate pattern and uterine activity due to uterine rupture. Paper speed is 3 cm/minute. The fetus was outside the uterus (extruded) and was born asphyxiated. When the uterus ruptures there may still be evidence of some contractions when the tocotransducer is used, but they will decrease in size and strength.

If the patient's uterus did not rupture, she may have dilated because vomiting seems to occur when women are dilated 7 to 8 cm or more. After you find that she is stable and the fetal heart rate pattern is not abnormal, reassure her that everything is progressing normally while you help her to change her soiled garments, bed linen, or linen protector, and clean the furniture or floor. Assess the cervix and fetal station if you suspect she is close to delivery. Document your findings and the emesis on the intake and output record.

MORE THAN ONE PASSENGER: MULTIPLE GESTATION

As an intrapartal nurse, you will see many women who have a multiple gestation. A multiple gestation is defined as two or more fetuses in the uterus. A multiple gestation may also be called a multiple pregnancy. It is more likely that you will have a patient who has twins than a patient who has triplets, quadruplets, or even more fetuses. If you have access to the prenatal record and the ultrasound reports, confirm the number of fetuses and placentas (see Exhibit 6.2).

ARE THEY ROOMMATES OR DO THEY HAVE PRIVATE ROOMS?

Now that you have read the ultrasound excerpt on Twin B, how many placentas were reported? In this case, there was only one and it was anterior in location. Therefore, there are monozygotic twins. There was also a dividing membrane (see Figure 6.15), which means that the fetuses are in their own amnions or sacs, and there is one chorion. The two amniotic sacs are divided by a layer of amniotic tissue. Usually when

> **Exhibit 6.2: Partial ultrasound report for Twin B.**
>
> - Type of gestation: Twin
> - Intrauterine pregnancy in vertex presentation
> - Fetal motion and organs seen
> - Fetal heart motion seen
> - Four-chamber fetal heart observed
> - Normal intracranial anatomy seen
> - Fetal body and limb movements observed
> - Fetal stomach observed
> - Fetal kidneys observed
> - Fetal bladder observed
> - Fetal spine observed
> - Fetal abnormalities observed: None seen at this time
> - Placenta location: Anterior
> - No evidence of placenta previa
> - Amniotic fluid within normal limits
> - Dividing membrane is seen

there is one placenta, the twins are identical in gender and genetics. There can also be both a male and female fetus when there is one placenta (due to the presence of a chimera), but it is rare. A chimeric fetus is the result of two or more genetically distinct cells that originated in different zygotes, then emerged in the same zygote. Chimera is also known as mosaicism.

If there are two placentas and separate amnions, the ultrasound report should include the location of both placentas. There will be no dividing membrane (see Figure 6.16), and each fetus would be enclosed in its own amniotic sac.

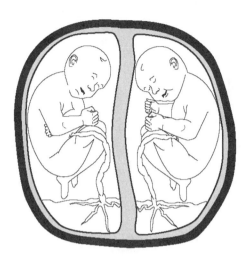

Figure 6.15: Monochorionic twins (one placenta) with a dividing membrane and two amniotic sacs.

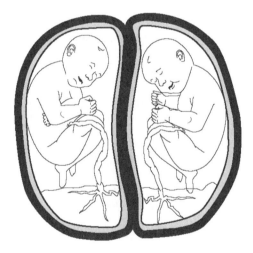

Figure 6.16: Dichorionic twins (two placentas). Each placenta has its own chorion and amnion.

DISCORDANT TWINS

Discordant growth means there is a significant difference (15% or more) in the estimated fetal weight of the twins. Discordant growth is suspected after an ultrasound examination of the twins and is confirmed after they are weighed in the nursery.

The placenta delivers nutrients to the umbilical vein (Pardi & Cetin, 2006). A problem with nutrient delivery may cause one or both twins to significantly differ in weight and size. Discordant growth increases the risk of an adverse outcome. Discordant twins may have discordant growth because there is one placenta (monochorionic) with vessel anastamoses that connect the circulation of both twins. This causes a twin-

to-twin transfer or transfusion of blood. The recipient twin will have polycythemia and polyhydramnios. The donor twin will have anemia and oligohydramnios. Both twins have an increased risk of death. When there is a monochorionic diamnionic pregnancy, fetoscopic laser coagulation may be done to disrupt these vessel connections.

The mother of discordant twins may be admitted for bed rest and intravenous hydration, and she may be scheduled for induction. You should listen to the mother. Ask her how she feels. One woman whose twin babies had discordant growth and oligohydramnios at 35 weeks of gestation said, "It felt to me as if the twins were rubbing bones against one another and it was sending a chill through my body." She also said, "I felt there was something wrong."

INTRAUTERINE GROWTH RESTRICTION

One or both twins may even be subject to intrauterine growth restriction (IUGR) and may have an estimated fetal weight below the 10th percentile for that gestational age. If the fetus is preterm, physicians may order bed rest in the hospital, with or without maternal hyperoxygenation (Battaglia et al., 1992, 1994; Bilardo, Snijders, Campbell, & Nicolaides, 1991; Visintine et al., 2006). In addition, Say, Gülmezoglu and Hofmeyr (2002) found that women who have an IUGR fetus and receive humidified oxygen via a tight-fitting face mask (long-term hyperoxygenation) have heavier babies at a higher gestational age than the babies of women who did not receive long-term oxygen therapy.

MONITORING TWINS

The best available tool for evaluation of fetal well-being is the electronic fetal heart rate monitor. Fetal monitoring of twins is a challenge. Fetal monitoring of three or more fetuses is very difficult. There are no clear standards of care related to monitoring three or more fetuses because usually two or more monitors will be needed and it may be impossible to confirm that all fetuses are being monitored. You just have to do the best you can if the physician or midwife wants you to monitor more than two fetuses. You should assess your equipment. Are there two ports for the ultrasound transducers? If so, the fetal monitor should be capable of monitoring twins. An ultrasound evaluation by the physician is usually the primary method of fetal surveillance in triplet or higher-order pregnancies (Eganhouse & Petersen, 1997).

Before you try to find the fetal heart rate, palpate the abdomen to locate the fetuses. You should also ask the mother where her twins were heard the last time they were assessed. If you can locate a twin's back, place the fetoscope, hand-held Doppler, or ultrasound transducer in that location and listen for the heart sounds (fetoscope) or heart rate. Differentiate the fetal heart rate from the maternal heart rate. Otherwise, listen to the mother and place your transducers over the location she reports her twins were last heard.

When you are monitoring twins, there should be two distinct fetal heart rate patterns and a separate tracing of the

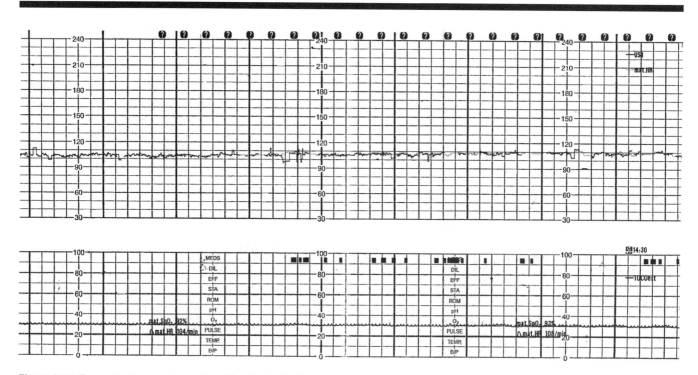

Figure 6.17: Example of cross-channel verification (coincidence detection) by the Philips fetal monitor. The maternal heart rate is being monitored with the ultrasound transducer and the pulse oximeter.

maternal heart rate (if you apply a device that will continuously print her heart rate). Different monitors have the ability to indicate that only one person is being monitored with two devices (see Figure 6.17). They also have a feature that allows you to distinguish the twins (see Figure 6.18).

Note the question marks printed at the top of the fetal heart rate channel. These question marks indicate that two devices are recording the same patient (the mother in this case). Devices that simultaneously recorded the maternal heart rate are the pulse oximeter for the fetal monitor and the ultrasound transducer. The question marks do not appear on the computer screen. Therefore, it is critical that you evaluate the paper printout, especially when you are monitoring twins or triplets. Remote monitoring, that is, at the nurses' station, may use different colors for each ultrasound transducer. The colors, however, do not confirm that there are two different fetal heart rates being recorded. You will need to see two distinct fetal heart rate patterns to be sure you are recording two fetuses (see Figure 6.18).

Discordant twins and IUGR fetuses are at risk for hypoxia (decreased oxygen delivery to their tissues) and metabolic acidosis (a low pH and a high level of lactic acid in their blood) (Pardi & Cetin, 2006). Expect a well-oxygenated fetus to have baseline (long-term) variability and accelerations (see Figure 6.18). If the baseline lacks variability and is fixed or flat (a silent pattern) without accelerations or decelerations, the fetus may be brain dead (Yogev, Ben-Haroush, Chen, & Kaplan,

2002). The neonate will be born hypotonic and unresponsive (Pardi & Cetin, 2006). Notify the physician if you see a silent pattern, even after only 10 minutes of monitoring. Assess maternal vital signs and fetal movement. Ask the mother when she last felt her baby or babies move and document your assessments and communications. Palpate for fetal movement and initiate intrauterine resuscitation measures as you await the physician's presence at the bedside.

Documentation example (with quadrants): Twin A on maternal left lower quadrant with FHR 140–150, LTV average with 15 × 15 acceleration. Twin B on maternal right upper quadrant with FHR 150 with absent variability, no accelerations, no decelerations. Mother to left side with tight-fitting face mask and oxygen at 10 L/minute. IV started in right hand. Lactated Ringers solution at 125 mL/hour. Dr. Nateperi paged.

Documentation example: Twin A baseline 144 to 150 bpm with accelerations to 160 bpm for 15 to 20 seconds. Variability moderate. Twin B baseline 140 to 145 bpm. Minimal variability with no accelerations and variable deceleration for 20 to 30 seconds down to 120 to 130 bpm. Dr. Duo called and asked to come to bedside to review tracing. Dr. Duo said she is on her way.

It may be helpful to periodically write "Twin A" and "Twin B" on the fetal monitor strip next to their corresponding fetal

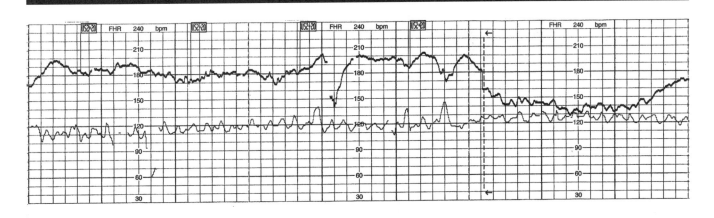

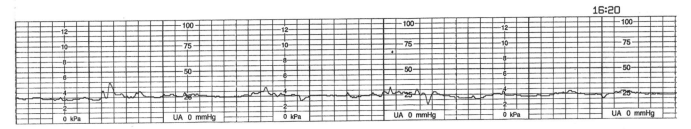

Figure 6.18: The twin offset or trace separation feature enables you to manipulate the fetal monitor and separate the twin tracings. In this case, the fetal monitor added 20 beats per minute to the tracing of the fetus being monitored with the ultrasound in port 1 (on the left side of the fetal monitor). It is impossible to offset the other twin's tracing. Learn how to enable this feature by reading the manufacturer's user guide.

heart rate pattern (unless your hospital protocol discourages this procedure). Some nurses mark the maternal abdomen with a small pen mark corresponding to the area where they could best monitor that twin. Thus when the monitors are removed, they can quickly find that location again. Some nurses will leave the tocotransducer and ultrasound transducers in place when they move the patient to the delivery room. That way the nurse is able to resume monitoring by reconnecting the cables into the fetal monitor. You must make sure you can differentiate the fetal heart rates from the maternal pulse. If there is no fetal monitor in the operating or delivery room, ask the charge nurse or another nurse to help you obtain a fetal monitor.

DELIVERY OF TWINS OR MULTIPLE FETUSES

Any time that twins or multiple fetuses will be delivered, it is best to deliver them in the operating room with a double set-up (ready for a cesarean section) and with a neonatal resuscitation team ready to receive the babies. Vaginal delivery of dichorionic twins is common when both twins are vertex, or the first twin is vertex and the second twin is breech. If the first twin is vertex and the second twin is in a transverse or oblique lie, the obstetrician will try to deliver the second twin vaginally after the first twin is delivered.

The second twin will be at a high station, and after the artificial rupture of the membranes, the umbilical cord may prolapse. If this occurs, an immediate cesarean section will have to be performed. If the two placentas are fused, the separation of the first twin's placenta may cause premature separation of the second twin's placenta, resulting in an abruption and the need for an immediate cesarean section.

DELIVERY OF MONOCHORIONIC TWINS

Monochorionic twins have higher morbidity and mortality than dichorionic twins (Lopriore et al., 2008). Monochorionic, monoamnionic twins are usually delivered by cesarean section.

Problems may arise if monochorionic, diamnionic twins are delivered vaginally. The first twin must be vertex. After delivery of the first twin, the placenta must remain intact for the second twin to receive adequate oxygenation. Even with an intact placenta, acute intrapartum fetoplacental transfusion may occur, and the second twin will rapidly deteriorate and be born severely hypovolemic and anemic (Uotila & Tammela, 1999). In addition, if the placenta they shared separates prematurely from the uterine wall, maternal and fetal blood loss may occur, thus resulting in the birth of a compromised second twin and maternal anemia.

You must continue monitoring the twins in the operating room prior to their birth. Be sure that both fetuses are recorded and that the remaining twin is recorded after delivery of the first twin. Be careful not to monitor the mother's heart rate after the birth of the first twin. You can place the first twin's ultrasound transducer on the maternal chest over her heart where it will detect and record a continuous tracing of her pulse. Compare that tracing with the tracing of the remaining twin. They should be different. If the patterns are not different, move the ultrasound until you find the second twin. Sometimes, a physician will use the ultrasound machine to locate the second twin's heart and observe the heart beating until that twin is delivered.

At delivery, the first baby born is identified as Baby A or Baby 1, and the second baby born is identified as Baby B or Baby 2. Consult your hospital's policy for identification of the newborn for guidance. If your hospital uses letters to identify the babies, what once was Fetus A may become Newborn B. This can be particularly confusing, especially when the fetuses were labeled "A" and "B" during all of the antepartal fetal monitoring tests during the pregnancy or during a prolonged hospitalization and labor. Some hospitals have colored identification bands for multiple fetuses, and the color corresponds to the order in which the fetus was delivered.

When multiple babies are born close together in a short amount of time, it is also helpful to have many attendants to assist with the care of the newborns and the correct identification of each newborn. You may also want to identify the placentas or cord segments with a plastic clamp that is marked with different-colored markers. A legend posted on the wall and the availability of colored markers will help you in this process. You will need to place a colored mark on the clamps and prepare the wrist and ankle bands ahead of time to avoid errors.

To receive the twins, you will need separate oxygen and suction equipment for resuscitation. Sometimes the babies are placed in one warmer, but it is best to have one warmer for each baby.

Frequently, the provider will want the twin placenta(s) to be sent to the pathology department. Your responsibility will be to collect the placenta(s), identify one of the cords (use a cord clamp) to indicate Twin A (Baby 1 or 2 depending on the birth order) or Twin B (Baby 1 or 2 depending on the birth order). Place the specimen in a container such as a plastic bucket with a lid. Complete a pathology request or requisition. Usually the request is for gross and microscopic examinations. Send the labeled specimen to the laboratory with the pathology request.

If you need to culture the placenta, swab the placenta prior to adding the fixative (formaldehyde). To collect the culture, separate the chorion from the amnion with your gloved hand and swab the interior lining with the sterile swab. Label the sample source as "fetal membranes" unless your only option using your computer program is "placenta." In some instances you may be requested to take a photograph of the placenta and/or cord, using a camera supplied by your hospital.

An aqueous solution of formaldehyde is referred to as "formalin." Formalin contains formaldehyde and water with a

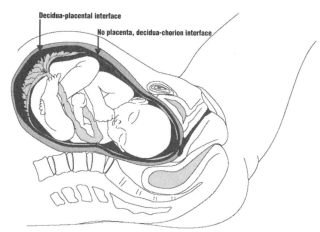

Figure 6.19: During pregnancy the decidua replaces the endometrial lining. The decidua is the maternal tissue between the uterus and the placenta. In the area without a placenta, the chorion-amnion lies adjacent to the decidua.

stabilizer, usually methanol. Formaldehyde is produced when methane is oxidized and it is found in automobile exhaust and tobacco smoke. It is therefore part of smog. Exposure to formalin can be harmful. It has been related to lung and nasopharyngeal cancer (Formaldehyde (CASRN 50-00-0, 2008). Therefore, if formalin is used as a tissue preservative, you should wear protective clothing, avoid breathing any fumes (wear a mask), and pour it over the placenta under a ventilation hood. In some hospitals in the United States, formalin is no longer found in the clinical setting because of the lack of a ventilation hood or other facilities to meet the Occupational Safety and Health Administration (OSHA) requirements.

THE PLACENTA AND PLACENTAL PATHOLOGY

The placenta and cord are formed in the fifth week of gestation. The placenta is a fetal organ that connects the fetus with the mother. The placenta is usually found next to the maternal decidua. Uterine arteries bring blood and oxygen to the uterus (see Figures 6.19 and 6.20). The level of oxygen in the umbilical vein (PO_2) is similar to, but lower than, the level of oxygen (PO_2) in the uterine veins (Pardi & Cetin, 2006).

CHORANGIOSIS

A condition related to fetal hypoxia is chorangiosis. Chorangiosis is diagnosed by the pathologist when there are 10 or more vessels in 10 or more areas of 3 or more random, noninfarcted placental samples, viewed using a 10× magnification. Normally there are no more than five fetal capillaries in each villus. The cause of chorangiosis may be related to diseases such as maternal diabetes or preeclampsia, drug use, or a urinary tract infection. Chorangiosis is also associated with

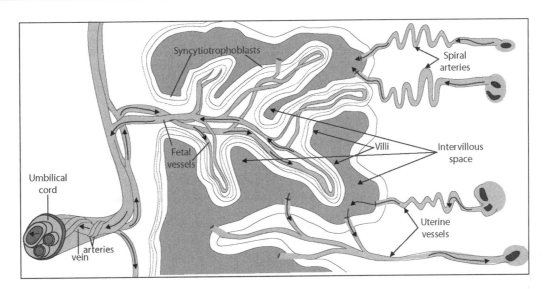

Figure 6.20: The placenta receives nutrients from the decidua as maternal spiral arteries bring blood and oxygen to the intervillous space. Oxygen passively diffuses through the syncytiotrophoblast cells into the fetal capillaries, where it is then transported to the fetus through the umbilical vein.

umbilical cord abnormalities such as one artery, abruption, placenta previa, chorangioma, amnion nodosum, and villitis (inflammation of the villi) from infections such as rubella, cytomegalovirus, and syphilis. Chorangiosis has been associated with congenital anomalies and low Apgar scores (De la Ossa, Cabello-Inchausti, & Robinson, 2001).

PLACENTAL PATHOLOGY

The placenta is the "historian" of the pregnancy and often holds clues that explain an unfavorable outcome of the pregnancy. It can reveal important information such as an abnormal number of fetal capillaries or changes in the villi suggestive of chronic hypoxia. Some hospitals have a protocol that indicates whether a placenta should be sent to pathology. The midwife or physician may also order an examination of the placenta (see Exhibit 6.3. and Figure 6.21).

The pathologist removes the membranes and cord prior to weighing the placenta. At term, the ratio between fetal and placental weight is around 6:1. A normal placenta weighs about 150 grams at 20 weeks of gestation, 375 grams at 30 weeks, and 400 to 600 grams at term. Assume the fetus weighed 3,500 grams at term, 3,500 divided by 600 is 5.8. That would be a normal fetal–placental ratio. A very large placenta (placentomegaly) is often found when the mother has diabetes or the baby has Beckwith-Wiedemann syndrome (Lage, 1994). A very small placenta may be found with chromosomally abnormal fetuses such as those exhibiting trisomy 21, or fetuses that are small for gestational age (SGA) (Pardi & Cetin, 2006).

Clinical example: At 32 weeks, a primigravid woman presented with preterm, premature rupture of the mem-

> **Exhibit 6.3: What to do when you send the placenta to the pathology department.**
>
> - Send a copy of the placental examination form.
> - Request both gross and microscopic examinations.
> - If available, send a copy of the delivery record or the labor/delivery summary.
> - Provide the neonatologist's or pediatrician's name.
> - Provide a reason for the submission.
> - Inform the pathologist of any other issues they should address.

branes. She is 5 feet 3 inches tall and weighs 142 pounds with a 20-pound weight gain. The amniotic fluid was clear. She was contracting every 5 to 10 minutes and was 4-centimeters dilated, 50% effaced, with a –1 station. Antibiotics and betamethasone were administered. Due to fetal tachycardia, delivery was by cesarean section. The Apgar scores were 9 and 9 at 1 and 5 minutes. The placental pathology revealed acute chorioamnionitis, syncytial knot hyperplasia, and chorangiosis. In this example, there were good Apgar scores but evidence of placental pathology.

CHORIOAMNIONITIS

Chorioamnionitis is an infection of the amnion and chorion. Chorioamnionitis is associated with fetal and maternal tachycardia and an elevation of the maternal temperature, including fever. Chorioamnionitis should be suspected when your pa-

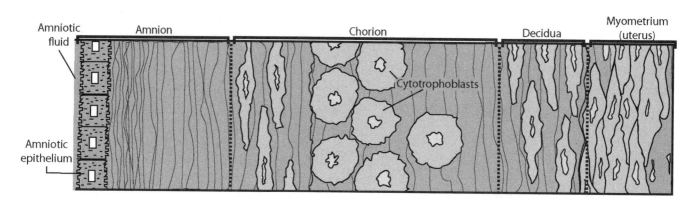

Figure 6.21: From right to left, note the different layers of tissue in the decidua-chorion interface. This image does not include the placenta, which lies between the chorion and the decidua. Fetal tissues are the amnion, chorion, and placenta. Maternal tissues are the decidua and the uterus.

tient has a fever of 100.4° F or 38° C, a heart rate of 120 bpm or higher, a fetal heart rate of 160 bpm or higher, or all three (Curtin, Florescue, Metlay, & Katzman, 2007).

SYNCYTIAL KNOTS

Syncytial knots are a localized accumulation of syncytiotrophoblast nuclei, which appear under the microscope as a clump of cells. Hypoxia causes syncytial knot hyperplasia. For example, maternal cigarette smoking is related to fetal and placental hypoxia and syncytial knots.

PLACENTA PREVIA

Placenta previa occurs when placental tissue is implanted over the internal cervical os. Factors associated with placenta previa include scarring of the uterus because of more than one pregnancy, the birth of multiple fetuses, a previous cesarean birth, a myomectomy (fibroid removal), or vigorous curettage.

There are three types of placenta previa: partial, marginal, or complete. A partial placenta previa occurs when only a portion of the internal os is covered with placental tissue. When only an edge of the placenta extends to the cervical os, it is called a marginal placenta previa. If the cervical os is completely covered by placental tissue, it is termed a complete previa (Lowdermilk, Perry, & Bobak, 2000).

You should read the prenatal ultrasound reports to find the location of the placenta. Ultrasound reports may also include an estimated fetal weight. Three-dimensional ultrasounds are more effective than two-dimensional ultrasounds in determining fetal weight at term, cervical length, and the likelihood of subsequent preterm delivery when there is an unusually short cervix or funneling of the cervix (Wiseman & Kiehl, 2007).

If your patient presents with vaginal bleeding, do not perform an examination of the cervix, especially if there is a known placenta previa. You do not want to puncture the placenta! Sometimes as the uterus grows in size, the placenta

that was over the cervical os is pulled up and away from the os. At the time of delivery, there may be no placenta previa, but there will likely be a low-lying placenta.

The site of the placenta, especially if it was low in the uterus, may bleed extensively after delivery. A tamponade balloon may be inserted into the uterus by the midwife or physician after delivery of the placenta in order to apply direct pressure on the internal wall of the uterus to stop the bleeding. The tamponade device and its use is discussed in chapter 3.

PLACENTA ACCRETA, INCRETA, AND PERCRETA

Placenta accreta is a partial or superficial invasion of the uterine wall by the placental trophoblast. Placenta increta is a deeper invasion of the uterine wall. Placenta percreta is perforation of the uterus by placental tissue (see Figure 6.22) (Lowdermilk, Perry, & Bobak, 2000). When there is an abnormal placental attachment, the placenta will not readily separate from the uterus after the baby is delivered. Consequently, the retained placental tissue will prevent the uterus from contracting to stop the bleeding from maternal blood vessels. Clots may form and hemorrhage may occur, creating a medical emergency. You must activate the emergency call light and expect to move the patient to the operating room. She may require a hysterectomy and blood transfusions.

PLACENTA INCRETA AND PERCRETA: FOLLOW-UP AND DELIVERY

Sophisticated ultrasound technology may reveal placentation (abnormal placental tissue invasion) before delivery. Suspected increta or percreta can be confirmed by magnetic resonance imaging (MRI) and, if present, a cesarean section will be planned. Because there is a high risk of hemorrhage, the possibility of preserving the uterus and avoiding a hysterectomy is increased if an interventional radiologist is available to insert catheters into the uterine arteries prior to the planned

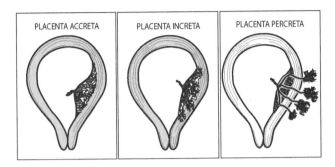

Figure 6.22: Abnormal placental implantation.

cesarean section. Cellulose pellets can be injected into these catheters to control the bleeding by restricting blood flow to the uterus.

Once the abnormal placentation is diagnosed, follow-up MRIs are used to monitor any sloughing off of placental tissue. This placental tissue is not removed in order to prevent massive internal bleeding and organ damage. If the placenta percreta tissue invades the bladder or bowel, other surgical specialists will be standing by during the cesarean section to repair or reconstruct the affected organs.

PLACENTAL ABRUPTION

Placental abruption is the premature separation of the placenta from the uterine wall. Maternal hypertension, smoking, poor nutrition, domestic violence, trauma after a motor vehicle accident, and blunt trauma to the maternal abdomen are all associated with placental abruption.

Placental abruption decreases fetal oxygen delivery. The placenta normally brings oxygen to the fetus via the umbilical vein and removes carbon dioxide from the fetus via the umbilical arteries. When the placenta separates, less oxygen will be delivered, and carbon dioxide will be retained. As a consequence, the fetus may develop respiratory acidosis and/or metabolic acidosis.

Symptoms of a placental abruption may include cramping or contractions, abdominal pain, vaginal bleeding, uterine tenderness, and an abnormal or nonreassuring fetal heart rate. If the abruption increases in size, the fetal heart rate will worsen (see Figures 6.23, 6.24, and 6.25). You should notify the physician or midwife promptly of your findings when you suspect a placental abruption and request a bedside evaluation.

UMBILICAL CORD LENGTH

The umbilical cord should grow from an average of 32 cm at 20 weeks of gestation to an average of 60 cm at 40 weeks of gestation. The length of the umbilical cord in 35,779 neonates was related to the mother's height, her prepregnancy weight, her weight gain, her socioeconomic status, and fetal gender (Naeye, 1985).

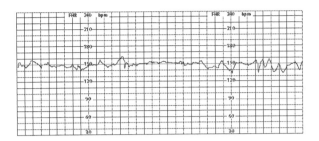

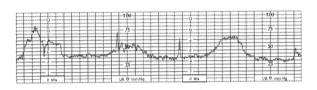

Figure 6.23: A secundigravida (second pregnancy) at 38 weeks of gestation and 1 cm/80%/–1 admitted with spontaneous rupture of the membranes and dark-red, bloody fluid. A 30 to 50% abruption was estimated at the cesarean section. Apgar scores were 2, 4, and 6 at 1, 5, and 10 minutes. Note the frequent contractions. Thrombin is a stimulus for uterine activity. Paper speed is 3 cm/minute.

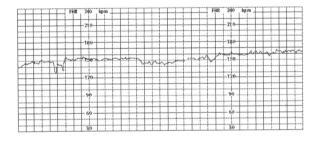

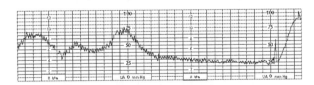

Figure 6.24: Some women who have preterm contractions or uterine irritability also have a placental abruption. The woman was a primigravida at 32 weeks of gestation with a blood pressure of 154/102, frequent contractions, and a closed cervix. Note the rising baseline (a sign of hypoxia). Paper speed is 3 cm/minute. Hypertension is associated with placental abruption. At the cesarean section, a 40% abruption was found. Apgar scores were 7 and 9 at 1 and 5 minutes.

The length of the cord is related to neonatal outcome. Short cords (≤ 40 cm at 40 weeks of gestation) were associated with neonatal hypotonia, jitters or tremulousness, abnormal crying, and an abnormal electroencephalogram. Short cords were also

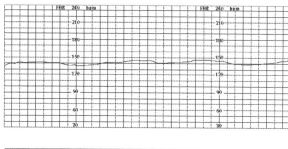

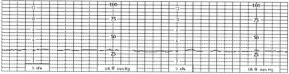

Figure 6.25: Placental abruption with recurrent late decelerations and absent variability. The baseline was near 145 bpm and rose above 150 bpm in the last minute. Paper speed is 3 cm/minute. Contractions are not well recorded at this time. The admission strip was reassuring and reactive. This is an ominous tracing because the lack of variability with late decelerations is related to metabolic acidosis and asphyxia. Delivery should be expedited.

related to low Apgar scores, low IQ values later in life, and neurologic abnormalities (Naeye, 1985).

Short cords (less than 32 cm or 12.6 inches) were associated with anomalies such as renal agenesis, pulmonary hypoplasia, placental abruption (probably when the fetus descended, the cord was pulled, which then pulled on the placenta and separated it from the uterine wall), and cord rupture (Welt, 1984).

A long cord at term is one that is greater than 70 centimeters (27.6 inches) in length (Pomeranz, 2004). Long cords are associated with fetal entanglements, true knots, and cord prolapse. Although many cases of cord prolapse cannot be anticipated prior to their occurrence, if the membranes are ruptured at a high station, there is an increased risk of a cord or limb prolapsing below the presenting part. A cord or limb prolapse may also be occult when it drops down beside the presenting part but is not felt by the person who examines the cervix.

RUPTURE OF THE MEMBRANES AND INFECTION OF THE PASSENGER
Human Immunodeficiency Virus
Human immunodeficiency virus (HIV) is not an absolute indicator for a cesarean section. In cases where there is a low HIV load, the incidence of maternal–fetal transmission is also low. If the woman has been given medication and her viral load is low, she should be given intravenous zidovudine (AZT) during labor, and the baby should be treated with AZT syrup in the nursery. If no AZT has been received during the pregnancy, there is a higher risk of maternal–fetal transmission during labor and delivery regardless of the mode of delivery.

The amnion is a bacteriostatic, not bacteriocidal, barrier. Once the membranes are ruptured, there is nothing stopping

the transmission of an ascending infection to the fetus. In the woman who is HIV positive, there is an approximately 2% increased risk of mother-to-child transmission of HIV for every hour since the membranes ruptured (Suy et al., 2007). Any increase in the mother-to-child transmission of HIV is considered too high. Artificial rupture of the membranes or application of a fetal spiral electrode, or both, should be avoided in a woman who is HIV positive, and even when the HIV status of the mother is unknown, unless the perceived benefit of the procedure outweighs the risks.

If the viral load is high, a cesarean section will be scheduled. Prior to the cesarean section, the HIV-positive woman should receive at least 2 hours of intravenous AZT. The World Health Organization recommends that HIV-positive women breastfeed their infants if the risk of starvation outweighs the risk of transmission of HIV to the infant. If there is no risk of starvation, however, breastfeeding is discouraged if the woman is HIV positive.

Herpes
Herpes can be transmitted to the fetus. If the membranes have ruptured prior to admission and there are recurrent genital herpes lesions, delivery should be expedited. If the membranes are intact, artificial rupture should be avoided as well as any invasive procedure, such as the insertion of a spiral electrode or an intrauterine catheter. The neonatal team should be advised of the recurrence of the maternal herpes lesions (*Management of Genital Herpes in Pregnancy*, 2007). Some clinicians apply a transparent dressing to cover herpes lesions in the groin area or near the introitus. There is no known research indicating that this prevents neonatal herpes transmission, but it causes no harm.

RUPTURE OF THE MEMBRANES AND PROLAPSE OF THE CORD
In addition to increasing the fetal risk of exposure to pathogens, artificial rupture of the membranes (AROM) increases the risk of an umbilical cord prolapse. Therefore, before you participate in the AROM be sure you know the HIV and herpes status of your patient and the fetal station. A high station, such as −2 or −3, increases the risk of a cord prolapse (see Figure 6.26). The practitioner who plans to rupture the membranes should explain the reason for the rupture and the patient should consent to this invasive procedure. You may be asked to push down gently on the uterine fundus with one hand while the midwife or physician ruptures the membranes. This procedure is called fundal stabilization, not fundal pressure.

Once the membranes are ruptured, the flow of amniotic fluid can move the umbilical cord down and out of the uterus. If the cord is visible after the rupture of the membranes, there is an overt or frank prolapse (Prabulos & Philipson, 1995). If the cord is not visible, but there is a dramatic change in the fetal heart rate pattern such as a prolonged deceleration or bradycardia, an occult cord prolapse should be suspected. When there is an occult cord prolapse, the umbilical cord is probably wedged between the fetal head and uterine wall (see Figure 6.27).

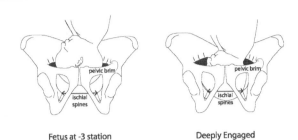

Fetus at -3 station   Deeply Engaged

Figure 6.26: When the fetal head is at a high station (dipping or floating), there is an increased risk of umbilical cord prolapse. Cord prolapse is less likely if the fetal head is deeply engaged.

In one study, the time from the diagnosis of the cord prolapse until delivery averaged 11 minutes, with a range of 5 to 15 minutes. In spite of this fairly short time interval, there were still unfavorable outcomes. Therefore, it was concluded that the time interval from diagnosis of the umbilical cord prolapse until the time of delivery may not be the only critical determinant of neonatal outcome (Prabulos & Philipson, 1995). Other factors may contribute to the amount of cord compression, such as the amount of Wharton's jelly. A thin umbilical cord is more easily compressed than a thick umbilical cord.

> **Documentation example:** Late entry for 0700: SVE 3/ 70%/-3. Amniotomy by CNM Hook. This RN responded to emergency call light. Overt cord prolapse noted. Fluid clear. FHR less than 80 bpm. Digital displacement by CNM. Bed moved to OR with continued digital displacement by CNM until patient draped. Dr. Cutnow, anesthesia provider, and NICU team called by charge nurse.

FUNIC PRESENTATION

When the umbilical cord lies in front of the fetal head, it can be felt through the membranes. Palpation of the umbilical cord through the membranes is called a funic presentation. A funic presentation can be confirmed by an ultrasound examination. If you suspect there is a funic presentation, immediately call the midwife or physician to the bedside. When there is a funic presentation, the fetus may have died prior to admission due to asphyxia from occlusion of the cord.

NUCHAL CORD

When the cord is wrapped around the baby's neck, it is usually below the nuchal notch on the back of the fetal head. This is called a nuchal cord. There may be one to eight loops of cord around the baby's neck. These loops may be tight or loose. A loose nuchal cord is easily reduced after the fetal head is out. An easily reduced, loose nuchal cord is one that slips over the baby's head. Document "loose nuchal cord × 1" or "loose nuchal cord × 2," etc. If there are more than two loops, record the number of loops in your delivery notes (see Figure 6.28).

A tight nuchal cord cannot be reduced at all. The baby will be delivered with the loop or loops of umbilical cord around the neck. The cord will be clamped in two places after delivery and carefully cut between the clamps. A team should be ready to begin neonatal resuscitation because a tight nuchal cord can significantly decrease fetal oxygen delivery.

A TRUE KNOT IN THE CORD

Occasionally you may note one or more true knots in the cord (see Figure 6.29). A tight knot may prevent oxygen and nutrients from reaching the developing fetus. Document "tight knot" or "loose knot" in your notes, along with the number of knots.

If the knot in the umbilical cord constricts blood flow, the fetus may be smaller than expected (due to the diminished delivery of nutrients) or may die from asphyxia and be stillborn.

If the fetus is normally grown, the knot was loose enough to allow nutrients and oxygen to reach the fetus. Expect to see meconium in the amniotic fluid and abnormal heart rate patterns when there is a true knot in the cord. Meconium-stained amniotic fluid and abnormal fetal heart rate patterns are more common with a true knot (7%) than when there is no true knot (3.6%) (Hershkovitz et al., 2001). One in 100 babies has a true knot in his or her umbilical cord (Sornes, 2000).

UMBILICAL CORD COILS

Umbilical cords may be normally coiled, hypocoiled, or hypercoiled. Cord coils are difficult to see with an ultrasound (Predanic, Perni, Chasen, Baergen, & Chervenak, 2005). You will need to look at the umbilical cord to determine if it is normally coiled, hypocoiled (flatter), or hypercoiled (more twisted) (see Figure 6.30). Cord length and the number of coils are related to the pH in the umbilical vein and arteries (Atala, Abrams, Bell, & Taylor, 1998). As the number of coils increases, the pH will be lower.

When the umbilical cord is hypocoiled (0.1 coils per centimeter) or hypercoiled (0.3 coils per centimeter) there are more moderate to severe variable decelerations (Strong, Jarles, Vega, & Feldman, 1994). Moderate variable decelerations last longer than 30 seconds, but less than 60 seconds, and do not usually drop below 70 bpm. Severe variable decelerations last 60 or more seconds and drop below 70 bpm (if the baseline is less than 160 bpm). Moderate to severe variable decelerations last longer than 30 seconds and drop below 70 bpm (if the baseline is less than 160 bpm), or last 60 or more seconds but do not drop below 70 bpm. Variable decelerations that were moderate to severe during the 90 minutes prior to delivery were associated with neonatal metabolic acidosis (Blackwell et al., 2001). The cord length and the number of cord coils were not measured.

DELAYED CORD CLAMPING

Waiting 2 to 3 minutes after birth to clamp the cord decreases the risk of neonatal anemia without increasing the risk of

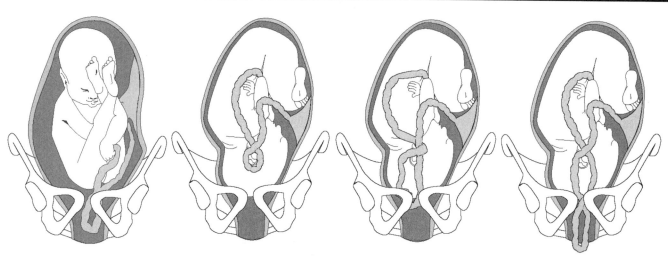

Figure 6.27: The risk of umbilical cord prolapse increases if the baby is small or breech, or if the head is not engaged. Viewed from left to right: frank breech with overt cord prolapse, occult cord prolapse, possible occult cord prolapse if cord cannot be felt at vaginal opening, and overt cord prolapse with cord exposure. If you are alone when there is an umbilical cord prolapse, call for help. Do not try to manipulate the cord. The amniotic fluid should keep it moist. Ask your patient to move into a knee–chest position or slightly lower the head of the bed and tilt her uterus to one side using a towel roll or pillow.

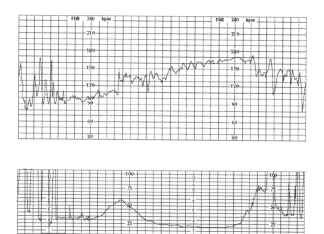

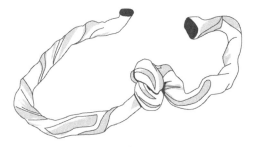

Figure 6.29: True knot in the umbilical cord.

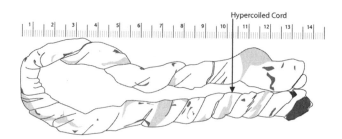

Figure 6.28: A primigravida at 41 weeks of gestation with oligohydramnios who was pushing with every other contraction. Apgar scores were 7 and 9 at 1 and 5 minutes. There were two loose loops of nuchal cord that were reduced after the head was out and prior to the birth.

Figure 6.30: Hypercoiled cord. Note there are two coils per centimeter. There should be one coil every 5 centimeters.

neonatal jaundice. The potential risk of delayed cord clamping is that more blood will infuse into the neonate, which can cause polycythemia. Neonates who have polycythemia may have tachypnea and they will be grunting. However, researchers did not find an increase in the incidence of neonatal tachypnea or grunting when cord clamping was delayed 2 to 3 minutes (Hutton & Hassan, 2007). With the increased incidence of cord blood banking (stem cell banking), delayed cord clamping is contraindicated because the placenta may be delivered before the midwife or physician collect the cord blood (stem cell) sample.

APGAR SCORES

Dr. Virginia Apgar first proposed the Apgar scoring tool in 1953 as a method to establish a list of objective signs pertinent

APGAR AND RESUSCITATION CHECKLIST

		POINTS			TIME AFTER BIRTH														
					1 minute			5 minutes			10 minutes			15 minutes			20 minutes		
		0	1	2	0	1	2	0	1	2	0	1	2	0	1	2	0	1	2
A	Appearance Color	Blue or Pale	Acrocyanotic	Completely Pink															
P	Pulse Heart Rate	Absent	< 100 minute	≥ 100 minute															
G	Grimace Reflex Irritability	No Response	Grimace	Cry or Active Withdrawal															
A	Activity Muscle Tone	Limp	Some Flexion	Active Motion															
R	Respiration Respiratory Effort	Absent	Weak Cry Hypoventilation	Good, Crying															
				TOTAL															

Check the boxes that apply	MINUTES																			
Resuscitation Events	1	2	3	4	5	6	7	8	9	10	11	12	13	14	15	16	17	18	19	20
Dry, clear airway																				
Stimulate, Reposition																				
Oxygen @_____ L/min																				
Bag & Mask Ventilations																				
ET Tube Size_____mm 2.5 3.0 3.5 4.0																				
Chest Compressions																				
Epinephrine 1:10,000																				
Volume Expanders																				
Naloxone (Narcan®)																				

Comments:

_____

_____

_____

_____

Recorder: _____   Date & Time: _____

Figure 6.31: Apgar and resuscitation checklist. Consult your hospital policies and procedures regarding documentation of the verbal orders for medications or volume expanders used during resuscitation.

to the newborn. Some people think of the Apgar score as evidence of a successful or failed resuscitation. The Apgar score is determined when the fetus is not being ventilated. Otherwise, the scores may be exaggerated. These exaggerated scores are known as "assisted Apgar scores."

The first Apgar score is determined at 1 minute of life, not at the time of birth. The second score is determined at 5 minutes of life, and every 5 minutes thereafter until a score of 7 is obtained or the baby is moved to the nursery.

Some infant warmers have a programmable Apgar timer. You should find out what kind of infant warmer is used in your birthing or delivery rooms and determine whether there is a timer and how to use it.

UMBILICAL CORD GASES

The collection and analysis of blood samples from the umbilical artery and the umbilical vein after delivery is designed to help the pediatrician decide if sodium bicarbonate is needed for neonatal resuscitation. However, pediatricians rarely use these values to treat the neonate.

Umbilical cord blood gases are analyzed to see if the results are normal, especially when there is a neonate who requires resuscitation (see Figure 6.32). Test results may be misleading if only one syringe of blood is obtained. If the one sample is from the umbilical vein, the blood-gas values reflect the ability of the placenta to deliver oxygen to the umbilical vein prior to delivery. A sample from the umbilical artery will reflect

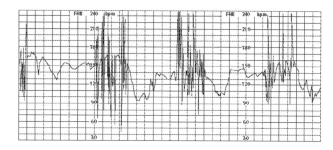

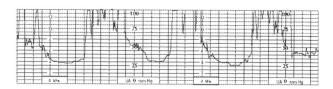

Figure 6.32: Primigravida at 39 4/7 weeks of gestation. Apgar scores were 4 and 8 at 1 and 5 minutes. There was thick meconium, a tight nuchal cord, and a loop of cord around the right arm. The umbilical artery gases were pH 7.00 PCO₂ 89.5 mm Hg PO₂ 6.4 mm Hg, and Base excess –12.6 mmol/L.

the fetal blood gases at the time of delivery. If two venous samples are drawn, you will see similar results. To determine whether one sample is venous and the other one is arterial, compare the color of the blood in the syringes. Umbilical cord venous blood is pinker than umbilical cord arterial blood.

UMBILICAL ARTERY BLOOD GASES

A cord artery pH of 7.00 or less is associated with metabolic acidosis. A PCO_2 higher than 60 mm Hg is associated with respiratory acidosis. A PO_2 less than 16 mm Hg is associated with hypoxia. A base excess less than –10 mmol/L is associated with metabolic acidosis. In the example in Figure 6.32, all of the umbilical artery values were abnormal, and the neonate was diagnosed with asphyxia.

> **Clinical example:** A woman who smoked 20 cigarettes a day but said she quit prior to the pregnancy arrived at the hospital in labor with a term fetus. She was underweight prior to her pregnancy. She was 4 feet 11 inches tall and gained 45 pounds during the pregnancy. Her fundal height was 36 cm and she had a fetus who was 39 weeks of gestation. Near 7:30 a.m., the admission test strip was normal and reactive. There was a baseline fetal heart rate in the 130 to 140 bpm range, with several accelerations that rose 15 or more bpm above the baseline. The accelerations lasted 15 or more seconds. There were no decelerations.
>
> At 1:00 p.m. she was 3-cm dilated, 80% effaced, and the fetus was at a –2 station. She was contracting every 2 to 3 minutes. Contractions lasted 60 to 70 seconds and she rated her pain as 8 on a 0 to 10 scale. Contractions

were palpated and recorded as moderate in their strength. A small amount of vaginal bleeding was noted at that time.

Between 1:00 p.m. and 2:30 p.m., there were 5 prolonged decelerations that dropped to 70 to 80 bpm and lasted 6 to 8 minutes each. The charge nurse was called into the room because the fetal heart rate dropped to 60 bpm after the fifth prolonged deceleration. At that time, the maternal pulse was near 90 bpm. The physician was called by the charge nurse to come to the hospital.

After that call, an emergency cesarean section was performed 1 hour later. The Apgar scores were 0 at 1 minute and 1 at 5, 10, 15, 20, and 30 minutes. Current neonatal resuscitation guidelines suggest stopping resuscitation after there are 10 minutes of asystole. The baby weighed 6 pounds 13 ounces and died later that day.

One cord blood sample was collected with a pH of 7.24 and a base excess of –7.8. It is probable that sample was from the umbilical vein not the umbilical artery. The placental pathology examination revealed the placenta weighed 304 grams. It was stained with meconium and the pathologist diagnosed acute chorioamnionitis and funisitis.

DRAW TWO SAMPLES: ONE FROM THE ARTERY AND ONE FROM THE VEIN

The neonatal status at the time of birth and the diagnosis of asphyxia in the nursery, confirm that the single cord sample was not an umbilical artery sample. It had to be drawn from the umbilical vein because the pH of 7.24 was too high and the base excess of –7.8 was normal, yet the neonate had Apgar scores of 0 to 1 for the first half hour of life and was diagnosed with asphyxia.

The small placenta created a condition of chronic placental insufficiency resulting in inadequate nutrient delivery to the fetus and inadequate fetal growth. Normal placental weight at term is usually 400 to 600 grams (Lage, 1994). In cases like this, it is important to obtain two cord blood samples, one from the artery and one from the vein, and to send the placenta for a pathologic examination. If a placental culture is needed, do not put formalin on the placenta.

To understand the baby's status at the time of birth, two syringes should be used to collect an arterial and venous sample from the cord. To determine if the blood is from the umbilical vein or the umbilical artery, lay the syringes on a piece of white paper or a white towel and compare the color of the blood. The pinker blood is venous, the darker blood is arterial.

The vein is a large, soft-walled vessel, whereas the arteries are smaller and wrapped around the vein. Use a tangential approach with the needle when you collect the blood. Draw blood first from the artery, if you can. If you draw blood from the vein, bleeding from the vein may obscure the artery. Once the blood is in the syringe, remove air bubbles. Remove the needle using a hemostat and cap the syringe. Discard the needle in a sharps container. Although it is not necessary to place the syringes on ice, personnel in the laboratory prefer receiving the labeled syringes in a plastic bag placed on ice. Cord blood gas values are stable in the syringe for 1 hour. If there is not sufficient blood in the cord for the samples, use placental vessels and draw the blood. The blood gases in the placental vessels are similar to those in the cord. Compare the color to determine if the source of the blood is arterial (darker) or venous (pinker).

CONCLUSIONS

Nurses, midwives, and physicians estimate fetal weight because it is important to anticipate how well the fetus will fit in the pelvis and descend for delivery. A nulliparous woman with a fetus at a −3 or higher station, or a very large fetus, creates a significant risk for a slow, protracted labor, an arrest of dilatation, and a cesarean section. A prolonged second stage of labor and a cesarean section should be anticipated if the fetal head is not at a 0 station (engaged) when the laboring woman is 7-cm dilated.

If there is a tight fit and the umbilical cord is compressed, there will usually be variable decelerations in the fetal heart rate during pushing and contractions. If there are accelerations with contractions and pushing, the fetus is most likely not being monitored, and it is the maternal heart rate accelerations that are probably being recorded. Nurses have to recognize this and move the ultrasound transducer or apply a spiral electrode to make sure the fetus is being monitored during labor.

Uterine rupture can occur in any woman who is receiving oxytocin. However, it is more common in women who have had a prior cesarean section, especially if they receive prostaglandins and/or oxytocin. Variable decelerations and unusual pain may herald a uterine rupture.

Twin gestations may be monochorionic or dichorionic. Usually monochorionic twins are identical in their appearance and gender. Rarely, a male and female will share one placenta if there is a chimera. Twins should be individually monitored during labor. Nurses must understand how to use and interpret the twin offset feature or coincidence detection feature of the electronic fetal monitor. A vaginal delivery can be expected if the first twin is vertex. A cesarean section is usually planned if the first twin is breech.

The placenta is fetal tissue. The placenta is also the historian of the pregnancy. Chorioamnionitis is an infection of the amnion and chorion. Maternal tachycardia and a temperature elevation are some of the signs of chorioamnionitis.

The placenta may be low in the uterus, even covering the cervical os (placenta previa). Placental tissue may grow into the uterus (placenta accreta or increta) or grow through the uterus (placenta percreta). Maternal hemorrhage may occur, and a hysterectomy or cesarean section may be required if there is abnormal placental implantation.

When the placenta separates from the uterus prematurely it is known as a placental abruption. The fetal heart rate pattern may worsen due to diminished oxygen delivery, and the mother may have cramping, contractions, vaginal bleeding, and pain.

Short umbilical cords are related to unfavorable outcomes and congenital malformations. Cord prolapse and cord entanglement are generally related to long cords. Some fetuses with a tight nuchal cord will need to be delivered before the cord is clamped and cut. A true knot in the cord may decrease fetal oxygenation or growth.

There should be one coil in the umbilical cord every 5 centimeters. Hypocoiled and hypercoiled cords increase the risk of metabolic acidosis. Delayed cord clamping increases the risk of neonatal polycythemia and jaundice.

Umbilical cord gases should be obtained from both the cord vein and the artery. An umbilical artery pH of 7.00 or less with a base excess less than −12 is associated with metabolic acidosis and an increased risk of neonatal brain damage.

REVIEW QUESTIONS

True/False: Decide if the statements are true or false.

1. The gynecoid pelvis is the most common female pelvis type.
2. Paternal height is not related to fetal weight.
3. Obese women have smaller babies than normal-weight women.
4. In a nulliparous woman who is 7-centimeters dilated, a fetal head at a −2 station is a normal finding.
5. Spontaneous uterine rupture can occur during oxytocin administration.
6. If a woman with an epidural has a history of a prior cesarean section and complains of persistent pain in her shoulder, she may have a uterine rupture.
7. In Figure 6.33, the twins would be identical or monozygotic.

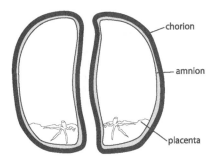

Figure 6.33

8. In Figure 6.34, twin fetuses would have a risk of cord entanglement.
9. There should be one coil of the umbilical cord every 5 centimeters.
10. Moderate and severe variable decelerations are more likely when the cord is hypocoiled or hypercoiled.

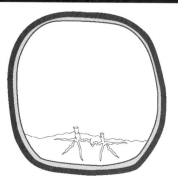

Figure 6.34

References

Aliyu, M. H., Salihu, H. M., Keith, L. G., Ehiri, J. E., Islam, M. A., & Jolly, P. E. (2005). High parity and fetal morbidity outcomes [Abstract]. *Obstetrics & Gynecology, 105,* 1045–1051.

American College of Obstetricians and Gynecologists. (2002). Induction of labor for vaginal birth after cesarean delivery. Committee Opinion Number 271. Washington, DC: Author.

Atalla, R. K., Abrams, K., Bell, S. C., & Taylor, D. J. (1998). Newborn acid-base status and umbilical cord morphology. *Obstetrics & Gynecology, 92,* 865–868.

Bastek, J., Elovitz, M., Pare, E., & Srinivas, S. (2007). Obstetric complications in obese, otherwise healthy women [Abstract]. *American Journal of Obstetrics and Gynecology, 197,* S96.

Battaglia, C., Artini, P. G., D'Ambrogio, G., Galli, P. A., Segre, A., & Genazzani, A. R. (1992). Maternal hyperoxygenation in the treatment of intrauterine growth retardation. *American Journal of Obstetrics and Gynecology, 167*(2), 430–435.

Battaglia, C., Artini, P. G., D'Ambrogio, G., Bencini, S., Galli, P. A., & Genazzani, A. R. (1994). Maternal hyperoxygenation in the treatment of mild intrauterine growth retardation: A pilot study. *Ultrasound in Obstetrics and Gynecology, 4*(6), 472–475.

Battista, L., Chung, J. H., Lagrew, D. C., & Wing, D. A. (2007). Complications of labor induction among multiparous women in a community-based hospital system. *American Journal of Obstetrics and Gynecology, 197,* 241.e1–241.e7.

Baylis, P. H. (1989). Regulation of vasopressin secretion. *Baillière's Clinical Endocrinology and Metabolism, 3*(2), 313–330.

Bekedam, D. J., Mulder, E. J., Snijders, R. J., & Visser, G. H. (1991). The effects of maternal hyperoxia on fetal breathing movements, body movements and heart rate variation in growth retarded fetuses. *Early Human Development, 27*(3), 223–232.

Bilardo, C. M., Snijders, R. M., Campbell, S., & Nicolaides, K. H. (1991). Doppler study of the fetal circulation during long-term maternal hyperoxygenation for severe early onset intrauterine growth retardation. *Ultrasound in Obstetrics and Gynecology, 1*(4), 250–257.

Blackwell, S., Field, S., Refuerzo, J., Hassan, S., Redman, M., & Naccasha, N. (2001). Pathologic acidemia at birth: Correlation with intrapartum electronic fetal heart rate patterns [Abstract]. *American Journal of Obstetrics and Gynecology, 184*(1), S98.

Bujold, E., Bujold, C., & Gauthier, R. J. (2001). Uterine rupture during a trial of labor after a one-versus two-layer closure of a low transverse cesarean [Abstract] *American Journal of Obstetrics and Gynecology, 184*(1).

Bujold, E., Bujold, C., Hamilton, E. F., Harel, F., & Gauthier, R. J. (2002). The impact of a single-layer or double-layer closure on uterine rupture. *American Journal of Obstetrics and Gynecology, 186*(6), 1326–1330.

Catanzarite, V., Cousins, L., Dowling, D., & Daneshmand, S. (2006). Oxytocin-associated rupture of an unscarred uterus in a primigravida. *Obstetrics & Gynecology, 108*(3, Part 2), 723–725.

Chan, W. Y., Wo, N. C., & Manning, M. (1996). Obstetrics: The role of oxytocin receptors and vasopressing V sub 1a receptors in uterine contractions in rats: Implications for tocolytic therapy with oxytocin antagonists. *American Journal of Obstetrics and Gynecology, 175*(5), 1331–1335.

Curtin, W., Florescue, H., Metlay, L., & Katzman, P. (2007). Evaluation of clinical signs for diagnosing histologic acute chorioamnionitis in the term parturient [Abstract]. *American Journal of Obstetrics and Gynecology, 197,* S68.

De La Ossa, M. M., Cabello-Inchausti, B., & Robinson, M. J. (2001). Placental chorangiosis. *Archives of Pathology and Laboratory Medicine, 125*(9), 1258.

Debby, A., Rotmensch, S., Girtler, O., Sadan, O., Golan, A., & Glezerman, M. (2003). Clinical significance of the floating fetal head in nulliparous women in labor. *Journal of Reproductive Medicine, 48*(1), 37–40.

Donnelly, V., Fynes, M., Campbvell, D., Johnson, H., O'Connell, R., & O'Herlihy, C. (1998). Obstetric events leading to anal sphincter damage. *Obstetrics and Gynecology, 92,* 995–961.

Eganhouse, D. J., & Petersen, L. A., (1997). Fetal surveillance in multifetal pregnancy. *Journal of Obstetric, Gynecologic, and Neonatal Nursing, 27,* 312–321.

Eogan, M. A., Geary, M. P., O'Connell, M. P., & Keane, D. P. (2003). Effect of fetal sex on labour and delivery: A retrospective review [Abstract]. *British Medical Journal, 326*(7381), 137.

Formaldehyde (CASRN 50-00-0). Retrieved July 8, 2008, from http://www.epa.gov/iris/_subst/0419.htm.

Fraser, D. M., & Cooper, M. A. (2003). *Myles textbook for midwives.* Edinburgh: Churchill Livingstone.

Fraser, W. D., Marcoux, S., Krauss, I., Douglas, J. K., Goulet, C., & Boulvain, M. (2000). Multicenter, randomized, controlled trial of delayed pushing for nulliparous women in the second stage of labor with continuous epidural analgesia. *American Journal of Obstetrics and Gynecology, 182*(5), 1165–1172.

Friedman, E. A., & Sachtleben, M. R. (1965a). Station of the fetal presenting. Part 1. Pattern of descent. *American Journal of Obstetrics & Gynecology, 93*(4), 522–529.

Friedman, E. A., Sachtleben, M. R. (1965b) Station of the fetal presenting. Part 2. Effect of the course of labor. *American Journal of Obstetrics & Gynecology, 93*(4), 530–536.

Friedman, E. A., Sachtleben, M. R. (1965c) Station of the fetal presenting. Part 3. Interrelationship with cervical dilatation. *American Journal of Obstetrics & Gynecology, 93*(4), 537–542.

Gyamfi, C., Juhuasz, G., Gyamfi, P., Blumenfield, Y., & Stone, J. L. (2006). Single-versus double-layer uterine incision closure and uterine rupture. *Journal of Maternal-Fetal and Neonatal Medicine, 19*(10), 639–643.

Hansen, S., Clark, S., & Foster, J. (2002). Active pushing versus passive fetal descent in the second stage of labor: A randomized controlled trial. *Obstetrics & Gynecology, 99,* 29–34.

Hershkovitz, R., Silberstein, T., Sheiner, E., Shoham-Vardi, I., Holcberg, G., & Katz, M. (2001). Risk factors associated with true knots of the umbilical cord. *European Journal of Obstetrics & Gynecology and Reproductive Biology, 98,* 36–39.

Hutton, E. K., & Hassan, E. S. (2007). Late vs. early clamping of the umbilical cord in full-term neonates. *Journal of the American Medical Association, 297*(11), 1241–1253.

Jensen, G. M., & Moore, L. G. (1997). The effect of high altitude and other risk factors on birthweight: Independent or interactive effects? *American Journal of Public Health, 87*(6), 1003–1007.

Kieffer, E. C., (2000). Maternal obesity and glucose intolerance during pregnancy among Mexican-Americans. *Paediatric Perinatal Epidemiology, 14,* 14–19.

Kieffer, E. C., Nolan, G. H., Carman, W. J., Sanborn, C. Z., Guzman, R., & Ventura, A. (1999). Glucose tolerance during pregnancy and birth weight in a Hispanic population. *Obstetrics & Gynecology, 94,* 741–746.

Kolderup, L. P., Laros, R. K. Jr., & Musci, T. J. (1997). Incidence of persistent birth injury in macrosomic infants: Association with mode of delivery. *American Journal of Obstetrics and Gynecology, 177*(1), 37–41.

Lage, J. M. (1994). The placenta. In C. Gompel & S. G. Silverberg (Eds.), *Pathology in gynecology and obstetrics* (pp. 448–512). Philadelphia: J. B. Lippincott.

Landon, M. B., Spong, C. Y., Thom, E., Hauth, J. C., Bloom, S. L., & Varner, M. W. (2006). Risk of uterine rupture with a trial of labor in women with multiple and single prior cesarean delivery. *Obstetrics & Gynecology, 108*(1), 12–20.

Lopriore, E., Stroeken, H., Sueters, A.M., Meerman, R.-J., Walther, F., & Vandenbussche, F. (2008). Term perinatal mortality and morbidity in monochorionic and dichorionic twin pregnancies: A retrospective study. *Acta Obstetricia et Gynecologica, 87,* 541–545.

Lowdermilk, D. L., Perry, S. E., & Bobak, I. M., (2000). *Maternity & women's health care.* St. Louis, MO: Mosby.

Lu, G., Rouse, D., Kimberlin, D., DuBard, M., Cliver, S., & Hauth, J. (2001). Obesity-attributable perinatal morbidity: Temporal trends [Abstract]. *American Journal of Obstetrics and Gynecology, 184*(1), S18.

Magnus, P., Gjessing, H. K., Skrondal, A., & Skjaerven, R. (2007). Paternal contribution to birth weight. *Journal of Epidemiology and Community Health, 55*(12), 873–877.

Management of genital herpes in pregnancy. Green-top Guideline No. 30. (2007). Royal College of Obstetricians and Gynaecologists.

Mazzone, M. E., & Woolever, J. (2006). Uterine rupture in a patient with an unscarred uterus: A case study. *Wisconsin Medical Journal, 105*(2), 64–66.

McDonagh, M. S., Osterweil, P., & Guise, J.-M. (2005). The benefits and risks of inducing labour in patients with prior caesarean delivery: A systematic review. *British Journal of Obstetrics and Gynaecology, 112,* 1007–1015.

Mishra, S. K., Morris, N., & Uprety, D. K. (2006). Uterine rupture: Preventable obstetric tragedies? *Australian and New Zealand Journal of Obstetrics and Gynaecology, 461,* 541–545.

Mongelli, M., & Gardosi, J. (2004). Estimation of fetal weight by symphysis-fundus height measurement. *International Journal of Gynecology & Obstetrics, 85,* 50–51.

Moore, L. G. (2003). Fetal growth restriction and maternal oxygen transport during high altitude pregnancy. *High Altitude Medicine & Biology, 4*(2), 141–156.

Morrison, J., Williams, G. M., Najman, J. M., & Andersen, M. J. (1991). The influence of paternal height and weight on birth-weight [Abstract]. *Australian and New Zealand Journal of Obstetrics and Gynaecology, 31*(2), 111–116.

Murphy, K., Shah, L., & Cohen, W. R. (1998). Labor and delivery in nulliparous women who present with an unengaged fetal head. *Journal of Perinatology, 18*(2), 122–125.

Naeye, R. L. (1985). Umbilical cord length: Clinical significance. *The Journal of Pediatrics, 107*(2), 278–281.

Nahum, G. G. (2005). *Estimation of fetal weight.* Retrieved March 23, 2006, from http://www.emedicine.com/med/topic 3281.htm.

Pardi, G., & Cetin, I. (2006). Human fetal growth and organ development: 50 years of discoveries. *American Journal of Obstetrics and Gynecology, 194,* 1088–1099.

Pomeranz, A. (2004). Anomalies, abnormalities, and care of the umbilicus. *Pediatric Clinics of North America, 51*, 819–827.

Prabulos, A.-M., & Philipson, E. H. (1998). Umbilical cord prolapse: Is the time from diagnosis to delivery critical? *Journal of Reproductive Medicine, 43*(2), 129–132.

Predanic, M., Perni, S. C., Chasen, S. T., Baergen, R. N., & Chervenak, F. A. (2005). Assessment of umbilical cord coiling during the routine fetal sonographic anatomic survey in the second trimester. *Journal of Ultrasound Medicine, 24*, 185–191.

Pryor, E. C., Mertz, H. L. O., Beaver, B. W., Koontz, G., Martinez-Borges, A., & Smith, J. G. (2007). Intrapartum predictors of uterine rupture. *American Journal of Perinatology, 24*(5), 317–321.

Samueloff, A., Langer, O., Berkus, M., Field, N., Xenakis, E., & Ridgway, L. (1994). Is fetal heart rate variability a good predictor of fetal outcome? *Acta Obstetricia et Gynecologica Scandinavica, 73*(1), 39–44.

Say, L., Gülmezoglu, A. M., & Hofmeyr, G. J. (2002). Maternal oxygen administration for suspected impaired fetal growth. *Cochrane Database of Systematic Reviews*, Issue 4. Art. No.: CD000137. doi: 10.1002/14651858.CD000137.

Shelton, R. L., Kinney, R. M., & Robertson, G. L. (1976). Emesis: A species-specific stimulus for vasopression (AVP) release [Abstract]. *Clinical Research, 24*, 531A.

Shin, K. S., Brubaker, K. L., & Ackerson, L. M. (2004). *American Journal of Obstetrics and Gynecology, 190*(1), 129–134.

Skupski, D. W., Rosenberg, C. R., & Eglinton, G. S. (2002). Intrapartum fetal stimulation tests: A meta-analysis. *Obstetrics & Gynecology, 99*, 129–134.

Sornes, T. (2000). Umbilical cord knots. *Acta Obstetricia et Gynecologica Scandinavica, 79*, 157–159.

Sousa, J. P., Miquelutti, M. A., Cecatti, J. G., & Makuch, M. Y. (2006). Maternal position during the first stage of labor: A systematic review. *Reproductive Health, 3*, 10–19.

Spencer, J. A., & Johnson, P. (1986). Fetal heart rate variability changes and fetal behavioural cycles during labour. *British Journal of Obstetrics and Gynaecology, 93*(4), 314–321.

Strong, T. H. Jr., Jarles, D. L., Vega, J. S., & Feldman, D. B. (1994). The umbilical coiling index. *American Journal of Obstetrics and Gynecology, 170*(1), 29–32.

Suy, A., Hernandez, S., Thorne, C., Lonca, M., Lopez, M., & Coll, O. (2007). Current guidelines on management of HIV-infected pregnant women: Impact on mode of delivery. *European Journal of Obstetrics & Gynecology*, doi:10.1016/j.ejogrb.2007.12.007.

To, W. W., Cheung, W., & Kwok, J. S. (1998). Paternal height and weight as determinants of birth weight in a Chinese population [Abstract]. *American Journal of Perinatology, 15*(9), 545–548.

Turner, M. J., Rasmussen, M. J., Turner, J. E., Boylan, P. C., MacDonald, D., & Stronge, J. M. (1990). The influence of birth weight on labor in nulliparas. *Obstetrics & Gynecology, 76*(2), 159–163.

Uotila, J., & Tammela, O. (1999). Acute intrapartum fetoplacental transfusion in monochorionic twin pregnancy. *Obstetrics & Gynecology, 94*, 819–821.

Visintine, J., Wood, D., Chanthasenont, A., Baxter, J., Weiner, S., & Berghella, V. (2006). Changes in the ductus venosus in fetuses with intrauterine growth restriction during maternal hyperoxygenation [Abstract]. *American Journal of Obstetrics and Gynecology, 195*(6), S215.

Walsh, C. A., & Baxi, L. V. (2007). Rupture of the primigravid uterus: A review of the literature. *Obstetrical and Gynecological Survey, 62*(5), 327–334.

Wang, Y.-L., & Su, T.-H. (2006). Obstetric uterine rupture of the unscarred uterus: A twenty-year clinical analysis. *Gynecologic and Obstetric Investigation, 62*, 131–135.

Welt, S. I. (1984). The fetal heart rate W sign. *Obstetrics & Gynecology, 63*(3), 405–408.

Wiseman, C. S., & Kiehl, E. M. (2007). Picture perfect. Benefits and risk of fetal 3D ultrasound. *MCN, 32*(2), 102–111.

Witter, F. R., Caulfield, L. E., & Stoltzfus, R. J. (1995). Influence on maternal anthropometric status and birth weight on the risk of cesarean delivery. *Obstetrics & Gynecology, 85*(6), 947–951.

Yogev, Y., Ben-Haroush, A., Chen, R., & Kaplan, B. (2002). Intra-uterine fetal brain death: Report of two cases and review of the literature. *European Journal of Obstetrics & Gynecology and Reproductive Biology, 105*, 36–38.

Zelop, C. M., Shipp, T. D., Repke, J. T., Cohen, A., Caughey, A. B., & Lieberman, E. (1999). Uterine rupture during induced or augmented labor in gravid women with one prior cesarean delivery. *American Journal of Obstetrics and Gynecology, 181*(4), 882–226.

7

Passageway

It is a long road from conception to completion.

—*Molière*

The pelvis is both the place of entrance and the passageway to birth. The type of pelvis and the estimated weight of the fetus should be recorded in the prenatal record. Read the prenatal record and look for the clinical pelvimetry notes. A gynecoid pelvis provides the most space for fetal descent. Even if the patient does not have a gynecoid pelvis and the estimated fetal weight is large, there are no tests to diagnose cephalopelvic disproportion (CPD) prenatally. Magnetic resonance imaging (MRI) of the pelvis was not helpful in predicting who needed a cesarean section due to CPD (Zaretsky et al., 2005).

The decision to deliver by cesarean section due to CPD is based on clinical judgment after considering each woman's constellation of facts. Nurses assess fetal descent to confirm the adequacy of the passageway. A delayed descent with the development of scalp swelling (caput) and a change in the shape of the fetal skull (molding) suggest that there is a problem with the fit of the passenger in the passageway. That is why it is important that nurses communicate the station, caput, and molding to the midwife or physician. If the nurse detects abnormal progress, he or she calls the obstetric provider to the bedside, and the obstetric provider evaluates the fetal–pelvic fit. If the obstetric provider suspects fetopelvic or cephalopelvic disproportion (CPD), the plan of care should change. If the patient's powers are inadequate, oxytocin augmentation may be ordered. If the powers are adequate, the plan may still include a cesarean section. In that case, the preoperative diagnosis will be "failure to progress."

THE MYTH OF SHOE SIZE

In the past, a myth in obstetrics was that a woman whose shoe size was smaller than size 5 had an increased risk of CPD and a cesarean section. We used to say, "small foot, small pelvis." It is now clear that it is not the patient's shoe size but her height that is related to an increased risk of a cesarean section. Short women are more likely to have an obstructed labor and a cesarean section (see Figure 7.1).

Women who were less than 5 feet tall had a high risk for cesarean section (Parsons, Winegar, Siefert, & Spellacy, 1989). When you escort the patient to the labor room, note her height. Ask her how tall she is. If you have a scale and can measure her height and weight, do so. Accurate information about her size helps the midwives and physicians determine medication dosages.

If the patient is 4 to 5 feet tall, you should be especially vigilant in following the progress of fetal descent. Keep the midwife or physician, or both, informed of labor progress and fetal descent. Short women (less than 5 feet 3 inches) have double the risk for cesarean section than taller women. Nulliparous, but not multiparous, women who are taller then 5 feet 5 inches have a decreased risk of cesarean section.

THE SACRED SPACE

Part of the passageway has been called the "birth canal" or "sacred space" (Bewley, 2005). The vagina and cervix are in the sacred space. The cervix must efface and dilate adequately for the fetus to leave the uterus. In some countries, unnecessary vaginal examination that was not required for the benefit of the patient was considered an assault (Bewley, 1992). Therefore, alternatives to learning how to assess dilatation, effacement, and station are needed. Pelvic models and other tools are available to meet these learning needs. If the patient consents to your examination while you are still learning to assess

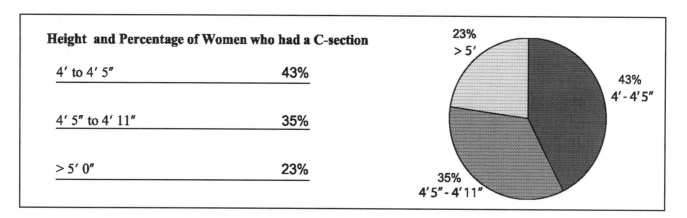

Figure 7.1: Height and percentage of women who had a cesarean section (Parsons et al., 1989). Percentages have been rounded up to total 101%.

dilatation, you can confirm your findings by using the fetal monitor paper as a ruler after you remove your glove and wash your hands (see Figure 7.2).

EFFACEMENT OF THE CERVIX

The closed cervix is usually about 3 cm long. Therefore, when it is 50% effaced it is half the usual thickness. At 50%, the cervix should be about 1-cm long. By measuring your index finger (see Figure 7.3), you should be able to insert it into the cervix (when it is sufficiently dilated) and estimate effacement. For example, if you find the cervix to be about 1-cm long, it is near 60 to 70% effaced. If it is about .5-cm long, it is near 80% effaced. When it is difficult to detect the cervix because it is extremely thin, it is 100% effaced. Sometimes it helps to move your gloved finger back and forth over the fetal head to find the cervix, especially when the patient is dilated more than 8 to 9 cm. Some providers use centimeters rather than a percentage when they document effacement.

To assist you in determining your finger length, place your hand across the minutes on the fetal monitor paper (see Figure 7.3). Measure your index finger on your examining hand. This will help you measure the length and effacement (thinning) of the cervix. Note the length of your index finger from its tip to 2.5 cm. This distance will be near the first joint. The distance from your fingertip to the second joint behind your knuckle is near 5 cm.

THE ISCHIAL SPINES

Now that you have measured your fingers, it should be easy to locate the ischial spines. To reach the ischial spines, the fetus must not be engaged in the pelvis. Insert your gloved fingers 5 to 6 cm into the introitus (vaginal opening). At the 3 o'clock and 9 o'clock positions you should find bony prominences. These are the ischial spines. The ischial spines may feel like pointed or rounded bones. Next, palpate the fetal skull with your fingertips. The distance between the tip of the

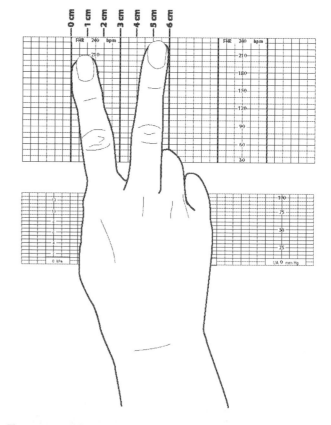

Figure 7.2: Using the fetal monitor paper immediately after a vaginal examination may help you decide the dilatation. In this case, the cervix was probably 6-cm dilated. Each cm of dilatation is equal to 20 seconds of time on the fetal monitor paper if the paper is set to advance from the electronic fetal monitor at 3 cm/minute.

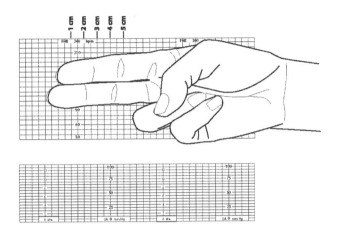

Figure 7.3: Use the fetal monitor paper as a guide to measure your fingers. Noting where 5 centimeters falls will aid you in assessing effacement and station. Station is discussed in the next chapter.

skull bone and the ischial spines determines the station. For example, if you estimate the tip of the skull to be 1 cm above the spines, the station is documented as −1. When the tip of the fetal skull, or the chin (in a face presentation), or the sacrum (in a breech presentation) are at the level of the ischial spines, the station is recorded as 0 (for 0 cm), which means level with the imaginary line between the ischial spines.

If the fetus is below the ischial spines, you will need to estimate the station by subtracting the distance from the vaginal opening to the fetal skull from the distance between the ischial spines to the vaginal opening, which is about 5 cm. Imagine you inserted your fingers 2 cm and felt the tip of the fetal skull. Subtract 2 from 5. The fetal station is +3. Or, if you insert your fingers approximately 3 cm into the introitus and then feel the tip of the skull, the distance of 5 cm minus 3 cm is 2 cm. The station will be recorded as +2.

> **Documentation example:** 3 cm/1 cm/−2.
> In this example, the cervix is dilated 3 cm, the cervix is felt to be 1-cm thick, and the station is −2 cm above the ischial spines.

> **Documentation example:** 5 cm/90%/0. In this example, the cervix is dilated 5 cm, is 90% thinned (effaced), and the tip of the fetal skull was at the level of the ischial spines or 0 station.

BIRTH EN CAUL

The fetus is surrounded by two membranes that are fused together. The amnion is the membrane closest to the fetus, and the chorion is the membrane next to the decidua and placenta. The fetus is surrounded by amniotic fluid, which is composed mostly of fetal urine. The baby can be born surrounded by the membranes and fluid with the placenta still attached to the uterine wall. This type of birth is documented

as an "en caul" birth. *Caul* means "bottom of the bag or sac" in French.

At the Royal Victoria Hospital in Montreal, Canada, en caul vaginal breech deliveries rather than cesarean sections of preterm fetuses who were less than 26 weeks of gestation resulted in higher cord pH values and 5-minute Apgar scores (Richmond, Morin, & Benjamin, 2002). In term gestations, if the membranes have not ruptured, they will bulge out of the vagina prior to birth of baby. The membranes might look like a water balloon or a light bulb. Don't be alarmed. Call the provider. The doctor or midwife will probably rupture the membranes and soon thereafter you should expect the baby to be delivered.

RUPTURE OF THE MEMBRANES

In 10% of pregnancies with a term fetus, and in 40% with a preterm fetus, the membranes rupture in advance of contractions (Pandey et al., 2007). This is called premature rupture of the membranes. Amniotic fluid may leak when biochemical changes have remodeled the collagen in the membranes and caused apoptosis (programmed cell death) (Pandey et al., 2007). If intact membranes are felt during a vaginal examination but there is fluid dripping out of the vagina, and there is a positive nitrazine or positive fern test, a high leak is probable. Some women experience the rupture of the membranes as a "pop" or a "fart" in the vagina. When there is little amniotic fluid visualized on the pad, this description of a pop may be helpful to communicate to the person who will be confirming rupture of the membranes. When there is a normal amount of amniotic fluid (500 to 1500 mL) within the membranes, a gross rupture will be easy to detect. There will have been a gush of fluid followed by continual leaking from the vagina. Once the fetal head is low in the pelvis, the release of amniotic fluid may decrease or stop.

Nurses assess and record the time the membranes ruptured and the color, amount, and odor of the amniotic fluid. They may record a spontaneous rupture (SROM or SRM) or an artificial rupture (AROM or ARM). The odor of the amniotic fluid has been described as musty or "like semen," or there may be no odor at all. You should document the color, amount, and odor of the amniotic fluid if there has been an artificial rupture of membranes or a spontaneous rupture of membranes. Continue to document the color, amount, and odor at least hourly throughout the duration of the labor, or with each vaginal examination or change of the linen protector, or both. A foul odor suggests the presence of an infection and should be reported to the midwife or physician.

Because of the risk of an ascending infection, maternal temperature will be assessed more frequently after the rupture of the membranes. Once her membranes have ruptured, her temperature needs to be assessed and recorded every 2 hours. More frequent temperatures may be taken when there is an elevation. Report a temperature elevation to the obstetric provider, especially if it is at or over 100.4° Fahrenheit or 38° Celsius (a fever).

Documentation example: SROM, moderate amount of clear fluid with streaks of blood, normal odor, FHR 155, 99.1, peri care given with soap and water. Dr. Alwaysthere notified.

PERINEAL CARE

Handwashing with soap and water removes bacteria. Washing with tap water and no soap only removes some viruses (Sickbert-Bennett et al., 2005). Therefore, perineal care should include soap and water. After washing the perineum, inspect the linen protector. Document the color, amount, and odor of any fluid on the pad. You should avoid the use of betadine solution for perineal cleansing because it can confuse the assessment of the color of amniotic fluid on the linen protector.

AMNIOINFUSION: INTAKE AND OUTPUT

If you need to measure the fluid leaving the uterus during an amnioinfusion, remove the pad first, then provide perineal care. Document the amount of uterine intake and output during an amnioinfusion. Separate this in your documentation from oral or intravenous intake and output. You can describe how saturated the pad is. To be more specific, weigh the wet pad. Subtract the weight of a dry pad. One milliliter (mL) of fluid weighs approximately 1 gram. Notify the provider of the color of the fluid or blood. If there is bleeding, is it bright red or dark red? Notify the provider of the characteristics and consistency of the bleeding. Are there clots or is the blood free flowing, intermittent, or continuous? Notify the provider of your estimation of the amount of blood.

Documentation example: Amnioinfusion at 100 mL/hr. Saturated chux with clear, nonfoul fluid.

Documentation example: Continuous bright red trickle of blood with dark red clots. Clots weighed 200 grams. Notified CNM Lavender of bleeding and blood loss.

Documentation example: AROM by Dr. Rightnough. Half of pad soaked with light-green meconium-stained fluid, normal odor. Bloody show noted and intermittent minimal bleeding after vaginal examination. 2/60%/−2. FHR 135 bpm with moderate variability and accelerations, and no decelerations. Peri wash done with soap and water. Dry Chux placed under patient.

ASCENDING INFECTIONS

Research has shown that there are approximately one billion bacteria-colony-forming units per gram of vaginal secretions (Casey & Cox, 1997). Bacteria proliferate in a moist environment. Other research has shown that prior to the first vaginal examination, there are from one to four types of microorganisms on the cervix. After a vaginal examination there were three to six types of microorganisms on the cervix, with or without ruptured membranes (Imseis, Trout, & Gabbe, 1999).

Women who have intercourse after the rupture of the membranes also have an increased risk of chorioamnionitis. In addition to vaginal examinations that introduce bacteria to the cervix, items placed in the vagina by undisclosed individuals or a delusional patient also increase the risk of an ascending infection. For example, breath mints, candy, a bag of cocaine, a cue ball, a baseball, a potato (even one growing leaves), and a $20 bill have been found in the vaginas of various women.

After rupture of the membranes there is no longer a bacteriostatic barrier to protect the fetus, placenta, and cord from infection. In this case, a sterile speculum examination can be nearly as accurate as a digital examination in estimating dilatation and effacement (Brown, Ludwiczsk, Blanco, & Hirsch, 1993; Munson, Graham, Koos, & Valenzuela, 1985). When the fetus is preterm and rupture of the membranes is suspected, a sterile speculum examination is preferred because an intrauterine infection shortens the latency period, the time from the preterm rupture of the membranes until the birth of the fetus. This latency period is different from the latent phase of labor.

Vaginal examination increases the risk of chorioamnionitis and neonatal sepsis. After rupture of the membranes, it is best to limit the number of examinations (Newton, Prihoda, & Gibbs, 1989; Soper, Mayhall, & Dalton, 1989). Somewhere near the seventh and eighth vaginal examination, the risk of neonatal infection significantly increases (McCaul IV et al., 1997; Seaward et al., 1998).

You should, therefore, communicate the number of vaginal examinations since the rupture of membranes when you give report to the incoming nurse. If you receive report, and this information is not provided, ask how many examinations have been done since the membranes ruptured. Assess your patient's temperature and monitor it closely until the time of birth. Notify the obstetric provider of signs of chorioamnionitis, such as a fever, foul-smelling amniotic fluid, uterine tenderness, and/or maternal tachycardia. Avoid the use of a spiral electrode if the woman is positive for group B streptococcus, hepatitis, or human immunodeficiency virus (HIV). The spiral electrode increases the risk of transmission of these diseases to the fetus.

BLEEDING IS NOT BLOODY SHOW

Vaginal bleeding is not the same as bloody show. It is important to distinguish bleeding from bloody show in written and spoken communications. Bloody show contains mucus released from the cervix prior to or early in labor when the cervix begins to dilate. Bloody show is a mixture of mucus from the mucous plug and blood from cervical capillaries. When the mucous plug has left the cervix and fallen into the toilet it looks like strings of mucus. The mucous plug may be removed from the cervix during an examination of the cervix. It is a sticky, grey-white, gelatinous substance and there may be streaks of blood in it. Document "bloody show" in your notes.

Documentation example: 1/50%/high, intact. Bloody show noted on examining glove.

Exhibit 7.1: Cardinal (main) movements of the fetus prior to and after birth.

- Descent, flexion, and internal rotation of the head
- Crowning, extension, and birth of the head
- Restitution of the head with internal rotation of the shoulders
- Birth of the baby

Vaginal bleeding, on the other hand, is blood that is not mixed with mucus. Bleeding is thin, watery, and bright red. Bleeding may be related to complications such as a placental abruption or a ruptured vasa previa. Therefore, when bleeding is noted, the obstetric provider should be informed. Documenting "heavy bloody show" to describe bleeding is inaccurate, improbable, and misleading. Bleeding is not a diagnosis, it is an observation. Therefore, nurses should chart bleeding in their notes just as they would chart the presence of bloody show. When vaginal bleeding occurs, describe and quantify blood loss.

Documentation example: Small amount of dark-red-brown bleeding noted on peri pad with two 2-cm clots. Vaginal examination deferred. Requested Dr. Here-innow evaluate bleeding.

Documentation example: With AROM by Dr. Ready-togo, large amount of bright-red continuous bleeding noted, approximately 200 mL, and FHR dropped to the 60s. Patient moved STAT to OR. (After delivery of the placenta, a ruptured umbilical cord vessel from vasa previa was noted.)

VAGINAL BIRTH: THE USUAL EXIT ROUTE

How you start out the race often determines how you will end the race. For example, if the fetus is too big to fit in the pelvis at the beginning of labor, it will obviously be too big to exit the pelvis through the sacred space. Since there are only two possible exit routes, a cesarean section will have to be performed.

DESCENT, FLEXION, AND INTERNAL ROTATION

Birth involves many fetal movements (see Exhibit 7.1). The fetus must first descend. Descent for a vaginal birth will be hindered if the fetal head is not flexed with the chin near the chest. If the hand is next to the fetal head, a compound presentation exists. This may delay or prevent a vaginal birth. Internal rotation is the process whereby the fetus rotates from an occiput posterior or transverse position to an occiput ante-

rior position. Some fetuses do not complete this step and are delivered in an occiput posterior position.

CROWNING, EXTENSION, AND BIRTH OF THE HEAD

Crowning occurs when the top of the fetal head is visible at the introitus and is not sliding back into the vagina after maternal pushing stops. Extension occurs when the head has passed under the pubic bone and the baby (in an occiput anterior position) lifts it chin from its chest and extends its head. When a baby is delivered in an occiput posterior position, its little nose is compressed and springs back into shape when the head extends and the chin lifts up from the chest.

RESTITUTION OF THE HEAD WITH INTERNAL ROTATION OF THE SHOULDERS

Restitution is what the head does next as it turns to one side. Internal rotation of the shoulders occurs at the same time as the shoulders move in the same direction as the baby's head. This is a critical time during the birthing process because one shoulder is under the pubic bone where it could become trapped, creating a shoulder dystocia.

BIRTH OF THE SHOULDERS AND BABY

If the anterior shoulder does not become trapped, the baby should deliver. If the anterior shoulder becomes trapped behind the pubic bone, shoulder dystocia will occur.

KEEP THE PATH OPEN

A full bladder blocks the exit. Your goal should be to keep the passageway open for descent and delivery. The bladder is located under the uterus (see Figure 7.4). Encourage your patient to urinate every hour or two and document the urine output. When you palpate a full bladder, it may feel like a sponge. A variety of situations may necessitate creativity in helping your patient empty her bladder. She may be confined to bed after an epidural or she may refuse to get up to the bathroom. She may also refuse catheterization, or there may be no order for catheterization. In any of these circumstances, ask her to void on the linen protector, a folded towel next to the perineum, or on a bedpan. Some women find the bedpan to be extremely uncomfortable. After she voids, wash her with soap and water or provide a soap-filled wash cloth and rinse the perineum. Provide a dry wash cloth. She may choose to pat herself dry or she may decide to forego this step. After an epidural or spinal-epidural, women may have an indwelling catheter, or there may be an order for intermittent catheterization.

PREPARE FOR VAGINAL DELIVERY

Inform the obstetric provider of changes in dilatation, effacement, station, and position, especially when there is a protraction disorder or your patient is getting closer to delivery. By the time your nulliparous patient is dilated 10 cm, you should have set up the delivery table and notified the obstetric pro-

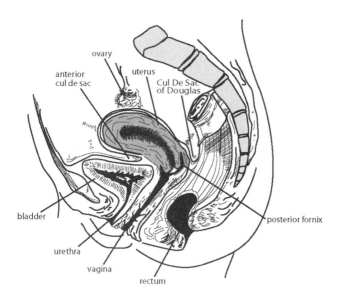

Figure 7.4: Note that the position of the bladder is under the uterus when the woman is in a supine position.

Exhibit 7.2: Preparation for delivery of a large fetus.

1. Notify the person who will be delivering the baby.
2. Inform the patient that additional steps and personnel may be involved.
3. Keep the charge nurse or supervisor informed of the clinical situation.
4. Anticipate use of McRoberts' maneuver and suprapubic pressure.
5. Alert additional medical personnel.
6. Confirm that step stool is in the delivery room and readily available.

---

vider. He or she may wish to be present and examine your patient before she begins to push.

The delivery provider should be readily available or in the room, especially if a large baby is anticipated (see Exhibit 7.2). When a multiparous woman is 6- to 7-cm dilated, it is a good idea to set up the delivery table at that time. Notify the obstetric provider so that he or she will be nearby when your patient reaches 10 cm.

McROBERTS' MANEUVER

McRoberts' maneuver can be used prior to the birth of a large baby or when shoulder dystocia is encountered. McRoberts' maneuver expands the passageway by straightening the sacrum relative to the lumbar vertebrae. With the woman in a near supine position or a supine position, flex her legs and

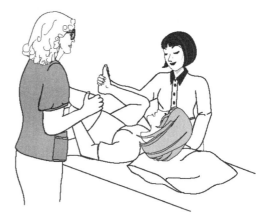

Figure 7.5: McRoberts' maneuver.

pull her knees toward her head (see Figure 7.5). The legs should also be abducted.

When a single maneuver does not resolve shoulder dystocia within 30 seconds, another maneuver should be attempted (Gurewitsch, 2007). Document the use of McRoberts' maneuver, or McRoberts' maneuver with suprapubic pressure, if both were used. You or another skilled nurse may need to use a step stool to position yourself to push down above the pubic bone (suprapubic pressure).

SHOULDER DYSTOCIA

Shoulder dystocia may persist even when gentle downward movement of the fetal head by the obstetric provider fails to deliver the shoulders (Mahlmeister, 2008). Shoulder dystocia has also been called "stuck shoulders" in verbal communications between health care providers. There is a heightened risk of posterior, not anterior, arm Erb-Duchenne palsy after normal labor and spontaneous delivery (Allen & Gurewitsch, 2005). Erb's palsy is more common in the anterior arm, however, after shoulder dystocia. Erb's palsy occurs because there is an injury to the nerves at the C5 and C6 level of the spine, which causes a temporary or permanent paralysis of muscles in the affected arm. If there is shoulder dystocia, document the time the baby's head was delivered and the time the entire baby was delivered.

SHOULDER DYSTOCIA DRILLS

As a labor and delivery nurse you may participate in shoulder dystocia drills, in which nursing skills and interventions will be demonstrated and practiced in a calm setting. Some hospitals use mannequins or simulators for this purpose. Shoulder dystocia drills improve communication and team performance (Fahey & Mighty, 2008).

OPERATIVE VAGINAL DELIVERY INCREASES THE RISK OF SHOULDER DYSTOCIA

The incidence of shoulder dystocia is lowest when no episiotomy was performed or no instruments were used prior to birth. Operative vaginal delivery with forceps or a vacuum extractor increases the risk of shoulder dystocia (Dandolu et al., 2005). Shoulder dystocia is also associated with a birth weight greater than or equal to 4,000 grams (Hackmon et al., 2007). Birth trauma and asphyxia are related to a birth weight of 4,500 to 4,999 grams (Zhang, Decker, Platt, & Kramer, 2008).

BE PREPARED

It is important to be prepared for shoulder dystocia with every birth. You must be mentally and physically ready to act quickly, especially when your patient is obese, diabetic, you suspect a large infant, or forceps or a vacuum extractor are used. A step stool should be in the room prior to delivery. The call light should be within your reach. There should be two nurses present prior to the birth. Verify that the person who can intubate the neonate is in the hospital and immediately available, or in the room if meconium is present and there is an abnormal or nonreassuring fetal heart rate pattern.

An emergency cesarean section will be performed when maneuvers are not successful in delivering the baby. The neonatal resuscitation team should be present to receive the newborn.

THE TURTLE SIGN

A turtle sign is when the fetal head delivers and then retracts tightly against the perineum. The turtle sign is a marker of shoulder dystocia that is usually observed during delivery by the midwife or physician. The obstetric provider may say, "I need McRoberts" or "I have shoulders" or "Shoulder dystocia — I need suprapubic pressure now." You should press the call light and call outside the room for help if you need additional nurses. The neonatal resuscitation team, the obstetric crew, and the anesthesia provider must be notified of the unanticipated shoulder dystocia if they are not in the room prior to delivery because of the potential need for a cesarean section and neonatal resuscitation.

SUPRAPUBIC PRESSURE

If shoulder dystocia occurs, you should perform and document use of McRoberts' maneuver and the application of suprapubic pressure. If you need to use both hands to provide suprapubic pressure (see Figure 7.6) and there are no other nurses to help you hold the leg, ask a family member to help keep her leg in a flexed, abducted position. You can make a fist and push down with your other hand or use the palm of one hand while pushing down with the other hand. This is similar to the pressure you would apply during chest compressions.

Another form of suprapubic pressure is when you use one hand to provide pressure to rotate the anterior shoulder (see Figure 7.7). You will need to know which direction the baby is facing and place your hand behind the anterior shoulder to roll the fetus away from the midline to a more oblique orientation. You should document the use of suprapubic pressure in your notes.

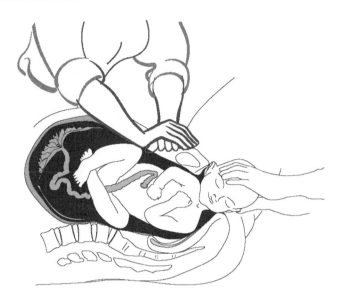

Figure 7.6: Suprapubic pressure using two hands. The lower hand is in a fist placed just above the pubic bone.

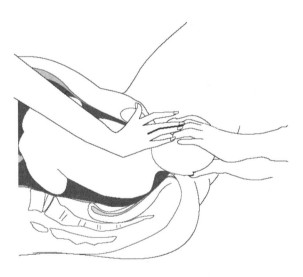

Figure 7.7: Posterolateral application of suprapubic pressure (external Rubin's maneuver). You will be pushing down above the pubic bone on the lower abdomen where you believe the anterior shoulder blade is located to roll the fetus toward the direction of its face.

THE GASKIN MANEUVER

If McRoberts' maneuver with suprapubic pressure does not help deliver the baby, you may be asked to assist the mother to her hands and knees. Using a hands-and-knees position to relieve shoulder dystocia is called the Gaskin maneuver (Mahlmeister, 2008). When a woman is on her hands and

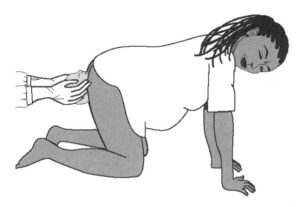

Figure 7.8: The Gaskin maneuver is named after Ina May Gaskin, a midwife.

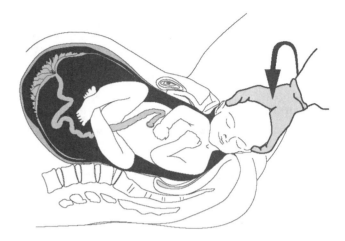

Figure 7.9: Zavanelli maneuver. The first part of this maneuver requires flexing the fetal head.

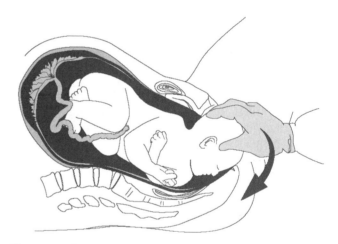

Figure 7.10: Zavanelli maneuver. The second part of this maneuver requires placing the fetus back into the vagina.

knees, the posterior shoulder should drop down due to gravity, which may expedite delivery. If the obstetric provider says, "Get her on all fours" or "Get her on her hands and knees" they are asking you to position her to use the Gaskin maneuver (see Figure 7.8). Summon help to change her position if she has had regional anesthesia or if she is obese. Ask the patient to help you as much as she can. After the delivery, document the use of the Gaskin maneuver in your summary notes.

WATCH THE CLOCK

Every minute matters when there is a shoulder dystocia. A shoulder dystocia should be resolved within 4 minutes to prevent the risk of an asphyxial insult. Asphyxial injury is likely if the shoulder dystocia lasts 6 to 8 minutes (Gurewitsch, 2007). Notify the physician of the time since the head was out. For example, you might say in a calm, firm voice, "Doctor, it's been 2 minutes," "Doctor it's been 3 minutes." You should call the physician or midwife by name to make sure he or she hears you.

MANUEVERS BY THE MIDWIFE OR PHYSICIAN

While you are providing suprapubic pressure, you may notice the midwife or physician placing his or her hand inside the vagina in an attempt to rotate the anterior shoulder or posterior shoulder. Sometimes he or she will break the fetal clavicle or the humerus. He or she may also perform a large episiotomy, often into the rectum. This is called an episioproctotomy.

SYMPHYSIOTOMY

When the 4th minute approaches, a skilled physician may elect to perform a symphysiotomy. This requires a local anesthetic and scalpel. The cartilage between the pubic bone is cut after numbing the skin. You will need to open and pour the lidocaine and place a sterile needle, a syringe, and a disposable scalpel with a stainless-steel blade on the delivery table. Usu-

ally these items are not kept in the room, but sometimes may be found in a drawer of the delivery table close to the sutures. After the baby is delivered, you will need to add sutures to the delivery table. You may need to add a needle holder and tissue forceps if they are not part of your basic vaginal delivery instruments.

ZAVANELLI MANEUVER

In the event the physician or midwife is unable to deliver the baby, he or she may choose to perform a Zavanelli maneuver, also known as a cephalic replacement, prior to the cesarean section (see Figures 7.9 and 7.10). When this occurs, the cord should not be clamped or cut. The baby is rotated, the head is flexed, and the baby is pushed back into the vagina.

Documentation example of a summary note after delivery: Head delivered at 1209 by Dr. Mityfein. Shoulder dystocia. Called for assistance. HOB flat and McRoberts' maneuver and suprapubic pressure applied by nurses Neu and Olde. See physician's notes for medical maneuvers. Patient moved to hands and knees at physician request. Shoulders and body delivered at 1216. See resuscitation notes of neonatal nurse and neonatal nurse practitioner.

Documentation example of a summary note after delivery: Head delivered by CNM Mei. Turtle sign. Called for help. Dr. Veryskilled and RN Imincharge responded. Patient placed in McRoberts' and lateral suprapubic pressure applied by physician. Head delivered at 0240, body delivered at 0246. Neonatal resuscitation crew notified and present prior to delivery.

DIFFICULT DELIVERY

A difficult delivery is an operative vaginal delivery or a delivery following shoulder dystocia. Usually difficult deliveries do not just happen, something abnormal precedes them. In 1975, Dr. John Studd wrote "normal babies of mature birth weight should not die during spontaneous labour if delay is recognized and corrected, if labour is monitored, and if difficult instrumental procedures are prohibited." A difficult delivery is a serious matter that can result in injury or death of the neonate. Theodore Roosevelt said "In any moment of decision, the best thing you can do is the right thing and the worst thing you can do is nothing." If the conditions are not right to perform an operative vaginal (difficult) delivery, do not remain silent. Any time an operative vaginal delivery is ordered, notify your charge nurse or house supervisor since the operating room must be immediately available for a cesarean section.

Difficult deliveries are associated with more injuries than normal spontaneous vaginal delivery. A difficult delivery might be a midpelvic vacuum extraction for cord prolapse with an abnormal fetal heart rate pattern. Difficult deliveries, more so than nondifficult deliveries, are associated with more third- and fourth-degree tears (18.2%) compared with 8.4% of nondifficult deliveries. Difficult deliveries compared with nondifficult deliveries had more episiotomies (75.6% versus 37.5%), blood loss of more than 500 mL (39.3% versus 11.5%), hospital stays of 5 or more days (14.7% versus 3%), more neonates requiring assisted ventilation (11.7% versus 5.3%), more neonatal hypotonia (9.6% versus 3.9%), and more babies with hypoglycemia (7.5% versus 3.4%) (Fraser et al., 2000).

MANUAL ROTATION

Most fetuses rotate to an occiput anterior position spontaneously by the time of delivery. When a fetus does not rotate to an occiput anterior position, the obstetric provider may manually or digitally rotate the fetal head. Manual rotation is performed with the examiner's hand. Digital rotation is

accomplished using fingertips to exert pressure on the fetal head to help it rotate from an occiput posterior position to an occiput anterior position (Reichman, Gdansky, Latinsky, Labi & Samueloff, 2007).

OPERATIVE VAGINAL DELIVERY: DOUBLE SET-UP

A double set-up means all of the instruments for both an operative vaginal delivery and an operative abdominal delivery are ready for use. A double set-up occurs in an operating room. An operative vaginal delivery may occur in a birthing room. If the forceps or vacuum extractor, or both, fails to deliver the fetus in the room, an immediate cesarean section will be needed. You should then mobilize other nurses to help you move the patient to the operating room.

VACUUM-ASSISTED VAGINAL DELIVERY

A vacuum-assisted vaginal delivery is also known as a ventouse delivery. The decision to use the vacuum extractor is the obstetric provider's responsibility. Labor and delivery nurses must know the indications and contraindications for use of the vacuum extractor and assist with the procedure as needed (see Exhibits 7.3, 7.4, and 7.5). If nurses believe the vacuum extractor is contraindicated, they should discuss their concerns with their charge nurse or supervisor and with the physician or midwife prior to the use of the vacuum extractor. Nurses are also responsible for observing the length of time the vacuum extractor is applied and removed, and the number of pop-offs.

Dr. Aldo Vacca (2004) wrote that vacuum-assisted delivery should not be used as a rescue procedure for the delivery of a severely compromised fetus. However, in some situations, the obstetric provider may believe a cesarean section will take longer to accomplish than a vacuum-assisted delivery. The obstetric provider may feel compelled to deliver the fetus vaginally. The decision to perform an operative vaginal delivery instead of a cesarean section will be based on the maternal and fetal condition, cervical dilatation, uterine contractions, fetal descent and position, molding of the fetal head, the adequacy of analgesia, and the experience of the obstetric provider who will be using forceps or a vacuum extractor (Doumouchtsis & Arulkumaran, 2008).

TWO KINDS OF VACUUM CUPS

The obstetric provider will usually say, "I need a vacuum." The nurse should provide the vacuum extractor only if the fetus is at or below 0 station and there are no contraindications to vacuum extractor use. The nurse also provides the correct vacuum cup based on the fetal position. If you do not know the fetal position, you should ask the obstetric provider, "What is the station and position?" Record the station and position at that time or in your summary notes for the delivery.

There are two cup shapes (see Figure 7.11). A posterior cup (on the right in Figure 7.11), can be used when the fetus is in any position because the handle bends. This makes it easy for the provider to place the cup over the flexion point near the

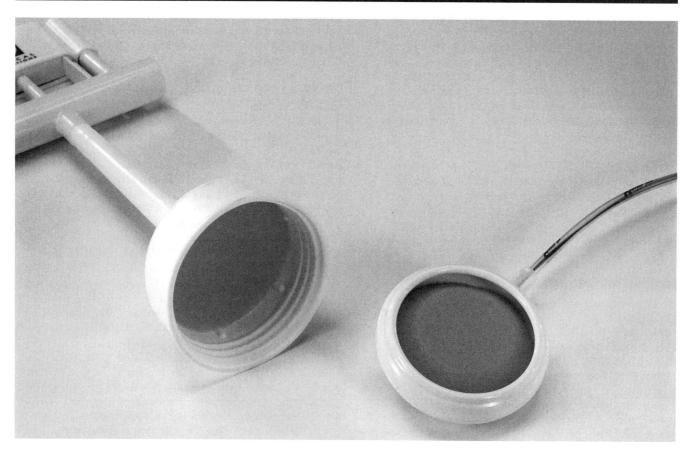

Figure 7.11: The bell-shaped cup (Kiwi™ Vacuum-Assisted Delivery System: ProCup) is on the left, and the posterior cup (OmniCup) is on the right. (Photograph courtesy of Clinical Innovations, Murray, Utah.)

posterior fontanel. The bell-shaped cup (on the left in Figure 7.11) has a stiff handle and is used if the fetus is in an occiput anterior position and the flexion point is easy to reach.

Locate and identify the types of vacuum extractors and cups used at your hospital. What is the shape of the cup? Is it shaped like a bell or trumpet, or is it shaped like a flat mushroom? The flat or mushroom-shaped cup is also known as a posterior cup. It is usually a rigid cup with a handle that bends near the cup. Posterior cups have a higher failure rate than soft cups (Johanson & Menon, 2000). Does the handle bend or is the handle stiff? Look at the gauge on the device. Is it in mm Hg or cm Hg? To deliver the proper suction, the vacuum will be pumped up to near 500 mm Hg! This is not a weak device. Imagine a blood pressure cuff on your arm pumping up to 500 mg Hg.

THE FLEXION POINT

The flexion point is approximately 3 cm in front of the posterior fontanel. Examples of posterior cups are the M-Style® Mushroom® MityVac® or the Kiwi™ OmniCup. The bell-shaped cup should only be used with occiput anterior positions in a low or outlet location because of its stiff handle and the location

of the flexion point (McQuivey, 2004). The provider should let you know if you hand him or her the wrong cup, but you are still responsible for documenting the fetal station and position, and for providing the appropriate equipment for each delivery.

SUDDEN DISENGAGEMENTS (POP-OFFS)

After the obstetric provider applies the vacuum extractor, he or she will pull on the handle during contractions, but not between contractions (McQuivey, 2004). Sometimes during traction, the vacuum extractor cup will disengage. This separation of the cup from the fetal scalp is called a "pop-off."

The number of pop-offs should not exceed the manufacturer's guidelines. Nurses must inform the obstetric provider after the last pop-off that meets the guidelines has occurred. For example, you might say, "Doctor, we now have two pop-offs. The operating room is available." Use of both a vacuum extractor and forceps increases the risk of fetal injury. Therefore, a nurse should not offer the physician or midwife forceps after he or she has used the vacuum extractor and has met, but not exceeded, the manufacturer's guidelines for pop-offs.

Exhibit 7.3: General rules for vacuum extractor use (Society of Obstetricians and Gynaecologists of Canada, 2004).

1. A valid indication for use should be documented prior to beginning procedure.
2. Verbal informed consent must be obtained from the patient prior to use.
3. An alternative plan for delivery should be in place.
4. The operating room crew and neonatal resuscitation team should be immediately available.
5. Limit pop-offs to 2 or 3 depending on the product (read the manufacturer's guidelines).
6. Empty the patient's bladder before use.
7. Limit total use of the vacuum to 15 to 20 minutes from the first application to its removal.
8. There must be descent of the fetus with every pull.
9. There should be no greater than 10 minutes of traction at maximal pressure.

Exhibit 7.4: Prerequisites and indications for vacuum extractor use (Vacca, 2004).

1. Tip of the skull (station) at or below 0
2. 10-cm dilatation
3. Near term or term gestation
4. No abnormal or nonreassuring fetal heart rate pattern. This is not a rescue device
5. Failure to deliver spontaneously following an appropriately managed second stage of labor
6. Maternal exhaustion or need to avoid expulsive efforts
7. Inadequate expulsive efforts

Exhibit 7.5: Contraindications for vacuum extractor use (McQuivey, 2004; Putta & Spencer, 2000; Society of Obstetricians and Gynaecologists of Canada, 2004).

1. 34 to 36 weeks of gestation or less
2. Fetal bleeding disorder or bone demineralization disorder
3. Unengaged fetal head
4. Incomplete cervical dilatation
5. Suspected cephalopelvic disproportion or macrosomia
6. Unknown position of the fetal head, a face or brow presentation or a nonvertex presentation
7. Lack of informed consent
8. Lack of operator skill

form the obstetric provider of fetal decelerations, bradycardia or tachycardia, or a decrease in or loss of variability. If the fetus suffers a bleed, you may see a flat, tachycardic baseline. The obstetric provider needs to know the fetal heart rate to make the decision to abandon the procedure and proceed to cesarean section.

DOCUMENT VACUUM EXTRACTOR USE

Both the obstetric provider and the nurse who assists with the procedure should write a summary note after delivery. Be sure that 10-cm dilatation is noted along with the fetal position and station prior to vacuum use. Document that the bladder was emptied before vacuum extractor use. Document the type of vacuum extractor used, for example, Kiwi™ OmniCup. Include in your summary note the time it was initially applied, the maximum pressure if you pumped it, and the time it was removed at the end of the procedure. You may also add whether the vacuum pressure was decreased or maintained between contractions or the number of contractions during which the vacuum was used. If there were pop-offs, the number should be documented. You should read your hospital policy, procedures, and protocol related to operative vaginal delivery.

Documentation example: Straight cath by this nurse at 1100 with approximately 100 mL of amber urine noted. At 1110, Kiwi posterior vacuum cup applied by Dr. Pully. Fetus +2, occiput posterior. Pulled over 5 contractions. Vacuum discontinued at 1130, one pop-off.

Documentation example: Mityvac bell-shaped cup placed on delivery table. ROA, +3 station prior to use. Baby delivered within 5 minutes of vacuum application. No sudden disengagements.

Documentation example: Posterior cup applied by Dr. Golightly at 0420. Fetus at 0 station at 0404. Physician

While the vacuum extractor is in use, you may be asked to release the pressure or the provider may use a quick-release button if a hand-held device is being used.

Pop-offs occur when there is incorrect cup placement, or prolonged or misguided traction (McQuivey, 2004). Pop-offs are related to rapid decompression that can cause injuries such as intracranial bleeds (Society of Obstetricians and Gynaecologists of Canada, 2004). Other complications of vacuum extractor use include cephalhematoma, subgaleal hemorrhage, skull fractures, and bleeds in the head and eyes (Doumouchtsis & Arulkumaran, 2008).

MONITOR THE FETUS

The scalp is the fetal defense to the resistance created by maternal tissue (Towner & Ciotti, 2007). If a vacuum extractor is applied to the fetal scalp, injuries may occur, including life-threatening bleeding. Nurses have the responsibility of monitoring the fetus during this procedure. Nurses also must in-reports fetal descent with each pull and fetus at +3 station prior to vacuum use. Vacuum applied between 0420 and 0440. Charge nurse Damadder at bedside. Forceps requested by physician, who was informed by the charge nurse that the OR is available. Patient moved to operating room at 0445.

Your summary note should include notification of your supervisor or charge nurse and names of the personnel who were present in the room during the operative vaginal delivery. You should also document the total number of minutes of vacuum extractor use and the length of time that the vacuum was at maximal pressure. The application of maximal pressure should be 10 minutes or less.

You must document your assessments of the neonate. Include the presence of a chignon, cephalhematoma(s), molding, overlapping sutures, and caput. Chignon is pronounced "sheen-yon" and comes from the French phrase "chignon du cou," which is where a woman would wear her hair in a bun. Note any neonatal bruises and their locations. Record the Apgar scores as well as the person who assigned them.

Documentation example after a vacuum-assisted delivery: Patient's questions answered by provider and patient consent obtained. Charge nurse called to room. 10/100%/+2, vertex ROP with mild caput per Dr. Vaqum. Kiwi posterior vacuum cup placed at 2102 by Dr. Vaqum. No pop-offs. Total time cup was on fetal head was 7 minutes over 3 contractions. Variable decelerations noted, lasting 40 to 50 seconds, dropping to 70 to 80 bpm during contractions with FHR baseline 150 to 155 bpm between contractions. Head delivered at 2108, birth at 2109. Infant handed to awaiting neonatal team. See newborn record and delivery record for additional details.

FORCEPS-ASSISTED VAGINAL DELIVERY

Instead of a vacuum extractor, the physician may call for forceps after obtaining verbal informed consent from the patient. The bladder should be emptied prior to the application of forceps. You should add a catheter and lubricant to the delivery table prior to use of a vacuum extractor or forceps. Usually the sterile lubricant is squeezed on the open sterile glove wrapper or directly onto the drape on the table.

Labor and delivery nurses should unwrap the sterile forceps and hand them to the physician or place them on the delivery table. You should find the location of forceps in your labor and delivery unit, note the various types, and learn the rules and contraindications for forceps use (see Exhibits 7.6 and 7.7).

Prior to handing a vacuum extractor or forceps to an obstetric provider, you should be familiar with his or her credentials. Ask your charge nurse or supervisor to show you where these privileges are listed. In some cases, a midwife or family prac-

---

Exhibit 7.6: General rules for use of forceps.

1. A valid indication for use prior to beginning procedure
2. 10 cm dilatation and at least a +2 station
3. Bladder emptied prior to use
4. Verbal informed consent obtained prior to use
5. Operating room crew and neonatal resuscitation team immediately available
6. Operating room available

Exhibit 7.7: Contraindications for forceps use (Society of Obstetricians and Gynaecologists of Canada, 2004).

1. Station unengaged (above 0)
2. Less than 10 cm of dilatation
3. Suspected cephalopelvic disproportion
4. Unknown position of the fetal head
5. Lack of verbal informed consent
6. Lack of operator skill

---

tice physician may be required to call an obstetrician for a consultation prior to operative vaginal delivery.

MIDFORCEPS AND LOW FORCEPS

The classification of a forceps delivery depends on the station of the fetal head when the forceps are applied. The three acceptable levels for forceps delivery are mid, low, and outlet. High forceps should never be done (Hankins & Rowe, 1996). A mid station is between 0 and +2 (McQuivey, 2004). Midforceps deliveries often require the physician to rotate the fetus. Unlike use of the vacuum extractor, where delivery is assisted during contractions, the physician can use forceps during and between contractions. Low forceps are applied to the fetal head when the station is between +2 or lower, but the fetal head is not yet on the pelvic floor. Outlet forceps are applied to a fetus whose scalp is crowning and visible at the introitus without separating the labia (American College of Obstetricians and Gynecologists, 2000).

If the physician stands to use the forceps, the pull will have less force on the fetus than if the provider is seated. The average traction force for women obstetrical residents who are standing is 45.5 pounds compared with 61.3 pounds when they are sitting. The average traction force exerted by male residents who are standing is 69.5 pounds, compared with 85.8 pounds when they are sitting (Leslie, Dispasquale-Lehnerz, & Smith, 2005).

The fetus is fragile and the use of forceps compresses the fetal head increasing the risk of a neonatal facial nerve injury, skull fractures, intracranial bleeding, anemia, and death (Doumouchtsis & Anulkumaran, 2008). In the rare event the physician desires high forceps (above a 0 station), you must advocate for a change in the plan of care. You or your charge nurse should calmly and quietly inform the physician that the operating room is available and the operating room crew is standing by for a cesarean section. Do not provide the forceps for a high forceps attempt. "Best practice" is to use either forceps or a vacuum extractor to facilitate birth, but not one followed by the other. If both are needed, there should be a clinically compelling and justified reason, and the pediatrician and neonatal resuscitation crew should be in the room at the time of birth. The use of both forceps and a vacuum extractor is associated with more neonatal injuries than when only one is used (American College of Obstetricians and Gynecologists, 2000; Mazza et al., 2008).

The physician should document the estimated fetal weight, the indications for the instrument delivery, and the fetal presentation and station prior to the use of a vacuum extractor or forceps (Mazza et al., 2008). Nurses should document the time the physician applied and removed the forceps. Nurses and physicians are part of the same team. By following a protocol that includes the information in Exhibits 7.6 and 7.7, injury should be prevented.

> **Documentation example:** Infant's head delivered at 0130 with Simpson's forceps by Dr. Fuerza. Delivery at 0131. Nuchal cord x 1, loose. Terminal meconium noted. Spontaneous cry. Forceps marks and bruising noted over both cheeks. Molding and slight caput. Placenta to pathology. Umbilical cord blood samples obtained by this nurse for cord blood gases.

FACTORS THAT INCREASE THE RISK OF A CESAREAN SECTION

Fibroids in the lower segment act like a boulder blocking the exit of the passenger and significantly increase the risk of cesarean section (Vergani et al., 1994). You should locate the ultrasound reports in the medical record and read them. It is important for you to note the presence and location of uterine fibroids because they can obstruct the pathway.

Maternal height and obesity are related to the risk of a cesarean section (see Exhibit 7.8). Women who are less than 5 feet 3 inches tall, and who are diagnosed with cephalopelvic disproportion are five times more likely to require a cesarean section than taller women. Nulliparous women who are overweight or obese prior to becoming pregnant also have an increased risk for a cesarean section compared with their normal-weight counterparts (see Exhibits 7.8 and 7.9) (Dempsey et al., 2005). Labor duration and the need for a cesarean section are related to fetal weight (Turner et al., 1990). The number of cesarean sections doubles from 4% for babies weighing 3,500 to 3,999 grams to 8% when the fetus weighs 4,000 to 4,999 grams.

Factors that predispose a woman to a cesarean section are multiple and factors besides the characteristics of the mother or baby affect the cesarean section rate (Chaillet & Dumont, 2006). Strategies and initiatives have been undertaken to safely

---

Exhibit 7.8: Weight classifications by BMI for adults (derived from Dempsey et al., 2005).

Weight Status	BMI	Recommended Weight Gain During Pregnancy
Underweight	< 18.5	28 to 40 lbs
Normal	18.5 to 24.9	25 to 35 lbs
Overweight	25 to 29.9	15 to 25 lbs
Obese	30 or more	15 lbs

Exhibit 7.9: Factors that increase the risk of a cesarean section.

1. Maternal height, especially women who were less than 5 feet tall*
2. Obesity**
3. Estimated fetal weight, especially more than 4,000 grams***
4. Extremes of neonatal birthweight****
5. Increasing neonatal head circumference****
6. Increasing maternal age****
7. Diabetes mellitus****
8. Epidural use, although some disagree****
9. Previous cesarean section****
10. Noncephalic presentation (breech, etc.)****

*Parsons et al., 1989
**Witter et al., 1995
***Farina et al., 1998, Kolderup et al., 1997 (Research was conducted in San Francisco, California)
****Patel et al., 2005 (Research was conducted in the United Kingdom)

---

decrease the cesarean section rate. Some hospitals use peer review, medical audits, and feedback to providers in an attempt to augment best practices and decrease the cesarean section rate. Other programs include quality improvement incentives using active management of labor protocols, continuity of care, and one-to-one nursing care during active labor (see Exhibit 7.10).

Low-risk orders (Exhibit 7.10, item 3) is vague, but probably means the woman and her fetus do not have an increased risk for injury during the pregnancy. Auscultation (item 8) means there is not continuous use of a fetal monitor and maternal immobilization. However, it does not mean electronic fetal monitoring cannot be used when decelerations or a tachycardic or bradycardic rate are detected by auscultation.

TIME-OUT PRIOR TO THE CESAREAN SECTION

When the cesarean section is not an emergency, reconfirmation of the patient's identity and a time-out procedure are im-

---

Exhibit 7.10: Factors that are related to lower cesarean section rates.

1. Admission when the cervix is ≥ 3 centimeters dilated*
2. Epidural placement at ≥ 4 centimeters*
3. "Low-risk" orders*
4. Doulas**
5. Induction**
6. Admission guidelines**
7. Use of the Friedman labor curve**
8. Auscultation**
9. Pain management**
10. Review cesarean sections (in committee)**
11. Intrauterine pressure catheter use***
12. Pitocin use***
13. Fetal scalp stimulation to evaluate fetal status***
14. Waiting an average of 5.2 hours to diagnose dystocia and proceed to cesarean section***

*Fernandez, Canterino, Dambeck, & McKeever, 1999
**Pinette & Blackstone, 1999
***Gilbert et al., 2000

---

portant. A time-out has become the standard of practice in some countries. Implants and special equipment (such as a pacemaker) should be mentioned to the operating room crew prior to the cesarean section. Some labor and delivery nurses hold the signed operative consent in their hands as a reminder of the planned procedure while they perform the time-out.

Example #1 of a cesarean section time-out in the operating room: RN: "What is your name and date of birth?" Patient: "My name is Cesara Tuday and I was born on April 1, 1988." RN: "I have confirmed that your name and date of birth on your identification band are correct. Patient: "Good." RN to Physician: "This is Cesara Tuday. She is having a primary cesarean section for a breech presentation. There is no tubal ligation planned today. She has no allergies and no special equipment. The site and side will be the abdomen."

Example #2 of a cesarean section time-out in the operating room: Physician: "I'm doing a primary cesarean section today on Mary Hadalittlelamb. We are not tying her tubes." RN: "I have verified her identity. She has no special equipment and no allergies."

Documentation example: 1145: Time-out completed prior to cesarean section.

UTERINE RUPTURE: AN UNPLANNED EXIT

Uterine rupture has been defined as "a disruption of the uterine muscle and peritoneum or a uterine muscle separation with extension to the bladder or broad ligament found at the time of cesarean delivery or laparotomy" (Landon et al., 2006). The risk of uterine rupture is associated with oxytocin augmentation, induction of labor, epidural anesthesia, and a period of less than 2 years since a previous cesarean section (Landon et al., 2006). Other researchers describe risk factors for uterine rupture as one or more of the following: a previous vertical or classical uterine incision, no previous vaginal delivery, induction of labor, oxytocin use, more than one cesarean delivery, stalled labor progress, and a thin lower uterine segment prior to labor (Bujold, Bujold, Hamilton, Harel, & Gauthier, 2002). If labor progress is stalled and there is mechanical dystocia, the passageway to birth may be through a hole in the uterus and a subsequent abdominal delivery by cesarean section.

With women who have a history of cesarean section or whose labor is being induced or augmented with oxytocin, you must be extra vigilant in monitoring the fetus and the uterus. Listen to the fetal voice by being attentive to changes in the heart rate pattern, fetal movement, and changes in the color of the amniotic fluid. Uterine rupture is accompanied by signs of fetal hypoxia, such as variable decelerations that increase in size, late decelerations, and bradycardia. There may be little to no vaginal bleeding. Closely observe the uterine activity pattern and act to decrease hyperstimulation. If the uterus ruptures when there is an intrauterine pressure catheter, contractions most likely will not be recorded. If the tocotransducer is in place, the "staircase sign" may indicate a uterine rupture. In that case, the graph line of each consecutive contraction is shorter in height than the preceeding one (Matsuo, Scanlon, Atlas, & Kopelman, 2008). If the patient has an epidural she may feel neck, shoulder, or jaw discomfort. If she reports feeling a "pop" she may have had a uterine rupture (Grotegut, Fitzpatrick, & Brancazio, 2008). If you suspect a uterine rupture, call for help immediately and institute intrauterine resuscitation measures.

REVIEW QUESTIONS

True/False: Decide if the statements are true or false.

1. Maternal height is related to labor progress and the risk of a cesarean section.
2. One millimeter of blood or fluid weighs approximately 1 gram.
3. The risk of ascending infection increases with the first vaginal examination.
4. Vaginal bleeding is synonymous with bloody show.
5. McRoberts' maneuver and suprapubic pressure are the first steps to relieve shoulder dystocia.
6. Forceps- and vacuum-assisted deliveries are relatively risk-free procedures.
7. Continuous labor support, pain management, and the use of a labor curve may lower the cesarean section rate.
8. Maternal obesity decreases the risk of a cesarean section.

9. Documentation for a vacuum-assisted vaginal delivery should include the type of vacuum used, total time on the fetal head, vacuum pressure, and the number of pop-offs.

10. Increasing uterine activity with each consecutive contraction is a sign of uterine rupture.

References

Allen, R. H., & Gurewitsch, E. D. (2005). Case reports. Temporary Erb-Duchenne palsy without shoulder dystocia or traction to the fetal head. *Obstetrics & Gynecology, 105,* 1210–1212.

American College of Obstetricians and Gynecologists. (2000). Operative vaginal delivery. Number 17. *Clinical management guidelines for obstetrician-gynecologists.* Washington, DC: Author.

Bewley, S. (1992). The law, medical students and assault. *British Medical Journal, 304,* 1551–1553.

Bewley, S. (2005). Who should be the guardians of women's "sacred space"? [Letter]. *American Journal of Obstetrics and Gynecology, 192,* 655–662.

Brown, C. L., Ludwiczak, M. H., Blanco, J. D., & Hirsch, E. E. (1993). Cervical dilation: Accuracy of visual and digital examinations. *Obstetrics & Gynecology, 81,* 215–216.

Bujold, E., Bujold, C., Hamilton, E. F., Harel, F., & Gauthier, R. J. (2002). The impact of a single-layer or double-layer closure on uterine rupture. *American Journal of Obstetrics and Gynecology, 186*(6), 1326–1330.

Casey, B. M., & Cox, S. M. (1997). Chorioamnionitis and endometritis. *Infectious Disease Clinics of North America, 11*(1), 203–222.

Chaillet, N., & Dumont, A. (2007). Evidence-based strategies for reducing cesarean section rates: A meta-analysis. *Birth, 34*(1), 53–64.

Dandolu, V., Lawrence, L. Gaughan, J.P., Grotegut, C., Harmanli, O. H., Jaspan, D., & Hernandez, E. (2005). Trends in the rate of shoulder dystocia over two decades. *Journal of Maternal, Fetal and Neonatal Medicine, 18*(5), 305–310.

Dempsey, J. C., Ashiny, Z., Qiu, C.-F., Miller, R. S., Sorensen, T. K., & Williams, M. A. (2005). Maternal pre-pregnancy overweight status and obesity as risk factors for cesarean delivery. *Journal of Maternal-Fetal and Neonatal Medicine, 17*(3), 179–185.

Doumouchtsis, S. K., & Arulkumaran, S. (2008). Head trauma after instrumental births. *Clinics in Perinatology, 35,* 69–83.

Fahey, J. O., & Mighty, H. E. (2008). Shoulder dystocia: Using simulation to train providers and teams. *Journal of Perinatal and Neonatal Nursing, 22*(2), 114–122.

Farina, A., Luzio, L. D., & Carinci, P. (1998). Birth injury and macrosomic fetuses: Association with mode of delivery [Letter]. *American Journal of Obstetrics and Gynecology, 178*(4), 867.

Fernandez, C. L., Canterino, J. C., Dambeck, S., & McKeever, J. (1999). Cesarean delivery rate reduction [Abstract].

American Journal of Obstetrics and Gynecology, 180(1, Part 2), S113.

Fraser, W. D., Marcoux, S., Krauss, I., Douglas, J. K., Goulet, C., & Boulvain, M. (2000). Multicenter, randomized, controlled trial of delayed pushing for nulliparous women in the second stage of labor with continuous epidural analgesia. *American Journal of Obstetrics & Gynecology, 182*(5), 1165–1172.

Gilbert, W. M., Melnikow, J., Romano, P., Schembri, M., Keyzer, J., & Kravitz, R. L. (2000). What processes of care during labor affect the cesarean section (C/S) rate? [Abstract]. *American Journal of Obstetrics & Gynecology, 182*(1, Part 2), S135.

Grotegut, C. A., Fitzpatrick, C. B., & Brancazio, L. R. (2008). A sudden pop. *American Journal of Obstetrics and Gynecology, 198*(3), 340.

Gurewitsch, E. D. (2007). Optimizing shoulder dystocia management to prevent birth injury. *Clinical Obstetrics and Gynecology, 50*(3), 592–606.

Gurewitsch, E. D., Kim, E. J., Yang, J. H., Outland, K. E., McDonald, M. K., & Allen, R. H. (2005). Comparing McRoberts' and Rubin's maneuvers for initial management of shoulder dystocia: An objective evaluation. *American Journal of Obstetrics and Gynecology, 192*(1), 153–160.

Hackmon, R., Bornstein, E., Ferber, A., Horami, J., O'Reilly Green, C.P., & Divon, M.Y. (2007). Combined analysis with amniotic fluid index and estimated fetal weight for prediction of severe macrosomia at birth. *American Journal of Obstetrics and Gynecology, 196,* 333–335.

Hankins, G. D. V., & Rowe, T. F. (1996). Operative vaginal delivery—Year 2000. *American Journal of Obstetrics and Gynecology, 175*(2), 275–282.

Imseis, H. M., Trout, W. C., & Gabbe, S. G. (1999). The microbiologic effect of digital cervical examination. *American Journal of Obstetrics and Gynecology, 180*(3, Part 1), 578–580.

Johanson R., & Menon, V. (2000). Soft versus rigid vacuum extractor cups for assisted vaginal delivery. *Cochrane Database of Systematic Reviews,* Issue 2. Art. No.: CD000446. doi: 10.1002/14651858.CD000446.

Kolderup, L. B., Laros, R. K., & Musci, T. J. (1997). Incidence of persistent birth injury in macrosomic infants: Association with mode of delivery. *American Journal of Obstetrics and Gynecology, 177*(1), 37–41.

Landon, M. B., Spong, C. Y., Thom, E., Hauth, J. C., Bloom, S. L., & Varner, M. W. (2006). Risk of uterine rupture with a trial of labor in women with multiple and single prior cesarean delivery. *Obstetrics and Gynecology, 108*(1), 12–20.

Leslie, K. K., Dispasquale-Lehnerz, P., & Smith, M. (2005). Obstetric forceps training using visual feedback and the isometric strength testing unit. *Obstetrics & Gynecology, 105*(2), 377–382.

Mahlmeister, L.R. (2008). Best practices in perinatal nursing: Risk identification and management of shoulder dystocia. *Journal of Perinatal & Neonatal Nursing, 22*(2), 91–94.

Matsuo, K., Scanlon, J. T., Atlas, R. O., & Kopelman, J. N. (2008). Staircase sign: A newly described uterine contraction pattern seen in rupture of unscarred gravid uterus. *Journal of Obstetrics & Gynaecological Research, 34*(1), 100–104.

Mazza, F., Kitchens, J., Akin, M., Fowler, D., Henry, E., & Landers, S. (2008). The road to zero preventable birth injuries. *Joint Commission Journal on Quality and Patient Safety, 34*(4), 201–205.

McCaul IV, J. F., Rogers, L. W., Perry, K. G., Martin, R. W., Albert, J. R., & Morrison, J. C. (1997). Premature rupture of membranes at term with an unfavorable cervix: Comparison of expectant management, vaginal prostaglandin, and oxytocin induction. *Southern Medical Journal, 90*(12), 1229–1233.

McQuivey, R. W. (2004). Vacuum-assisted delivery: A review. *Journal of Maternal-Fetal and Neonatal Medicine, 16*, 171–179.

Munson, L. A., Graham, A., Koos, B. J., & Valenzuela, G. J. (1985). Is there a need for digital examination in patients with spontaneous rupture of membranes? *American Journal of Obstetrics and Gynecology, 153*, 562–563.

Newton, E. R., Prihoda, T. J., & Gibbs, R. S. (1989). Logistic regression analysis of risk factors for intra-amniotic infection. *Obstetrics & Gynecology, 73*(4), 571–575.

Pandy, V., Jaremko, K., Moore, R. M., Mercer, B. M., Stetzer, B., & Kumar, D. (2007). The force required to rupture fetal membranes paradoxically increases with acute in vitro repeated stretching. *American Journal of Obstetrics and Gynecology, 196*, 165.e1–165.e7.

Parsons, M. T., Winegar, A., Siefert, L., & Spellacy, W. N. (1989). Pregnancy outcomes in short women. *Journal of Reproductive Medicine, 34*(5), 357–261.

Patel, R. R., Peters, T. J., Murphy, D. J., & ALSPAC Study Team. (2005). Prenatal risk factors for Caesarean section: Analyses of the ALSPAC cohort of 12,944 women in England. *International Journal of Epidemiology, 34*, 353–367.

Pinette, M. G., & Blackstone, J. (1999). Rapid reduction of cesarean deliveries [Abstract]. *American Journal of Obstetrics and Gynecology, 180*(1, Part 2), S113.

Putta, L. V., & Spencer, J. P. (2000). Assisted vaginal delivery using the vacuum extractor. *American Family Physician, 62*, 1316–1320.

Reichman, O., Gdansky, E., Latinsky, B., Labi, S., & Samueloff, A. (2008). Digital rotation from occipito-posterior to occipito-anterior decreases the need for cesarean section. *European Journal of Obstetrics & Gynecology and Reproductive Biology, 136*, 25–28.

Richmond, J. R., Morin, L., & Benjamin, A. (2002). Extremely preterm vaginal breech delivery en caul. *Obstetrics & Gynecology, 99*(6), 1025–1030.

Seaward, P. G., Hannah, M. E., Myhr, T. L., Farine, D., Ohlsson, A., & Wang, E. E. (1998). International multicenter term PROM study: Evaluation of predictors of neonatal infection in infants born to patients with premature rupture of membranes at term. Premature rupture of membranes. *American Journal of Obstetrics & Gynecology, 179*(3, Pt. 1), 635–639.

Sickbert-Bennett, E. E., Weber, D. J., Gergen-Teague, M. F., Sobsey, M. D., Samsa, G. P., & Rutala, W. A. (2005). Comparative efficacy of hand hygiene agents in the reduction of bacteria and viruses. *American Journal of Infection Control, 33*(2), 67–77.

Society of Obstetricians and Gynaecologists of Canada. (2004). Guidelines for operative vaginal birth. Number 148. *International Journal of Gynecology & Obstetrics, 88*, 229–236.

Soper, D. E., Mayhall, G., & Dalton, H. P. (1989). Risk factors for intraamniotic infection: A prospective epidemiologic study. *American Journal of Obstetrics and Gynecology, 161*(3), 562–568.

Studd, J. (1975). Identification of high-risk labours [Letter to the editor]. *British Medical Journal*, 702.

Towner, D. R., & Ciotti, M. C. (2007). Operative vaginal delivery: A cause of birth injury or is it? *Clinical Obstetrics and Gynecology, 50*(3), 563–581.

Turner, M. J., Rasmussen, M. J., Turner, J. E., Boylan, P. C., MacDonald, D., & Stronge, J. M. (1990). The influence of birth weight on labor in nulliparas. *Obstetrics & Gynecology, 76*(2), 159–163.

Vacca, A. (2004). Vacuum-assisted delivery: Practical techniques to improve patient outcomes. *OBG Management*, S1–12.

Vergani, P., Ghidini, A., Strobelt, N., Roncaglia, N., Locatelli, A., Lapinski, R. H., & Mangioni, C. (1994). Do uterine leiomyomas influence pregnancy outcome? *American Journal of Perinatology, 11*(5), 356–358.

Witter, F. R., Caulfield, L. E., & Stolzfus, R. J. (1995). Influence of maternal anthropometric status and birth weight on the risk of cesarean delivery. *Obstetrics & Gynecology, 85*(6), 947–951.

Zaretsky, M.V., Alexander, J. M., McIntire, D. D., Hatab, M. R., Twickler, D. M., & Leveno, K. J. (2005). Magnetic resonance imaging pelvimetry and the prediction of labor dystocia. *Obstetrics & Gynecology, 106*(5, Part 1), 919–926.

Zhang, X., Decker, A., Platt, R. W., & Kramer, M. S. (2008). How big is too big? The perinatal consequences of fetal macrosomia. *American Journal of Obstetrics and Gynecology, 198*, 527–519.

8

Presentation, Station, and Position

Be always sure you're right.
—Davy Crockett

PRESENTATION

Labor should progress toward a vaginal delivery if the fetus is in the right presentation, at the right station, and in the right position. Presentation is the part of the fetus that lies over the pelvic inlet and is expected to be delivered first. Presentation is confirmed by an ultrasound examination or palpation of the presenting part with your gloved fingers during a vaginal examination. The three types of presentation are: head first (cephalic), pelvis first (breech), and shoulder first (transverse lie) (see Figures 8.1, 8.2, and 8.3). The most common presentation is a cephalic presentation. When the fetal head is palpated during a vaginal examination, it is recorded as a "vertex" presentation. The word *vertex* means the "highest point, top, acme, apex, or peak" of an object. A vertex presentation is synonymous with a cephalic presentation.

COMPOUND PRESENTATION

A compound presentation (see Figures 8.4 and 8.5) involves the prolapse of one or more limbs next to the presenting part. A hand, arm, foot, or leg may be felt next to the head or buttocks during a vaginal examination. Compound presentations are rarely found during spontaneous labor. They are more common after artificial or premature rupture of the membranes, especially if the fetus is at a high station. They are also found in cases of preterm labor or when pelvic masses displace the presenting part.

There are two types of compound presentation. The first is called a cephalic presentation with prolapse of the upper limb or lower limb. In other words, the arm or leg drops down next to the head or buttocks (see Figure 8.4). Prolapse of the lower limb next to the fetal head occurs when the leg is flexed at the hip and the leg is straight at the knee. The baby is essentially bent in half. The second type of compound presentation is called a breech presentation with prolapse of the hand or arm (see Figure 8.5).

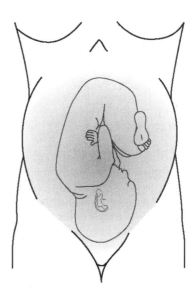

Figure 8.1: Cephalic presentation.

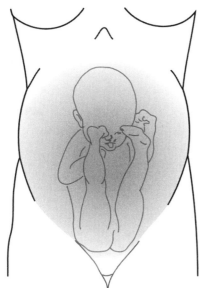

Figure 8.2: Breech presentation.

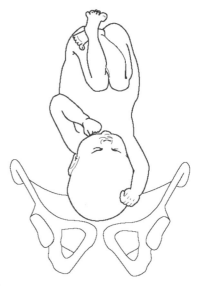

Figure 8.4: Compound cephalic presentation with prolapse of the upper limb (head and hand presenting). This is the most common compound presentation.

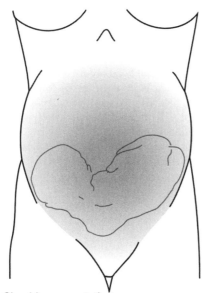

Figure 8.3: Shoulder presentation.

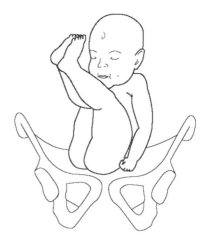

Figure 8.5: Compound breech presentation with prolapse of the hand.

The risks to the fetus of a compound presentation include umbilical cord prolapse, umbilical cord compression, circulatory compromise in the prolapsed limb, and bruising of the prolapsed limb. If the hand is next to the neck, and there is a nuchal cord, the hand may be pressing on the umbilical cord. If you feel fingers next to the baby's head or buttocks during the vaginal examination, notify the midwife or physician immediately. If the hand has not prolapsed past the baby's head, he or she will try to make the hand retract. If the hand or arm prolapses past the presenting part, a vaginal delivery will probably not be possible. In that case, a cesarean section will be performed.

Following are examples of presentations, including a vertex presentation (head first) (see Figure 8.6), a brow presentation (head first with the forehead leading the way) (see Figure 8.7), and a face presentation (see Figure 8.8). A brow or face presentation may occur when there is a very tight fit and the fetus does not have enough room to flex its head and bring its chin down to its chest. Sometimes, these babies will have to be delivered by cesarean section.

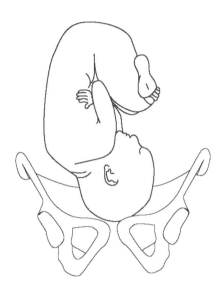

Figure 8.6: An attitude of flexion with a cephalic presentation.

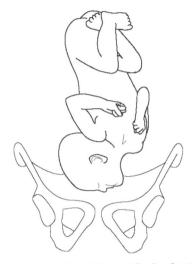

Figure 8.8: Face presentation with an attitude of extension.

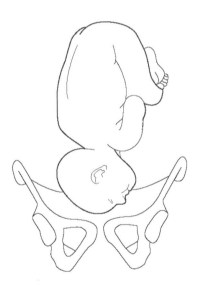

Figure 8.7: Brow presentation with an attitude of extension.

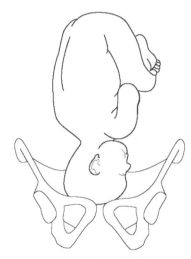

Figure 8.9: Military attitude with a cephalic presentation.

ATTITUDE

"Attitude" is the position of the head in a cephalic presentation. Attitude may be flexion, military, or extension. Attitude is determined by the relationship between the fetal chin and chest. When the fetal chin is near the chest, the attitude is called flexion (see Figure 8.6). When the fetal head is neither flexed nor extended, it is called a military attitude (see Figure 8.9). A military attitude may delay descent or cause an arrest of descent because a larger surface is presenting. The fetus may also have an attitude of extension when a brow or face is presenting (see Figures 8.7 and 8.8).

Passage of the brow is slow and often traumatic to the mother. Perineal and rectal lacerations are inevitable because of the large diameter of the fetal presenting part. If a brow presentation is detected early in labor, the physician may be able to flex the fetal head, which should speed up labor and decrease the risk of maternal trauma. If you feel part of the fetal face or an angle instead of a dome, there may be a brow presentation. Notify the midwife or physician of your findings and inform your charge nurse or supervisor.

FACE PRESENTATION

If you feel a round small lump, with or without something fluttering beneath your finger, you are probably feeling the baby's eye. If you feel two little holes or a protruding lump you may be feeling the fetal nostrils or nose. If you feel a small opening and insert your fingers and feel sucking on your fingers, you have found the fetal mouth. If that occurs, you know the fetus is well oxygenated! Anything that feels bumpy or lumpy is not a normal finding. Immediately inform the midwife or physician of your findings. Let your charge nurse or supervisor know that you have felt something unusual and that you have called the obstetric provider.

A face presentation may require a change in the plan of care, including delivery by cesarean section. Expect the midwife or physician to examine the fetal presenting part. If they find the fetal chin is anterior or pointing towards the top of the pelvis, the head will be in a position of extension. In that position vaginal birth is often possible. However, when the mentum (chin) is posterior and persists in that position, the fetus cannot deliver vaginally and a cesarean section is required (see Figure 8.10).

> **Documentation example:** 4/80%/–1 with nose palpated. Dr. Standandeliver notified of face presentation and she stated she would come to the bedside as soon as possible.

> **Documentation example:** 6/90/0. Unable to determine presenting part, felt small soft lump on exam. Dr. Standandeliver notified of VE and is on her way from office.

LIE

Lie is the relationship of the long axis of the fetus to the long axis of the mother. A longitudinal lie is the most common and

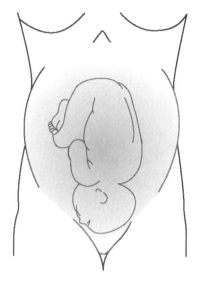

Figure 8.11: Longitudinal lie.

occurs when the fetal and maternal spine are parallel (see Figure 8.11). A transverse or oblique lie occurs when the spine (long axis) of the fetus is perpendicular or oblique to the spine (long axis) of the mother (see Figure 8.12).

TRANSVERSE LIE

Fetuses in a transverse lie must be delivered by cesarean section. The immediate concern when a woman presents in labor

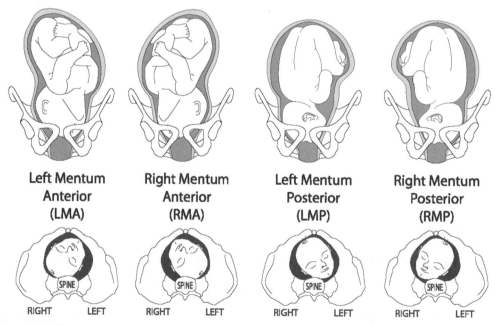

Figure 8.10: Face presentations with positions of LMA, RMA, LMP, and RMP.

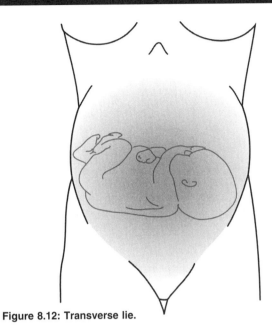

Figure 8.12: Transverse lie.

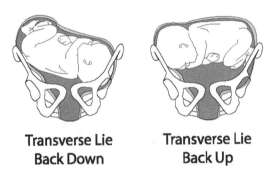

| Transverse Lie Back Down | Transverse Lie Back Up |

Figure 8.13: Transverse lie with back down and back up.

with a transverse lie is the risk of prolapse of the umbilical cord if the membranes rupture and the fetus is back up (see Figure 8.13). It is important to know if the fetus is back up or back down. When the transverse lie is back down with a fundal placenta, there may be less risk of a cord prolapse. Another risk of a transverse lie is that in the back-down fetus, the shoulder may descend and be mistaken for the vertex, which would delay the diagnosis of a transverse lie.

By performing Leopold's maneuvers, a vaginal examination, or both, a transverse lie can be confirmed. Report your findings of a transverse lie immediately to the midwife or physician and to your charge nurse or supervisor.

Documentation example: Suspect transverse lie following Leopold's maneuvers. Unable to palpate vertex on vaginal exam. Membranes intact with bulging bag of waters. Dr. Deliverme notified and Charge Nurse Geewiz informed.

Documentation example: Unsure of presenting part. Mother reports feeling fetal kicking on left side. Last examination in prenatal record was cephalic presentation. Estimate fetal weight by palpation as very large. Suspect transverse lie based on Leopold's maneuvers. CNM Heertohelp was informed of findings. Charge Nurse Whaddayouneed also notified.

LEOPOLD'S MANEUVERS

Leopold's maneuvers are used to determine the presentation, attitude, lie, and position of the fetus in the uterus (see Figure 8.14). The first maneuver helps you identify what is in the fundus. The second maneuver helps you determine the fetal lie and locate the fetal back. The third maneuver helps you determine the presenting part. After the second and third maneuver you will know where to place the fetoscope, stethoscope, ultrasound transducer, or hand-held Doppler device to assess the fetal heart rate. The fourth maneuver is the most difficult. This maneuver should help you determine the fetal attitude and whether or not the fetus is engaged (0 station). During the fourth maneuver your hands progress down toward the pubic bone. When your fingers meet the fetal forehead and occiput you should be able to determine the fetal attitude. As you move your hands down the side of the fetal head, if your fingers meet, the fetal head is not in the pelvis. If your hands diverge, the fetus has descended into the pelvis. Ask an experienced nurse, midwife, or physician to demonstrate Leopold's maneuvers. Ask them for feedback when you perform these four maneuvers.

When you practice Leopold's maneuvers, the location of the fetal back will also be the location of the fetal occiput. If the occiput is near the maternal left side, you have a left occiput (LO) position. If you think you can feel the fetal feet, legs, or knees and your laboring patient has strong lower back pain, the baby is probably in an occiput posterior (OP) position. Your vaginal examination should help you confirm the fetal presenting part and fetal position.

By performing Leopold's maneuvers, you should be able to recognize a fetus in a breech presentation and avoid laboring a woman who is admitted for induction with a malpositioned fetus. When you suspect a breech presentation, notify the provider as soon as possible. This presentation may require a change in the plan of care if the plan included a vaginal delivery.

Documentation example: 6/90%/−1 on admission exam. No vertex felt. Suspect breech presentation. Dr. Deliverusall notified of vaginal examination findings and stated he is on the way to the hospital.

Documentation example: 8/80%/0 after epidural. Soft fetal part noted on exam. Dr. Deliverusall notified.

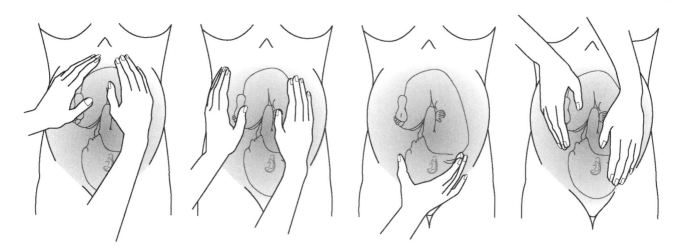

Figure 8.14: Leopold's maneuvers from left to right, including the first, second, third, and fourth maneuver.

STATION

Station is the distance of the presenting part from the level of the ischial spines. A zero station indicates the tip of the presenting part is at the level of the ischial spines. A minus (-) station indicates the tip of the presenting part is above the ischial spines. A plus (+) station indicates the tip of the presenting part is below the ischial spines. When there is a cephalic presentation, station is determined by measuring the distance in centimeters (cm) between the leading bony point of the skull and the level of the ischial spines (American College of Obstetrics and Gynecology, 2000). A minus station is recorded as −1, −2, −3, or high because it is impossible for most practitioners to reach a station that is 4 or 5 centimeters above the ischial spines. A plus station is recorded as +1, +2, +3, +4, and +5 cm (see Figure 8.15). Usually the baby is crowning at a +6 station. Instead of "+6" the word "crowning" is written in the nursing notes. The fetal head is crowning when it is seen at the vaginal opening or introitus and stays there with every contraction. In other words, it does not retract between contractions. Delivery usually occurs within minutes of crowning.

POSITION

To determine the fetal position, you will need to identify the denominators on the presenting part. The denominator is the occiput, the sacrum, or the chin. You will consider the maternal right or left side of the pelvis, and the anterior, posterior, or transverse sides of the pelvis. For example, if the occiput is near the left side of the pelvis and near the top or anterior aspect of the pelvis, the position is recorded as LOA for "left occiput anterior." If the chin (face presentation) is near the maternal right side of the pelvis and towards the back or posterior aspect of the pelvis, the position will be recorded as RMP for "right mentum posterior."

Before you can determine the position of a cephalic presentation, you need to know the anatomy of the fetal skull (Figure

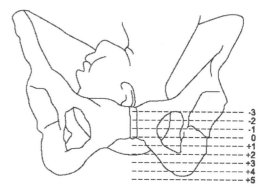

Figure 8.15: Classification of station. In a cephalic presentation, the distance between the tip of the skull to the level of the ischial spines is measured to determine the fetal station.

8.16). The anterior fontanel is in the shape of a diamond with four suture lines leading toward it. The posterior fontanel has a triangular shape, with three suture lines leading toward it. The frontal bones and frontal suture are in front of the anterior fontanel. The parietal bones are on the sides of the skull and are where cephalhematomas occur. The occipital bone is on the back of the head and this is the part of the head that usually delivers first. The sagittal suture is the longest and the easiest to find when you touch the fetal head. When the parietal bones overlap with head molding, this suture line will be felt as a ridge.

If the fetal scalp is swollen there is caput. If you feel caput and molding, record those findings in your notes. Station is the location of the tip of the skull bone in relation to the level of the ischial spines. Do not use caput to determine the station. Some providers use "C" to indicate "complete" for 10-cm dilatation, 100% effacement, or both.

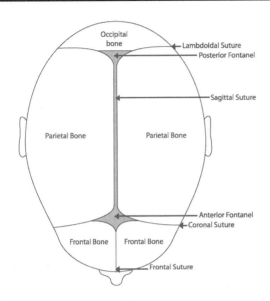

Figure 8.16: Fetal skull with sutures.

Documentation example: 7/100%/0 with molding and caput at +1. Contractions every 2 to 2 1/2 minutes for 60 to 90 seconds, moderate with soft resting tone.

Documentation example: 8/C/+1 with molding and caput at +2.

Documentation example: C/C/+2 with molding and caput at +3. Pushing with contractions every 2 to 3 minutes.

If you can follow the sagittal suture to the anterior or posterior fontanel, you should know where the occiput is and record the fetal position. If you are still not sure of the fetal position, perform Leopold's maneuvers. If you are confident that you have accurately determined the fetal position, record it in your notes. For example, you might write LOP for "left occiput posterior" or LOT for "left occiput transverse" (see Figure 8.17). When a fetus is in an occiput posterior (OP) or occiput transverse (OT) position, there may also be coupling of uterine contractions with the first contraction being stronger (taller on the graph) than the second contraction. The second contraction may follow the first contraction with little to no time between the two.

Left occiput anterior (LOA) is a common position prior to delivery. The fetal head is flexed with the posterior part of the vertex leading the way. The posterior fontanel and the occiput are palpable during the vaginal exam (see Figure 8.18). Sometimes the posterior fontanel is compressed and you will not be able to feel a triangle.

Posterior fetal positions are less common at the time of delivery. These babies are looking up when they are born.

Women with a fetus in a posterior position will complain of a backache. The fetal occiput is pressing against the maternal lumbosacral spine. When the fetus is posterior, the occiput is higher than when the fetus is in an occiput anterior (OA) position. In a left occiput position (LOP), the fetal back is on the maternal left side, and the occiput is near the maternal spine (see Figure 8.19). In addition, during Leopold's maneuvers you may palpate fetal kicking or feel the feet, legs, or arms on the maternal right side. The fetal spine will be on the maternal left side. When the fetal head is palpated during a vaginal examination, the posterior fontanel will be found to the maternal left and near her spine.

In a right occiput anterior (ROA) position, the fetal back is located on the maternal right side. Fetal parts may not be easily palpated during Leopold's maneuvers because the fetal parts are under the baby toward the maternal spine. The occiput leads the way, is near the anterior aspect of the pelvis, and the posterior fontanel may be felt on the maternal right side during a vaginal examination (see Figure 8.20).

In a right occiput transverse (ROT) position, the fetal back is located on the maternal right side. Fetal feet, arms, or legs may be palpated on the maternal left side. The occiput leads the way and the sagittal suture should be easily felt if she is at least 5-cm dilated. It will be between her left side and right side (see Figure 8.20).

In a right occiput posterior (ROP) position, the fetal back is located on the maternal right side, towards the maternal spine. Fetal small parts should be easily palpated on the maternal left side. The mother may report feeling fetal kicking on her left side. The posterior fontanel will be on the maternal right side (see Figure 8.20).

THE POSITION IF THE FETUS IS BREECH

Breech is a type of presentation. The position of the breech presentation is determined by the location of the fetal sacrum to the maternal pelvis. In a left sacrum anterior (LSA) position the fetus is sitting in the uterus with its spine and sacrum located near the maternal left side and under the anterior aspect of the maternal pelvis (see Figure 8.21).

When the fetus is sitting with its spine towards the maternal left side and the back of the pelvis, the position is left sacrum posterior or LSP (see Figure 8.22).

If a fetus is in breech presentation, such as left sacrum transverse (see Figure 8.23), you might accidentally examine the fetal anus and think it is the cervix. Push on the presenting part. Does it feel soft or hard? The buttocks is soft, the head is hard. Notify the midwife or physician of your findings after you perform Leopold's maneuvers to confirm the breech. If you enter the anus, you may find meconium on your gloved fingertip. It is always a good habit to look at your glove after a vaginal examination and record the amount, color, and odor of amniotic fluid or the presence of blood-streaked mucus (bloody show), bleeding, or meconium.

CLASSIFICATIONS OF BREECH PRESENTATION

In addition to position, breech presentations are classified based on the position of the fetal legs. These classifications

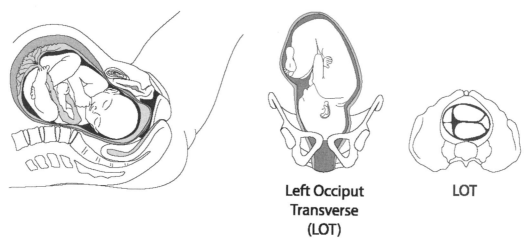

Figure 8.17: LOT position. Note the fetal occiput is on the maternal left side and the baby is lying on its left side in the uterus.

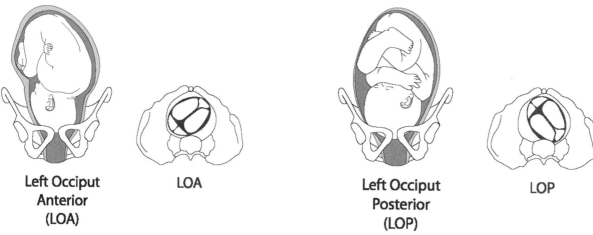

Figure 8.18: Left occiput anterior.

Figure 8.19: Left occiput posterior.

are: a complete breech, a frank breech, a kneeling breech, a single-footling breech, and a double-footling breech (see Figure 8.24). A complete breech is when the legs are flexed. A frank breech is when the legs are extended with the feet near the head of the fetus. A kneeling breech is when the knees are presenting. A footling breech is when one or both feet present below the buttocks. To assess the fetal position, determine the location of the fetal back and sacrum.

You will usually feel the fetal buttocks on your exam in either a complete or frank breech presentation. A complete breech has legs that are flexed at the hips and bent at the knees. A frank breech has extended legs that are flexed at the hips and straight at the knees. A kneeling breech has legs that are not flexed at the hips but are bent at the knees. Fetal knees may feel like one or two "nubby bumps" during the vaginal

examination. A single-footling breech has only one leg flexed at the hip. A doubling-footling breech will have straight legs.

If you see a foot hanging out of the vagina, it is highly likely there is a single footling breech! The cord may not be far behind it. You should put the patient in bed, don a sterile glove, and check for cord prolapse after you have pulled the emergency cord and called for help. If the fetus is a footling breech, the foot may not be exposed. You might feel something wiggling against your fingers during the vaginal examination. This is probably the fetal toes. Confirm that what you feel is not soft like an umbilical cord. The cord should be pulsating, the toes would be wiggling.

If you find a footling breech during a vaginal examination, you may have a stress reaction. This is not the time for flight. Ask a family member or friend of the patient to pull the

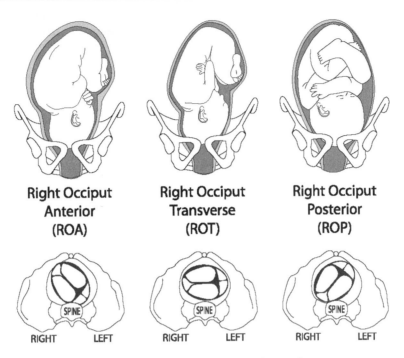

Figure 8.20: Right occiput anterior, transverse, and posterior.

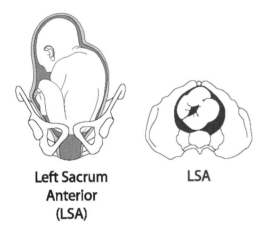

Figure 8.21: Left sacrum anterior position.

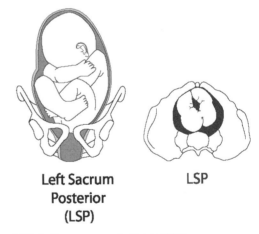

Figure 8.22: Left sacrum posterior position.

emergency cord, if they are present, or call out for help. If there is a prolapsed cord with a foot presenting, digital displacement (lifting up on the buttocks) is not necessary because the cord is probably not being significantly compressed. Remember to recognize, vocalize, and mobilize. Once you have recognized the problem and called for help, you need to mobilize other nurses to start an intravenous (IV) line if it is not already present. Ask them to call the physician and the operating room crew. They will also need to prepare the operating room for a cesarean section.

MECONIUM

Meconium develops in the fetus between the 10th and 16th week of gestation and is composed of secretions, cells, bile, pancreatic juices, mucus, blood, amniotic fluid, swallowed lanugo, and vernix (Folsom, 1997; Houlihan & Knuppel, 1994; Srinivasan & Vidasagar, 1999). There are about 60 to 200 grams of meconium in the term fetal intestine (Wiswell, 1997). Pre-term fetuses who are less than 36 weeks of gestation rarely release meconium. Mature or near-term fetuses are more likely to release meconium.

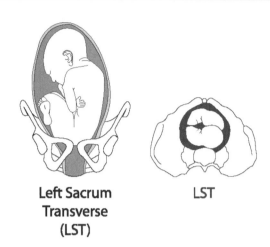

Left Sacrum Transverse (LST)

LST

Figure 8.23: Left sacrum transverse position.

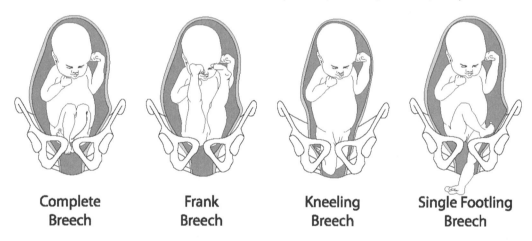

Complete Breech   **Frank Breech**   **Kneeling Breech**   **Single Footling Breech**

Figure 8.24: Complete, frank, kneeling, and single-footling breech presentations.

2005). If you see meconium in the amniotic fluid, you should inform the midwife or physician of the color, amount, and consistency, along with other pertinent information about the mother, her fetus, and uterine activity.

WHY IS MECONIUM RELEASED IN UTERO?

A hypoxic event may precede the release of meconium into the amniotic fluid. Stimulation of the vagus nerve is also associated with anal sphincter relaxation and the release of meconium (Grignaffini et al., 2004).

Near-term, term, and postterm fetuses release meconium more often than preterm fetuses. Hypoxic fetuses of mothers who smoke cigarettes or mothers diagnosed with hypertension, diabetes, respiratory or cardiovascular disease, pre-eclampsia, or eclampsia are also more likely than nonhypoxic fetuses to release meconium. Intrauterine growth restriction, oligohydramnios, and abnormal fetal heart rate patterns have also been found to be related to the release of meconium (Gelfand, Fanaroff, & Walsh, 2004).

Meconium is not just a colorful addition to labor. Meconium is a significant risk factor because it is related to fetal and neonatal injury. Meconium-stained amniotic fluid (MSAF) is associated with cerebral palsy in term and preterm human fetuses (Blackwell et al., 2004). Fetuses who are 36 weeks or younger in the presence of meconium-stained amniotic fluid were more likely to die and have a 1-minute Apgar score less than 3, and a 5-minute Apgar score less than 7 (Mazor et al., 1998). Even though some researchers have reported that meconium only occurs in one in five labors, do not be fooled into thinking its presence is not a risk factor.

It has been reported that midwives from nonhospital settings, who observed dark, thick, or particulate meconium, recognized the risks associated with meconium and transferred their patients to the hospital. They also requested an intrapartum consultation from a physician (Simkin & Ancheta,

In 1979, researchers found that motilin, which causes peristalsis, was four times greater in the plasma of neonates who had fetal distress than in normal term neonates (Lucas, Christofides, Adrian, Bloom, & Aynsley-Green, 1979). Corticotropin-releasing hormone (CRH) may also be related to the stress-induced stimulation of the distal regions of the bowel and the release of meconium (Ahanya, Lakshmanan, Rehan, Bronshtein, & Ross, 2007; Richard, Ross, Sugano, Ho, & Lakshmanan, 2007).

There may be a genetic reason why some fetuses release meconium and others do not. Black women from East and North Africa had more fetuses who released meconium than the babies of women from India or the Middle East. The release of meconium was not found with additional signs of fetal compromise (Sedaghatian, Othman, Rashid, Ramachandran, & Bener, 2004).

THE COLOR OF MECONIUM

The color of meconium is related to the time it was released or the presence of gastroschisis, or both. For example, recently released meconium is thick, blackish green, or dark green. It will have particulate matter in it and will be viscous. Fetuses whose intestines are exposed (gastroschisis) will have amniotic fluid stained with a lime, chartreuse, or golden color. Greenish tan, muddy-brown, and light-tan meconium occurs when the meconium has been in the uterus longer than 6 hours (Sienko & Altshuler, 1999). After 12 to 14 hours, vernix will be stained and may be a yellow or tan color (Ahanya, Lakshmanan, Morgan & Ross, 2004). Yellow meconium is old meconium. Therefore, you should document the color and consistency of the meconium. Once the baby is born, document any staining of the neonatal skin, cord, or nails.

THE CONSISTENCY OF MECONIUM

Meconium in the amniotic fluid can be thin or thick. Some researchers also use the word "moderate" to describe the consistency of meconium. Thin meconium is green- or yellow-tinged without particulate matter. Thin meconium-stained amniotic fluid will often be watery. Moderate meconium may have some particulate matter and looks like split pea soup (without the peas). Moderate meconium may be green or yellow. Thick meconium is usually dark green and viscous with particulate matter (Simsek, Celen, Islimye, Danisman, & Buyukkagnici, 2008). Some nurses have classified this as "clumps" or "chunks" of meconium.

It is best to describe the consistency and color of meconium in your notes. "Moderate" may be misinterpreted to be an amount rather than a consistency. It is better to be descriptive. You may describe the meconium as "split-pea soup" instead of using the word "moderate."

> **Documentation example:** Light yellow and thin MSAF noted after SROM.

> **Documentation example:** "Split-pea soup" light-green MSAF, no particles.

> **Documentation example:** Light-yellow meconium-stained amniotic fluid. No foul odor. Linen protector half saturated. FHR 130s with accelerations and no decelerations. Fetal movement palpated by this nurse.

HYDROTHERAPY: IS MECONIUM A CONTRAINDICATION?

In some hospitals, the presence of meconium is a contraindication for the use of hydrotherapy, but in other hospitals water immersion is allowed if there is light meconium. Hydrotherapy is a safe practice. Meconium will float to the surface and should pose no risk to the woman or her fetus. You may want to remove any meconium with a gloved hand, a small net, or a towel. External fetal and uterine monitoring with submersible transducers may be used if they are available and if continuous monitoring was orderd.

> **Documentation example:** AROM at 0740 with particulate meconium. Continuous fetal monitoring with telemetry while soaking in tub. FHR baseline 145 to 155 bpm with accelerations to 155 to 160 bpm and occasional variable decelerations.

THE MESSAGE OF MECONIUM

When the fetus releases meconium the message is "Watch me closely." When meconium is present in the fluid prior to a scheduled cesarean section, more neonates have asphyxia than when there is no meconium (Pi, Zhu, & Huang, 2003). What this means is that the nurse must be vigilant because bad things happen when meconium is present. Examine the fetal heart rate pattern closely during labor for signs of fetal hypoxia. Act to oxygenate the fetus when necessary, and report your findings in a timely manner to the obstetric provider.

Even when women have been initially classified as low risk, the presence of meconium makes them high risk. It has been documented that women who had no identified risk factors and who were in labor with a fetus between 37 and 42 weeks of gestation with meconium in the amniotic fluid were more likely to have a baby who had severe acidemia, low Apgar scores, and meconium aspiration syndrome (Ziadeh & Sunna, 2000). Prolonged exposure to meconium can impair oxygen delivery to the fetus due to vasoconstriction of placental and cord vessels (Blackwell et al., 2004). Meconium may also be present when the fetus has cardiovascular malformations or erythroblastosis (Fujikura & Klionsky, 1975).

MONITORING THE FETAL HEART RATE

If there is moderate or thick meconium-stained amniotic fluid during labor, continuous fetal monitoring throughout labor and delivery is recommended (Ahanya, Lakshmanan, Morgan, & Ross, 2004). If there is thick, old (yellow or tan) meconium and a persistently nonreactive, fixed, and flat fetal heart rate pattern, the fetus may already be brain damaged (Phelan & Ahn, 1994) (see Figure 8.25).

> **Documentation example:** Spontaneous rupture of the membranes prior to admission. Reports decreased fetal movement for 24 hours. 5-cm spot of yellow-stained amniotic fluid on Chux with foul odor noted. Fetal heart rate 150 bpm and fixed. To right side, oxygen on at 10 L/minute with nonrebreather mask. IV started in left cephalic vein with lactated Ringer's solution now at 125 mL/hr. Dr. Beritethere and Charge Nurse Omygoodness notified. Requested physician come to room immediately.

A normal fetal heart rate pattern in the presence of meconium indicates fetal well-being at that time (see Figure 8.26). In this figure the term fetus released meconium and is well oxygenated evidenced by accelerations. Expect fetal oxygen

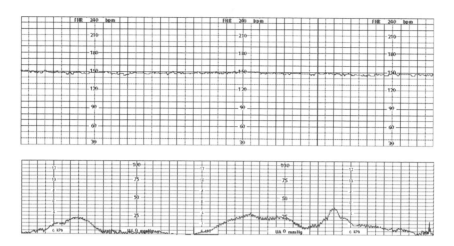

Figure 8.25: Thick meconium, breech presentation at 40 weeks of gestation. After the administration of terbutaline, a cesarean section was performed. Paper speed is 3 cm/minute. Apgar scores were 1, 4, and 8 at 1, 5, and 10 minutes of age. The neonate was diagnosed with hypoxic ischemic encephalopathy (brain damage).

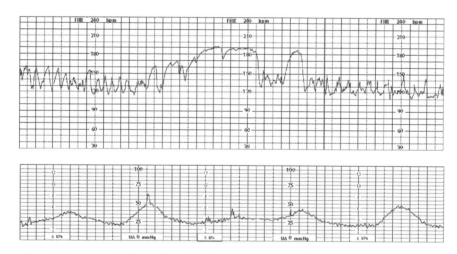

Figure 8.26: Thick meconium, vertex presentation at 40 weeks of gestation with large accelerations and moderate to marked (long-term) variability prior to the accelerations. A cesarean section was performed later in the day after a prolonged deceleration. Apgar scores were 9 and 10 at 1 and 5 minutes. Note uterine hyperstimulation. Oxytocin should be discontinued when the interval between contractions is less than 1 minute in duration. Paper speed is 3 cm/minute.

saturation (SpO$_2$) to be lower when there is an abnormal or nonreassuring fetal heart rate pattern (Grignaffini et al., 2004).

FETAL TOLERANCE OF LABOR

Absent or nearly absent variability, and the lack of accelerations on the admission test strip, during labor, or during the 30 minutes prior to delivery, may reflect fetal intolerance with a strong risk of an adverse outcome. There is a myth that the presence of long-term variability means the fetus is tolerant of the hypoxic stress created by contractions. Long-term vari-

ability is *not* the sole indicator of fetal well-being (Samueloff et al., 1994). Accelerations are needed to rule out metabolic acidosis and they should be present every 90 minutes or less.

MECONIUM AND CHORIOAMNIONITIS: IS THERE A CONNECTION?

Meconium is related to a decrease in the zinc level in the amniotic fluid. At one time it was thought that meconium, with or without a decreased zinc level, might increase the risk of infection (Ahanya, Lakshmanan, Morgan, & Ross, 2004). In one study in which there was meconium in the amniotic fluid, chorioamnionitis was diagnosed in 8% of the placentas compared with 4% when there was no meconium (O'Reilly-Green & Divon, 1998). In 2007, researchers failed to show a direct connection among meconium, chorioamnionitis, and endometritis (Panichkul, Boonprasertmd, Komolpismd, Panichkul, & Caengow, 2007).

There was an increase in the incidence of chorioamnionitis when women had an amnioinfusion to dilute thick meconium. But amnioinfusion to dilute thick meconium is no longer advocated because amnioinfusion does not decrease the incidence of meconium aspiration syndrome. The rate of chorioamnionitis with endometritis was 16% in the amnioinfusion group but only 8% in women without an amnioinfusion (Spong, Ogundipe, & Ross, 1994). Endometritis may not be related to amnioinfusion for thick meconium (Moen, Besinger, Tomich, & Fisher, 1995). However, chorioamnionitis is related to the presence of an epidural. Thirteen percent of women with an epidural had chorioamnionitis compared with 2.2% of women who did not have an epidural (Soper, Mayhall, & Froggatt, 1996).

NEONATAL CARE RELATED TO MECONIUM

Meconium aspiration usually occurs in utero. Since suction of the oropharynx and nasopharynx after delivery of the head does not reduce the incidence of meconium aspiration syndrome, the practice of suctioning prior to the birth is no longer advised (Stringer, Brooks, King, & Biesecker, 2007).

An infant exposed to meconium in utero may need endotracheal suctioning after birth. If the neonate is not breathing, intubation and endotracheal suctioning of moderate or thick meconium should occur prior to positive pressure ventilation (Manganaro, Mami, Palmara, Paolata, & Gemelli, 2001; Wiswell & Henley, 1992). Intubation and endotracheal suctioning for thin meconium is neither helpful nor required. Failure to intubate and suction for thin meconium was not related to the need for oxygen or the 5-minute Apgar score (Liu & Harrington, 1998). A neonatal team educated in neonatal resuscitation improves neonatal outcomes and there should be fewer neonates diagnosed with asphyxia (Duran, Aladağ, Vatansever, Süt, & Acunaş, 2008). Therefore, anyone who participates in neonatal resuscitation should have the knowledge and skills to do so.

> **Documentation example:** Thick meconium with birth of head. Baby delivered, placed in warmer. No stimulation. Intubated by CNNP (certified neonatal nurse practitioner) Readyandwaiting, no meconium found below the vocal cords. See resuscitation notes.

> **Documentation example:** Previously clear fluid now light-green meconium stained with no particles noted. FHR 155 bpm. Reported MSAF to Dr. Neverfaraway.

> **Documentation example:** Particulate, thick meconium noted with AROM. Charge Nurse Gottaloveme and

nursery personnel notified, 10F suction catheter set up, and meconium aspirator placed in neonatal radiant warmer.

MECONIUM ASPIRATION

Neonatal pneumonia may occur when meconium is aspirated. Meconium inhibits phagocytosis and may cause the death of alveolar macrophages in the lower respiratory tract. In vitro, meconium also decreases phagocytosis by neutrophils. Macrophages and neutrophils are white blood cells. Phagocytosis is the process whereby white blood cells consume bacteria (Craig, Lopez, Hoskin, & Markham, 2005). The presence of meconium can inhibit the consumption of bacteria and heighten the risk of infection.

Permanent lung injury can occur when meconium is aspirated. Oxygen free radicals or superoxides are released from alveolar macrophages that are exposed to meconium. These macrophages also produce proteins called cytokines. Cytokines are inflammatory markers. The two cytokines related to lung injury are platelet activating factor (PAF) and tumor necrosis factor-alpha (TNF-α) (Berdeli et al., 2004; Tripathi, Saili, & Dutta, 2007).

Childhood asthma diagnosed by the age of 2 has been found to be related to meconium aspiration (Vasquez-Nava, 2006). Fetal and neonatal demise after in utero meconium exposure is related to fetal pneumonia, neonatal bronchopneumonia, and inflammation of the umbilical cord, which is called "funisitis." Fetal and neonatal demise after in utero meconium exposure is also associated with chorioamnionitis, injury of cord vessels (including ulceration), and chorioamnionitis without funisitis (Burgess & Hutchins, 1996).

AMNIOINFUSION AND MECONIUM ASPIRATION

Meconium aspiration is the result of in utero gasping with inhalation of meconium into the fetal lungs (Ahanya, Lakshmanan, Morgan, & Ross, 2004; Usta, Mercer, Aswad, & Sibai, 1995). Meconium aspiration obstructs airways and causes surfactant dysfunction (Lucas, 2002). Meconium aspiration syndrome (MAS) includes atelectasis with severe impairment of pulmonary gas exchange, surfactant inactivation, persistent pulmonary hypertension, and inflammation (Gadzinowski, 1998; Hilgendorff et al., 2006).

Researchers hoped that MAS could be prevented with amnioninfusion, the infusion of a crystalloid solution such as normal saline into the uterus during labor. Amnioinfusion with a 600 to 800 mL normal saline bolus delivered quickly or at 15 mL/minute, followed by 3 mL/minute, seemed to be related to a decrease in the number of babies who had MAS (Hofmeyr et al., 1998). Hofmeyr (2002) reviewed 12 well-designed studies and found that amnioinfusion reduced the thickness of the meconium in the amniotic fluid, the number of variable decelerations, the number of cesarean sections, the incidence of MAS, the incidence of neonatal hypoxic ischemic encephalopathy, neonatal ventilation, and admission to the neonatal intensive care. However, the current thinking is that prevention of MAS is impossible. The results of a study from 56 medical centers in 13 countries support this conclusion (Fraser et al., 2005). Amnioinfusion in the presence of thick meconium without variable decelerations is no longer recommended.

MECONIUM AND DAMAGE TO THE PLACENTA AND CORD

It takes 4 to 12 hours for meconium to diffuse into the lumens of placental and umbilical cord vessels (Altshuler, 1995). If meconium reaches the inside of the umbilical vein, it causes the vein to constrict (Pickens, Toubas, Hyde, & Altshuler, 1995). Meconium particles that enter the umbilical vein may be transported to the fetal brain and cause vasospasm and ischemic injury in the brain (Blackwell et al., 2004). Prolonged exposure to meconium may induce injury and necrosis of the placenta and umbilical cord vessels due to vasoconstriction and hypoperfusion (Sienko & Altshuler, 1999). The pathologist may find large, ovoid, or round macrophages in the placenta that are filled with yellow, brown, or green meconium, or any combination thereof. There may be umbilical cord ulcerations or placental vascular necrosis, or both (Altshuler, Arizawa, & Molnar-Nadasdy, 1992; King et al., 2004). Chorionic vessel necrosis may also be found (King et al., 2004).

In the past, it was believed that formalin should not be used as a fixative as it might change the pathologic analysis of a meconium-stained placenta. However, even if formalin washes the meconium off the placental surface, the pathologist will look deeper (a microscopic examination) to decide how long the placenta has been exposed to meconium and any damage resulting from exposure to meconium.

CONCLUSIONS

Nurses who work in labor and delivery must assess the fetal presentation, attitude, lie, and station, and the position of the fetus. Leopold's maneuvers are important to assist nurses in determining these characteristics. It takes time to develop the skills to perform Leopold's maneuvers.

A compound presentation increases the risk of an umbilical cord prolapse or umbilical cord compression, fetal circulatory problems, and bruising. A brow presentation increases the duration of labor and increases the risk of maternal perineal trauma. If a fetus is in a breech position or transverse lie, there is an increased risk of an umbilical cord prolapse, especially when the fetus is back up with a transverse lie.

The presence of meconium is a risk factor that is related to infection, placental and umbilical cord damage, and neonatal injury or death. Nurses who see meconium in the amniotic fluid should inform the obstetric provider of its color, consistency, and any foul odor. They should remain vigilant in observing the fetal heart rate pattern for abnormal findings. If there are abnormal findings, labor and delivery nurses must act immediately to improve fetal oxygenation and decrease uterine activity, and to communicate their assessments and actions to the midwife or physician so that the plan of care can be modified.

REVIEW QUESTIONS

True/False: Decide if the statements are true or false.

1. In Figure 8.27, the fetus has a vertex position and a left occiput transverse presentation.
2. In Figure 8.28, the fetal face is facing the maternal right side.
3. A frank breech presentation is when the fetus presents buttocks first with the fetal legs fully extended.
4. If the vertex is at a station near or lower than +5, the fetus is usually crowning.
5. Golden or lime-green meconium may be associated with gastroschisis.
6. "Moderate meconium" is a clear and complete description of its consistency.
7. It is recommended that amnioinfusion be used to dilute meconium-stained fluid.
8. Meconium-stained amniotic fluid increases the risk of neonatal acidemia, infection, and asphyxia.
9. Meconium aspiration usually occurs in utero.
10. The placenta and umbilical cord may be damaged by exposure to meconium.

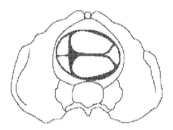

LOT

Figure 8.27

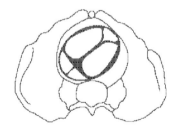

LOA

Figure 8.28

References

Ahanya, S. N., Lakshmanan, J., Morgan, B. L. G., & Ross, M. G. (2004). Meconium passage in utero: Mechanisms, consequences, and management. *Obstetrical and Gynecological Survey, 60*(1), 45–56.

Ahanya, S., Lakshmanan, J., Rehan, V., Bronshtein, E., & Ross, M. (2007). Hypoxia induced in utero meconium passage is mediated via corticotrophin releasing hormone in a novel fetal rat model [Abstract]. *American Journal of Obstetrics and Gynecology, 197*, S151.

Altshuler, G. (1995). Placental insights into neurodevelopmental and other childhood diseases. *Seminars in Pediatric Neurology, 2*, 90–99.

Altshuler, G., Arizawa, M., & Molnar-Nadasdy, G. (1992). Meconium-induced umbilical cord vascular necrosis and ulceration: A potential link between the placenta and poor pregnancy outcome. *Obstetrics & Gynecology, 79*(5, Part 1), 769–766.

American College of Obstetrics and Gynecology. (2000). *Operative vaginal delivery.* ACOG Practice Bulletin No. 17: Washington, DC: Author.

Berdeli, A., Akisu, M., Dagei, T., Akisu, C., Yalaz, M., & Kultursay, N. (2004). Meconium enhances platelet-activating factor and tumor necrosis factor production by rat alveolar macrophages [Abstract]. *Prostaglandins, Leukotrienes, and Essential Fatty Acids, 71*(4), 227–232.

Blackwell, S. C., Hallak, M., Hotra, J. W., Refuezo, J., Sokol, R. J., & Sorokin, Y. (2004). Prolonged in utero meconium exposure impairs spatial learning in the adult rat. *America Journal of Obstetrics and Gynecology, 190*, 1551–1556.

Brown, C. L., Ludwiczak, M. H., Blanco, J. D., & Hirsch, C. E. (1993). Cervical dilation: Accuracy of visual and digital examinations. *Obstetrics & Gynecology, 81*, 215–216.

Burgess, A. M., & Hutchins, G. M. (1996). Inflammation of the lungs, umbilical cord and placenta associated with meconium passage in utero: Review of 123 autopsied cases. *Pathology in Research and Practice, 192*(11), 1121–1128.

Casey, B. M., & Cox, S. M. (1997). Chorioamnionitis and endometritis. *Infectious Disease Clinics of North America, 11*(1), 203–222.

Craig, S., Lopez, A., Hoskin, D., & Markham, F. (2005). Meconium inhibits phagocytosis and stimulates respiratory burst in alveolar macrophages. *Pediatric Research, 57*, 813–818.

Duran, R., Aladağ, N., Vatansevere, U., Süt, N., & Acunaş, B. (2008). The impact of neonatal resuscitation program courses on mortality and morbidity of newborn infants with perinatal asphyxia. *Brain Development, 30*, 43–46.

Folsom, M. (1997). Amnioinfusion for meconium staining: Does it help? *American Journal of Maternal/Child Nursing, 22*(2), 74–79.

Fraser, W., Hofmeyr, J., Lede, R., Faron, G., Alexander, S., & Goffimet, F. (2005). An international randomized controlled trial of amnioinfusion for thickly meconium stained amniotic fluid [Abstract]. *American Journal of Obstetrics and Gynecology, 193*, S3.

Fujikura, T., & Klionsky, B. (1975). The significance of meconium staining. *American Journal of Obstetrics and Gynecology, 121*(1), 45–50.

Gadzinowski, J. (1998). Contemporary treatment options for meconium aspiration syndrome [Abstract]. *Croation Medical Journal, 39*(2).

Gelfand, S. L., Fanaroff, J. M., & Walsh, M. C. (2004). Meconium stained fluids: Approach to the mother and the baby. *Pediatric Clinics of North America, 51*, 655–667.

Grignaffini, A., Soncini, E., Ronzoni, R., Piazza, E., Anfuso, S., & Vadora, E. (2004). Meconium-stained amniotic fluid and fetal oxygen saturation measured by pulse oximetry during labour. *Acta Bio Medica Ateneo Parmense, 75*(Suppl.), 45–52.

Hilgendorff, A., Doerner, M., Rawer, D., Leick, J., Trotter, A., & Ebsen, M. (2006). Effects of a recombinant surfactant protein-C based surfactant on lung function and the pulmonary surfactant system in a model of meconium aspiration syndrome. *Critical Care Medicine, 34*(1), 203–210.

Hofmeyr, G. J. (2002). Amnioinfusion for meconium-stained liquor in labour. *Cochrane Database of Systematic Reviews.* Issue 1. CD000014.

Hofmeyr, G. J., Gümezoğlu, A. M., Buchmann, E., Jowarth, G. R., Shaw, A., & Nikodem, V. C. (1998). The collaborative randomized amnioinfusion for meconium project (CRAMP): 1. South Africa. *British Journal of Obstetrics and Gynaecology, 105*(3), 304–308.

Houlihan, C., & Knuppel, R. (1994). Meconium-stained fluid: Current controversies. *Journal of Reproductive Medicine, 39*(11), 888–897.

Imseis, H. M., Trout, W. C., & Gabbe, S. G. (1999). The microbiologic effect of digital cervical examination. *American Journal of Obstetrics and Gynecology, 180*(3, Part 1), 578–580.

King, E. L., Redline, R. W., Smith, S. D., Kraus, F. T., Sadovsk, Y., & Nelson, D. M. (2004). Myocytes of chorionic vessels from placentas with meconium-associated vascular necrosis exhibit apoptotic markers. *Human Pathology, 35*(4), 412–417.

Liu, W. F., & Harrington, T. (1998). The need for delivery room intubation of thin meconium in the low-risk newborn: A clinical trial. *American Journal of Perinatology, 15*(12), 675–682.

Lucas, A., Christofides, N. D., Adrian, T. E., Bloom, S. R., & Anysley-Green, A. (1979). Fetal distress, meconium and motilin. *Lancet, 2*, 718.

Lucas, G. N. (2002). Management of meconium-stained amniotic fluid (MSAF) and the meconium aspiration syndrome (MAS). *Sri Lanka Journal of Child Health, 31*, 118–121.

Manganaro, R., Mami, C., Palmara, A., Paolata, A., & Gemelli, M. (2001). Incidence of meconium aspiration syndrome in term meconium-stained babies managed at birth with selective tracheal intubation. *Journal of Perinatal Medicine, 29*, 465–468.

Mazor, M., Hershkovitz, R., Bashiri, A., Maymon, E., Schreiber, R., & Dukler, D. (1998). Meconium stained amniotic fluid in preterm delivery is an independent risk factor for perinatal complications. *European Journal of Obstetrics, Gynecology, and Reproductive Biology, 81*(1), 9–13.

McCaul IV, J. F., Rogers, L. W., Perry, K. G., Martin, R. W., Albert, J. R., & Morrison, J. C. (1997). Premature rupture of membranes at term with an unfavorable cervix: Comparison of expectant management, vaginal prostaglandin, and oxytocin induction. *Southern Medical Journal, 90*(12), 1229–1233.

Moen, M. D., Besinger, R. E., Tomich, P. G., & Fisher, S. G. (1995). Effect of amnioinfusion on the incidence of postpartum endometritis in patients undergoing cesarean delivery. *Journal of Reproductive Medicine, 40*(5), 383–386.

Munson, L. A., Graham, A., Koos, B. J., & Valenzuela, G. J. (1985). Is there a need for digital examination in patients with spontaneous rupture of membranes? *American Journal of Obstetrics and Gynecology, 153*, 562–563.

Newton, E. R., Prihoda, T. J., & Gibbs, R. S. (1989). Logistic regression analysis of risk factors for intra-amniotic infection. *Obstetrics & Gynecology, 73*(4), 571–575.

O'Reilly-Green, C., & Divon, M. Y. (1998). Oligohydramnios and meconium as predictors of neonatal outcome in prolonged pregnancy [Abstract]. *American Journal of Obstetrics and Gynecology, 178*(1, Part 2), S46.

Panichkul, S., Boonprasertmd, K., Komolpismd, S., Panichkul, P., & Caengow, S. (2007). The association between meconium-stained amniotic fluid and chorioamnionitis or endometritis. *Journal of the Medical Association of Thailand, 90*(3), 442–447.

Phelan, J. P., & Ahn, M. O. (1994). Perinatal observations in forty-eight neurologically impaired term infants. *American Journal of Obstetrics and Gynecology, 171*, 424–431.

Pi, P. X., Zhu, F. F., & Huang, J. (2003). Meconium-stained amniotic fluid and intra-amniotic infection [Abstract]. *Hunan Yi Ke Da Xue Xue Bao, 28*(6), 648–650.

Pickens, J., Toubas, P. L., Hyde, S., & Altshuler, G. (1995). In vitro model of human umbilical venous perfusion to study the effects of meconium staining of the umbilical cord. *Biology of the Neonate, 67*(2), 100–108.

Richard, J. D., Ross, M., Sugano, S., Ho, B., & Lakshmanan, J. (2007). Mechanisms of fetal meconium passage: Anatomical and biochemical localization of CRF-R1 receptors in fetal rat gastrointestinal tract [Abstract]. *American Journal of Obstetrics and Gynecology, 197*, S12.

Samueloff, A., Langer, O., Berkus, M., Field, N., Xenakis, E., & Ridgway, L. (1994). Is fetal heart rate variability a good predictor of fetal outcome? *Acta Obstetricia et Gynecologica Scandinavica, 73*(1), 39–44

Seaward, P. G., Hannah, M. E., Myhr, T. L., Farine, D., Ohlsson, A., & Wang, E. E. (1998). International multicenter term PROM study: Evaluation of predictors of neonatal infection in infants born to patients with premature rupture of membranes at term: Premature rupture of membranes. *American Journal of Obstetrics and Gynecology, 179*(3, Part 1), 635–639.

Sedaghatian, M. R., Othman, L., Rashid, N., Ramachandran, P., & Bener, A. B. (2004). An 8-year study of meconium stained amniotic fluid in different ethnic groups. *Kuwait Medical Journal, 36*(4), 266–269.

Sienko, A., & Altshuler, G. (1999). Meconium-induced umbilical vascular necrosis in abortuses and fetuses: A histopathologic study of cytokines. *Obstetrics & Gynecology, 94*(3), 415–420.

Simkin, P., & Ancheta, R. (2005). *The labor progress handbook* (2nd ed.). Oxford, England: Blackwell Publishing.

Simsek, A., Celen, S., Islimye, M., Danisman, N., & Buyukkagnici U. (2008). A long-standing incomprehensible matter of obstetrics: Meconium-stained amniotic fluid, a new approach to reason. *Archives of Gynecology and Obstetrics.* doi 10.1007/s00404-008-0607-2.

Soper, D. E., Mayhall, G., & Dalton, H. P. (1989). Risk factors for intraamniotic infection: A prospective epidemiologic study. *American Journal of Obstetrics and Gynecology, 161*(3), 562–568.

Soper, D. E., Mayhall, C. G., & Froggatt, J. W. (1996). Characterization and control of intraamniotic infection in an urban teaching hospital. *American Journal of Obstetrics and Gynecology, 175*(2), 304–310.

Spong, C. Y., Ogundipe, O. A., & Ross, M. G. (1994). Prophylactic amnioinfusion for meconium-stained amniotic fluid. *American Journal of Obstetrics and Gynecology, 171*(4), 931–935.

Srinivasan, H., & Vidyasagar, D. (1999). Meconium aspiration syndrome: Current concepts and management. *Comprehensive Therapy, 25*(2), 82–89.

Stringer, M., Brooks, P. M., King, K., & Biesecker, B. (2007). New guidelines for maternal and neonatal resuscitation. *Journal of Obstetric, Gynecologic, and Neonatal Nursing, 36*, 624–635.

Tripathi, S., Saili, A., & Dutta, R. (2007). Inflammatory markers in meconium induced lung injury in neonates and effect of steroids on their levels: A randomized controlled trial. *Indian Journal of Medical Microbiology, 25*(2), 103–107.

Usta, I. M., Mercer, B. M., Aswad, N. K., & Sibai, B. M. (1995). The impact of a policy of amnioinfusion for meconium-stained amniotic fluid. *Obstetrics & Gynecology, 85*(2), 237–241.

Vazquez-Nava, F. (2006). Asthma symptoms under two years old after suffering meconium aspiration syndrome. *Journal of Allergy and Clinical Immunology, 117*(2), S155.

Wiswell, T. E. (1997). Meconium staining and the meconium aspiration syndrome. In D. K. Stevenson & P. Sunshine

(Eds.), *Fetal and neonatal brain injury: Mechanisms, management, and the risks of practice* (pp. 539–563). New York: Oxford University Press.

Wiswell, T. E., & Henley, M. A. (1992). Intratracheal suctioning, systemic infection, and the meconium aspiration syndrome. *Pediatrics, 89*(2), 203–206.

Ziadeh, S. M., & Sunna, E. (2000). Obstetric and perinatal outcome of pregnancies with term labour and meconium-stained amniotic fluid. *Archives in Gynecology and Obstetrics, 264*(2), 84–87.

9

Powers: Stimulation and Hyperstimulation

Power produced by the contracting uterus is a prerequisite for vaginal birth. The once quiescent uterus transforms into a powerful contracting muscle. The previously firm cervix is modified, collagen is rearranged, water enters the cells, and the cervix softens in preparation for it to thin and open (Feltovich et al., 2005). The successful change from a firm (unripe) cervix to a soft (ripe) cervix will decrease the risk of a cesarean section (Grobman et al., 2007).

Behind these changes are genetic and biochemical events that are only partially understood. The S100A9 gene in the pregnant uterus and at least 17 other genes found in the amnion seem to be related to the onset of labor (Kim et al., 2007; Muleba et al., 2004). It is known that progesterone maintains uterine quiescence by repressing the influx of calcium into uterine contractile cells. Progesterone also regulates prostaglandin receptors in the cervix (Hinton, Grigsby, Pitzer, Brockman, & Myatt, 2005a, 2005b; Ruddock et al., 2007). The amnion may play a role in the withdrawal of progesterone, and progesterone receptors in the amnion appear to increase near term (Oh et al., 2005). As the level of progesterone wanes, the level of estrogen increases, thus decreasing uterine resistance to oxytocin. The plasma level of oxytocin and the prostaglandins E_2 and $F_{2\alpha}$ also increase, causing an increase in the frequency and strength of contractions (Yamaguchi, Cardoso, & Torres, 2007).

THE PHYSIOLOGY OF LABOR: UPREGULATION

The processes that prepare the uterus to contract during labor have been divided into three parts: upregulation, activation, and stimulation. Upregulation initiates the transition of the uterus from a quiescent state to a state in which rhythmic contractions can occur. During upregulation the cervix is invaded by neutrophils (Bugg, Crocker, Baker, Johnston, & Taggart, 2005). Neutrophils release proteins called cytokines. The cytokine interleukin (IL)-1β induces the production of the enzymes cyclooxygenase (COX-2) and matrix metalloproteinase (MMP-9) from the cells of the cervix. COX-2 and MMP-9 are needed to convert arachidonic acid in the cervix and uterine cell walls to prostaglandins (COX-2) and to break down the collagen in the cervix (MMP-9) (Astle, Newton, Thornton, Vatish, & Slater, 2007; Choi, Oh, Kim, & Roh, 2007).

During upregulation, the uterus also receives a signal from the fetal lungs. The signal comes from a surfactant protein (SP-A) from alveolar cells, which is present when the fetal lungs mature (Condon, Jeyasuria, Faust, & Mendelson, 2004). The level of the enzyme protein kinase Cβ increases and is related to the strength of uterine contractions (Yasuda et al., 2007). The placenta produces corticotropin-releasing hormone (CRH), which regulates the relaxation of the contracting uterus (Grammatopoulos, 2007; Smith, 2007). If the woman smokes, the placenta releases CRH. Nicotine also stimulates the adrenal glands to release norepinephrine, which can cause vasoconstriction and stimulate the uterus to contract (Justus, Arora, Sandhu, & Hobel, 2005).

ACTIVATION

After upregulation, the activation phase or preparatory phase begins. During this phase, uterine muscle cells change from a quiescent state to a contractile state during which genes that permit the uterus to contract during labor are expressed. Prostaglandin E_2 and $F_{2\alpha}$ and prostaglandin receptors increase in the uterus. Oxytocin receptors and gap junctions increase in number in the uterine cells (Shmygol, Gullam, Blanks, &

Thornton, 2006). Gap junctions allow ions with an electric charge to move from one cell to another so that the cells communicate and contract simultaneously.

STIMULATION

Spontaneous contractions of smooth muscle cells in the uterus can occur without neural or hormonal stimuli (Garfield, Maner, MacKay, Schlembach, & Saade, 2005). The synchronous contraction of uterine smooth muscle cells requires a "pacemaker" with an electric command. Apparently these pacemakers are functioning a few days before the onset of labor contractions because researchers have found a surge of uterine activity 3 days before the onset of spontaneous labor (Leman, Marque, & Gondry, 1999). Uterine irritability may occur in women who have a preterm gestation. After three days (or less) these women move into spontaneous labor.

PACEMAKER CELLS

Pacemaker cells are like the conductor of an orchestra. The conductor tells the orchestra when to begin, when to strengthen the sound, and when to diminish the sound. However, instead of one sole conductor of the orchestra, there are billions of pacemaker cells distributed throughout the body (corpus) of the uterus (Garfield, Maner, MacKay, Schlembach, & Saade, 2005). In laboring women, these pacemaker cells generate electrical bursts to trigger contractions and increase the frequency of contractions. There are no pacemaker cells, however, in the cervix (Garfield, Maner, MacKay, Schlembach, & Saade, 2005; Shafik, El-Sibai, & Shafik, 2004).

Depolarization and repolarization of pacemaker cells generates bursts or spikes of action-potential events (Allix et al., 2008; Garfield et al., 2005; Rihana, Lefrancois, & Marque, 2007; Shmygol, Gullam, Blanks, & Thornton, 2006). Action-potential events occur in single- and multiple-voltage spikes that can last more than 1 minute (Garfield, Maner, MacKay, Schlembach, & Saade, 2005). A single-voltage spike initiates contraction of the uterine cell. Multiple-voltage spikes increase the duration and strength of the contraction of the uterine cells (Maul, Maner, Olson, Saade, & Garfield, 2004).

Action-potential electrical activity is low and uncoordinated early in the pregnancy and becomes more intense and synchronized later in the pregnancy. Action-potential events peak at term gestation (Garfield, Maner, MacKay, Schlembach, & Saade, 2005). Closer to term or at term, when the uterine cells contract in unison, they will generate the power needed for labor and delivery (Smith, 2007).

OXYTOCIN

Oxytocin is a potent uterotonic agent and an endogenous neuropeptide that is released from the posterior pituitary gland into maternal plasma. During pregnancy, labor, and delivery, women secrete oxytocin from their posterior pituitary gland into their bloodstream in two to three spurts or pulses every 10 minutes (Dawood, 1989). The decidua also produces oxytocin during late gestation (Arthur, Taggart, & Mitchell, 2007).

Oxytocin binds with oxytocin receptors in the decidua and amnion, triggering the production of prostaglandins such as prostaglandin E_2 (Fuchs, Fuchs, Husslein, & Soloff, 1984; Makino, Zaragoza, Mitchell, Yonemoto, & Olson, 2007; Pavan et al., 2000). Oxytocin transiently increases the resting tone between contractions and it increases the strength and duration of contractions (Smith, 2007). Oxytocin released during nipple stimulation may cause uterine hypercontractility with an increased uterine tone (Lenke & Nemes, 1984; Schellpfeffer, Hoyle, & Johnson, 1985; Yamaguchi, Cardoso, & Torres, 2007). Nipple stimulation has been used to induce contractions and may not cause uterine hypercontractility if a strict protocol is followed (Kavanagh, Kelly, & Thomas, 2005). You should find out whether your hospital has a protocol for a nipple-stimulation/uterine-contraction stress test.

Oxytocin also binds with receptors in the uterine arteries causing vasoconstriction (Vedernikov, Betancourt, Wentz, Saade, & Garfield, 2006). This may decrease blood flow and oxygen delivery to the placenta and fetus.

During labor, oxytocin in the maternal plasma has two sources: the mother and her fetus. The fetal contribution averages 2.75 mU/minute, and the maternal contribution ranges between 2 and 4 mU/minute (Dawood, 1989; Dawood, Ylikorkala, Trivedi, & Fuchs, 1979; Dawood, Wang, Gupta, & Fuchs, 1978; Khan-Dawood & Dawood, 1984). At the time of delivery, the level of oxytocin in the maternal plasma rarely exceeds 8 mU/minute (Dawood, 1989; Dawood, Ylikorkala, Trivedi, & Fuchs, 1979; Khan-Dawood & Dawood, 1984).

CALCIUM

Oxytocin indirectly stimulates the release of calcium from intracellular stores (Bursztyn, Eytan, Jaffa, & Elad, 2007; Collins, Idriss, & Moore, 1995). The rise of intracellular calcium precedes the interaction between actin filaments and myosin in the uterine cells (Blanks et al., 2007; Woodcock, Taylor, & Thornton, 2006). Myosin is a protein that converts energy from adenosine triphosphate (ATP) to generate force from, and movement of, the smooth muscle cells of the uterus.

ADENOSINE TRIPHOSPHATE (ATP)

In vitro and in vivo administration of ATP stimulated uterine cell contractions, potentiated prostaglandin $F_{2\alpha}$-evoked contractions, and increased the rate of cervical ripening and dilation (Ziganshin et al., 2005). Researchers also found that women who are preeclamptic have higher levels of ATP than healthy women (Bakker, Donker, Timmer, van Pampus, & van Son, 2007; Bakker & Faas, 2007). Some nurses will tell you they have found that women with preeclampsia dilate faster than women who do not have preeclampsia. Perhaps ATP is related to their observations.

PROSTAGLANDINS

Prostaglandins are produced by almost every tissue in the body, but the prostaglandins most important to labor are the prostaglandins E_2 and $F_{2\alpha}$. Both produce uterine contractions, however, prostaglandin E_2 is needed to soften the cervix (O'Brien, 1995). Prostaglandin $F_{2\alpha}$ increases the calcium sensitivity of uterine cells, and influences the contraction and relaxation of uterine cells (Woodcock, Taylor, & Thornton, 2006).

ANXIETY, FEAR, AND DEPRESSION

Women who are anxious or fearful have a high level of catecholamines in their plasma. The catecholamine epinephrine may enter the fetal circulation triggering fetal tachycardia.

Women who smoke cigarettes or who are fearful, anxious, or depressed have a high level of the catecholamine norepinephrine in their plasma (Field et al., 2007). Norepinephrine binds with alpha-receptors in the uterus to stimulate contractions. These contractions usually do not dilate the cervix. Beta$_2$-receptors in the uterus bind with uterine relaxants such as the medication terbutaline (Brethine®), to decrease the number of contractions (Csonka et al., 2007; Grammatopoulos, 2007).

Norepinephrine may cause vasoconstriction, which may then cause a profound decrease in uterine blood flow to the uterus. This decrease in blood flow may affect the delivery of oxygen to the placenta and fetus. Anxiety may also be related to spasms in the spiral arteries contributing to partial separation of the placenta (Ascher, 1978). Therefore, nurses should act to decrease anxiety and fear in the mother in order to reduce placental and fetal complications. Depression may need medical intervention and the physician may need to prescribe an antidepressant.

ASSESSMENT OF UTERINE ACTIVITY: PALPATION

A gentle hand on the abdomen may be all that is needed to palpate the uterus during and between contractions. The duration of the contraction is as important as the relaxation between contractions. If there is a distance between your hand and the uterus, try pressing deeper or lift the panus and palpate under it to get closer to the uterus.

Women in preterm labor may not perceive contractions (Lawson, Dombrowski, Carter, & Hagglund, 2003). They may report cramping, a groin ache, thigh pain, or a low backache. You should palpate and place the tocotransducer low on the abdomen if her fetus is preterm.

The strength or quality of palpated contractions may be classified as mild, moderate, or strong. Some nurses use the word "firm" or "hard" to describe strong contractions. Mild contractions are felt when your hand easily indents the abdominal tissue during gentle palpation. Some practitioners think that mild contractions feel similar to pressing on one's cheek. Moderate contractions feel more like the nose; they are slightly indentable. Strong contractions feel hard like a forehead. The uterus will be hard and unindentable. Press your own cheek, nose, and forehead to gain a sense of the feel of mild, moderate, and strong contractions.

Palpation, however, is an inaccurate way to determine the strength of contractions. Physicians and nurses were only correct 56% of the time when they thought there was a mild contraction, 28% of the time when they thought there was a moderate contraction, and, 68% of the time when they thought there was a strong contraction compared with simultaneous intrauterine pressure readings (Arrabal & Nagey, 1996). If you use palpation to assess uterine activity without the aid of an electronic fetal monitor waveform, document your assessment of the frequency, duration, and strength of the contractions, and the resting tone of the uterus.

> **Documentation example**: Contractions every 3 to 4 minutes, mild to moderate lasting 40 to 60 seconds, resting tone soft.

> **Documentation example**: Complains of urge to push. 9 cm/100%/+1. Contractions palpate strong every 3 minutes, lasting 70 to 80 seconds with soft resting tone between contractions. Encouraged to breathe through contractions and discussed she is not ready to push because she is not 10-cm dilated.

EXTERNAL UTERINE MONITORING: THE TOCOTRANSDUCER

To assist in your evaluation of uterine activity, you may use an external monitor called a tocotransducer (toco) or an internal monitor called an intrauterine pressure catheter (IUPC). The method chosen to assess uterine activity depends on the clinical situation and the availability of personnel skilled in the insertion of an intrauterine pressure catheter (Allman & Steer, 1993).

The word *tocotransducer* is derived from the Greek word *tokos*, which means "childbirth." The tocotransducer has also been called a tocodynamometer. It is pressure sensitive. Avoid placing the tocotransducer too high on the uterus because it can slide up and flip over, and then it is monitoring her gown! Periodically move the tocotransducer to increase maternal comfort.

If pressure is applied to the surface of the tocotransducer, a hill or peak is produced on the fetal monitor paper. If pressure is withdrawn from the tocotransducer, a valley or a drop from a peak of the contraction hill will be recorded. The goal is to create a hill when there is a contraction. To do this, place the tocotranducer near the top of the uterus (fundus). The fundus usually pushes forward during a contraction. If the fetus kicks, pressure may be applied to the tocotransducer and you will see a spike or spikes on the recording. If she vomits, you may see multiple short spikes. If she pushes, the spikes may look like pickets in a picket fence. If she is snoring, there may be a jagged appearance to the uterine activity tracing. When she is breathing, you may see up and down movements in the recording.

INTRAUTERINE PRESSURE CATHETER (IUPC)

Contractions may also be recorded with a specially designed intrauterine catheter placed inside the amniotic sac after the rupture of the membranes. An IUPC may be a transducer-tipped catheter with a microchip in the tip, or a sensor-tip catheter with an air-filled balloon in the tip.

The transducer-tipped IUPC is attached to the cable, and the cable is plugged into the electronic fetal monitor prior to insertion. Transducer-tipped IUPCs are equilibrated to room air prior to insertion. This is called zeroing. This equilibrates the pressure-sensitive computer chip in the tip to the pressure in room air. Once it is inserted, there should be 5 to 25 mm Hg of resting tone.

The sensor-tipped (ballon-tipped) catheter (Koala®) does not have a microchip in the tip. Instead, the pressure-sensitive computer chip is in the cable. The cable is plugged into the electronic fetal monitor and zeroed either before or after the IUPC is inserted. After confirming there was no flashback of blood in the IUPC (which would indicate an extraovular insertion), the IUPC is attached to the cable. You will have to learn about the specific type of IUPC at your hospital. Read the entire IUPC package and any other literature your hospital has available. You should also read your hospital's policy, procedure, and protocol related to IUPC insertion. In some states of the United States, a registered staff nurse may insert an IUPC following validation of competency.

EXTRAOVULAR INSERTION

Extraovular insertion occurs when the IUPC is inadvertently inserted between the uterine wall and the membranes (extraovular) instead of into the amniotic sac (see Figure 9.1). Evidence of an extraovular placement will be the lack of a uterine waveform or a reversed waveform (like a valley instead of a hill), or a blunt or damped waveform. If the Koala® IUPC or any other IUPC with a clear window is inserted into the extraovular space, there will usually be a flashback of blood that you will see in the IUPC, as well as a blunt waveform with an elevation in the resting tone on the printout, usually near 30 mm Hg.

If there is an extraovular insertion of the IUPC, the IUPC must be removed and another one inserted at a different location. Any IUPC can be inserted into the extraovular space. This is not related to the skill of the person who inserted the IUPC, it just happens.

> **Clinical example**: Dr. Intrau inserted a sensor-tipped IUPC and there was an immediate flashback of blood. There was also a blunt contraction waveform with a resting tone recorded at 30 mm Hg. The nurse stated, "Doctor, we have an extraovular insertion." The physician immediately removed the IUPC. The tocotransducer was reapplied until a new IUPC was obtained. After the new IUPC was obtained, it was inserted into the uterus and the waveform indicated an intrauterine insertion. An amnioinfusion of a bolus of 500 mL normal saline was infused into the uterus, followed by 80 mL/hour via an infusion pump to cushion the umbilical cord.

Occasionally, an intraovular transducer-tipped IUPC will produce a blunt waveform when the computer chip in it is

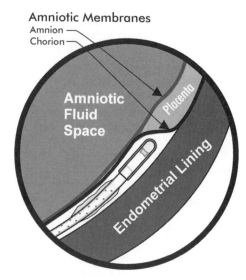

Figure 9.1: Extraovular insertion of an intrauterine pressure catheter between the uterine wall and membranes surrounding the fetus. (Image courtesy of Clinical Innovations, LLC, Murray, Utah.)

obstructed. Roll the IUPC 180 degrees to see if you can move the tip away from the obstruction. If the waveform changes from a blunt hill to a peaked hill, you successfully removed the obstruction. If it does not change the waveform, there probably is an extraovular insertion and the IUPC should be removed. To confirm an intraovular IUPC placement, ask your patient to cough. There should be a spike in the IUPC waveform and a normal resting tone (less than 25 mm Hg) with a peaked contraction waveform during contractions.

UTERINE ACTIVITY WAVEFORMS

Contractions affect the fetus. Adequate monitoring of uterine activity is a prerequisite for proper analysis of the fetal heart rate pattern (Bakker & van Geijn, 2008). In addition to palpation, nurses analyze the uterine activity waveform produced by the electronic fetal monitor (EFM) and classify contraction patterns based on the images they see. Some of the contraction waveforms nurses may see include uterine irritability, prolonged contractions, normally spaced contractions, coupling, and tachysystole. Uterine irritability occurs when contractions are created by physiologic factors caused by an infection and prostaglandin production, dehydration with the release of antidiuretic hormone (vasopressin), or bleeding and the presence of thrombin in the uterus.

THE ANATOMY OF A CONTRACTION WAVEFORM

Contractions have a beginning, a peak (acme), and an end (see Figure 9.2). The time between contractions is called the interval. Resting tone is the state of the uterus during the interval. The resting tone may palpate firm or soft. It is unlikely

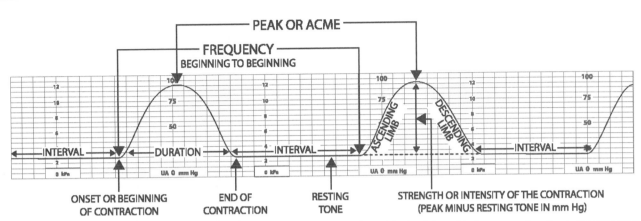

Figure 9.2: The ascending limb, peak, and descending limb of a contraction with the interval between contractions. Resting tone is assessed during the interval. If the interval is less than 60 seconds, there is an abnormal resting tone.

that the uterus following an interval lasting less than 1 minute will have a soft resting tone.

Contraction frequency is timed from the beginning of one contraction to the beginning of the next contraction, except in the case of coupling or tripling. With coupling or tripling there will be two or three contractions with little rest between them. With coupling or tripling, frequency is timed from the beginning of the first contraction in the series to the beginning of the first contraction in the next series.

LOW-AMPLITUDE, HIGH-FREQUENCY WAVES

The image of uterine irritability is low-amplitude, high-frequency (LAHF) waves. Uterine irritability is not the same as tachysystole (high-amplitude, high-frequency waves). When there is uterine irritability there are contractions but they are usually brief (less than 30 seconds in duration), weak, and frequent, that is, there is little to no interval between the contractions (see Figure 9.3).

Uterine irritability may have a waveform of high-amplitude, high-frequency waves, but the duration of the contractions will be close to 20 seconds. Usually contractions during labor that change the cervix are 30 or more seconds in duration. Women who have little subcutaneous tissue and fat are more likely to have high-amplitude, high-frequency waves when they have uterine irritability, and they are monitored with a tocotransducer.

Women who have uterine irritability may not feel the contractions or they may feel cramps. If they feel pain, there may be a placental abruption. Uterine stimulants should be discontinued until the cause of the uterine irritability is determined. Notify the obstetric provider when you observe uterine irritability. In addition to a placental abruption, uterine irritability may occur when women are dehydrated or when they have an infection. Thrombin is the stimulant for contractions when there is a placental abruption. Thrombin activates receptors in the uterus called protease-activated receptors or PARs.

PAR-1 activation in the human uterus exerts a significant uterotonic effect (Allen, O'Brien, Friel, Smith, & Morrison, 2007).

Documentation example: Uterine irritability. Complains of cramping and low backache. Reports burning with urination. Temperature 99.6. Fetal heart rate 140 to 150 bpm, moderate variability, acceleration to 160 for 40 seconds, no decelerations. SVE: FT/thick/high. Notified Dr. Tanksfurcallin of this assessment. Orders received.

COUPLING OR DOUBLING OF CONTRACTIONS

The waveform of coupling of contractions is illustrated in Figure 9.4. The first contraction in the set is longer than the second (shorter and weaker) contraction. When there is coupling, the interval between the two contractions is shorter than 1 minute. However, the interval between the sets of contractions should be longer than 1 minute to allow fetal oxygen to be replenished. Some people call coupling "doubling" or "camelback contractions" or "biphasic contractions." When labor is augmented with oxytocin, coupling occurs almost twice as often as in spontaneous labor or induced labor. In augmented labors, coupling reflected ineffective uterine function (Gyselaers, Vansteelant, Spitz, Odendaal, & Van Assche, 1991).

Documentation example: Coupling every 6 minutes with contractions 80 to 100 seconds, peak pressure 50 to 75 mm Hg with resting tone near 20 mm Hg.

Coupling of contractions has also been found in longer labors and is associated with an increased cesarean section rate in nulliparous women (Oppenheimer et al., 2002). The fetal position in these longer labors was not determined. The incidence of uterine coupling increases as maternal age increases. Coupling of contractions in older women may also

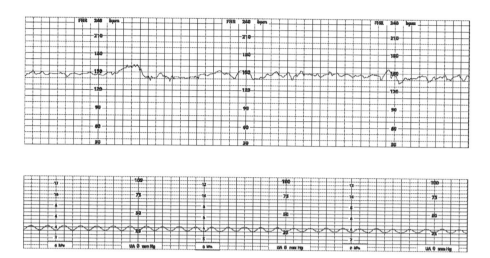

Figure 9.3: Uterine irritability is usually reflected by the waveform of low-amplitude, high-frequency waves. Occasionally a thin woman will have a waveform with high-amplitude, 20-second contractions close together.

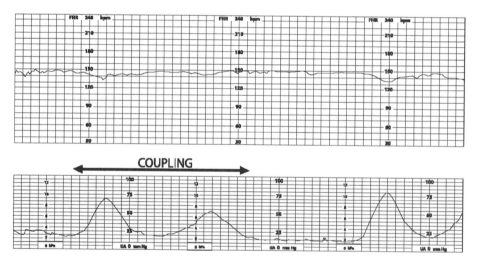

COUPLING

Figure 9.4: Coupling of contractions often occurs when the fetus is occiput posterior or has a persistent occiput transverse position, or during augmentation.

be associated with an increased risk of a cesarean section (Smith et al., 2007).

HIGH-AMPLITUDE, LOW-FREQUENCY WAVES

During labor, cervical dilation will occur if there are 11 to 12 contractions each hour, or approximately two contractions every 10 minutes (see Figure 9.5). As delivery approaches, there may be 21 to 23 contractions an hour, or approximately 3 to 4 contractions every 10 minutes (Lindgren, 1973).

Documentation example: Contractions every 2 to 2 1/2 minutes for 60 seconds, moderate to strong, and soft between contractions. Fetal heart rate 140s with average variability (alternate documentation is baseline 145 with moderate variability).

SPONTANEOUS PROLONGED CONTRACTIONS

Only two case reports were found related to spontaneous prolonged contractions where contractions lasted more than

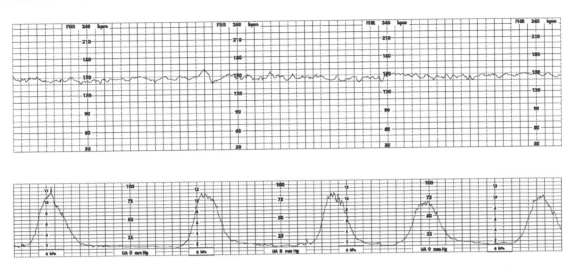

Figure 9.5: Contractions during early labor at 3 cm/80%/–2. In this example, there are adequate contractions to dilate the cervix (at least two in 10 minutes).

2 minutes (Meniru et al., 2002; Sieprath, Koninckx, & Van Assche, 1986). These abnormally long contractions were classified by the authors as essential, prolonged, and hypertonic, or "essential hypertonus." They seemed to be related to deciduitis with chorioamnionitis and funisitis in the first case report, and there was no identified cause in the second case report.

HIGH-AMPLITUDE, HIGH-FREQUENCY WAVES

Uterine activity is abnormal if the interval between contractions is less than 1 minute. Unlike uterine irritability, contractions of high amplitude and high frequency will usually last longer than 20 to 30 seconds. They may palpate as mild, moderate, or strong. High-amplitude, high-frequency waves have been called "tachysystole" or "hyperstimulation." Tachysystole is the waveform. Hyperstimulation is what happens to the uterine cells to produce tachysystole.

More than five contractions in 10 minutes is considered abnormal (see Figure 9.6). The cause of this abnormal uterine activity may be physiologic or the presence of a uterine stimulant.

Although the dose of oxytocin in the example in Figure 9.6 is not extreme (10 mU/minute), it is too high for the uterus. The oxytocin dose must be titrated to produce fewer than five contractions in 10 minutes and should be decreased, if necessary, to maintain less than five contractions in 10 minutes.

A HYPERSTIMULATED UTERUS BY OXYTOCIN

A hyperstimulated uterus may have fewer than five contractions in 10 minutes, but the interval between contractions is less than 1 minute (see Figure 9.7). Another word used to describe long, strong contractions is "tetanic." An overdose of oxytocin may cause this type of uterine activity.

The half-life of oxytocin ranges from 3 to 4 minutes to as long as 15 minutes. After discontinuing the oxytocin infusion, wait 30 minutes for the uterine contractions to space out and for the exogenous oxytocin to be fully metabolized. During that time you should assess and record the fetal heart rate and uterine activity. If there are no contraindications, infuse a bolus of intravenous fluid (500 to 1000 mL) to diminish the number of contractions and then assess the cervix. If the patient is dilated 5 cm, she may no longer need a uterine stimulant. Notify the midwife or physician of your assessments, actions, and evaluation of the maternal and fetal status.

MONTEVIDEO UNITS

In 1960 Drs. Caldeyro-Barcia and Poseiro of Montevideo, Uruguay, called the pattern of more than five contractions in 10 minutes "tachysystolia" (uterine hyperactivity). Usually when there was tachysystolia there were also more than 250 Montevideo Units (MVUs). However, MVUs are not the same thing as tachysystole. A hyperstimulated uterus may, however, have 240 or more MVUs with a waveform of five or more contractions in 10 minutes, or long contractions with less than a 1-minute interval between contractions.

Montevideo Units are calculated by subtracting the resting tone (in mm Hg) from the peak pressure (in mm Hg) for each contraction in a 10-minute period and adding up those values. The pressure at the peak of the contraction minus the pressure when the uterus is at rest is called "intensity" or "active pressure." For example, if the peak pressure is 70 mm Hg and the resting tone is 20 mm Hg, the intensity or active pressure is 50 mm Hg. If there are three contractions in 10 minutes and the active pressures are 60, 50, and 40, there are 150 MVUs (see Figure 9.8). Another way to calculate MVUs is to take the average peak pressure and subtract the average resting tone

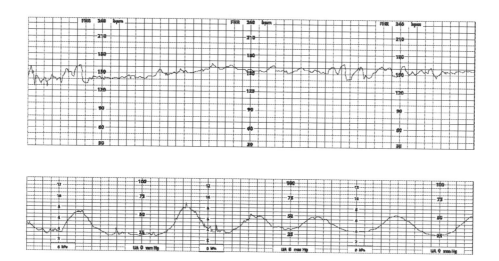

Figure 9.6: High-amplitude, high-frequency waves (tachysystole) due to hyperstimulation of the uterus from the infusion of exogenous oxytocin. The cervix was 5 cm/100% effaced. The oxytocin infusion should be decreased or discontinued until there are four or fewer contractions every 10 minutes.

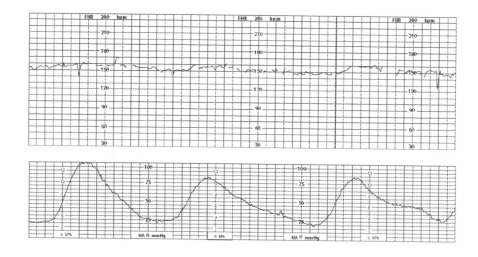

Figure 9.7: Uterine hyperstimulation in a nulliparous woman who was receiving an overdose of oxytocin (42 mU/minute). If you encounter this type of uterine activity, the oxytocin should be immediately discontinued because this abnormal uterine activity significantly increases the risk of fetal hypoxia and acidemia.

and multiply that value by the number of contractions in 10 minutes. Some nurses calculate MVUs each half hour when an IUPC is in place. Note, however, that MVUs cannot be calculated when a tocotransducer is used to assess uterine activity.

It was once believed that a calculation of 350 MVUs was the maximum acceptable and that oxytocin should be discontinued when there were 350 MVUs (Caldeyro-Barcia & Poseiro,

1960). Bakker and van Geijn (2008) found that an average of 236 MVUs during the last hour of the first stage of labor preceded the birth of a baby with a normal umbilical artery pH of ≥ 7.12. An average of 261 MVUs preceded the birth of a baby with a low umbilical artery pH (≤ 7.11). Instead of 350 MVUs, oxytocin should be decreased or discontinued when there are 240 mm Hg during the last hour of the first stage of labor. Of course, oxytocin can be decreased or discontinued

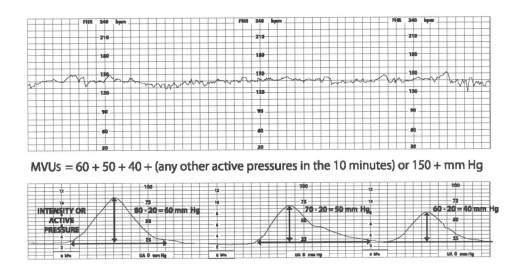

MVUs = 60 + 50 + 40 + (any other active pressures in the 10 minutes) or 150 + mm Hg

Figure 9.8: Calculation of Montevideo Units (MVUs).

any time contractions are too strong or too frequent, or if the fetus is intolerant.

During the second stage of labor, Bakker and van Geijn (2008) found an average of 402 MVUs preceded the birth of a baby born with a normal umbilical artery pH, but 442 MVUs preceded the birth of a baby with a low umbilical artery pH. To avoid fetal and neonatal acidemia, you should discontinue oxytocin if the MVUs are near 400 during the second stage of labor. In fact, most women do not need oxytocin at all during the second stage of labor.

UTERINE REVERSAL PATTERN

When the external tocotransducer is placed on the maternal abdomen over the uterus, the fetus or that portion of the uterus under the tocotransducer may move away from the tocotransducer during contractions. When this occurs, the pressure on the tocotransducer diminishes and a reversal pattern will appear (see Figure 9.9). If the mother is sleeping, do not move the tocotransducer! The contractions can still be counted, they are just upside down.

If the mother is awake, however, you should move the tocotransducer to a new location. Pick a location where the uterus pushes on the tocotransducer during a contraction. Palpate the abdomen during a contraction to locate that part of the uterus that pushes forward and place the tocotransducer at that spot.

> **Documentation example:** Uterine reversal pattern noted. Tocotranducer adjusted. Patient turned to right side due to variable decelerations with contractions. Baseline 150 bpm. No accelerations, minimal variability.

MATERNAL CARDIAC FUNCTION AND FETAL OXYGENATION

Uterine contractions increase maternal myocardial oxygen demand, right ventricular preload, mean arterial pressure, pul-

monary artery pressure, and pulmonary artery wedge pressure (Witcher & Harvey, 2006). An increase in maternal oxygen demand and consumption may decrease oxygen that would otherwise be available for the uterus, placenta, and fetus. Oxytocin increases tension in the uterine arteries, which decreases perfusion of the placenta, thus decreasing oxygen delivery to the fetus (Vedernikov, Betancourt, Wentz, Saade, & Garfield, 2006). Blood flow and oxygen delivery to the uterus are reduced during contractions.

Maternal blood flow to the placenta decreases during contractions because the uterine muscle squeezes spiral arteries, which then decreases blood flow to the placenta and venous outflow from the placenta (East, Dunster, & Colditz, 1998). Because of the decrease in blood flow and oxygen delivery to the placenta and fetus, contractions can cause fetal hypoxia and acidemia (Bakker, Kurver, Kuik, & van Geijn, 2007; Graham, 2007). Fetal arteriolar oxygen saturation (SaO_2) decreases 5 to 10% during contractions. The lowest level is found 92 seconds after the contraction peak (McNamara & Johnson, 1995). Fetal hemoglobin oxygen saturation (SpO_2) reached its lowest level 50 seconds after the contraction ended (East, Dunster, & Colditz, 1998). With this in mind, if the time between contractions is less than 1 minute, the fetus basically doesn't have time to "catch its breath" by having its oxygen replenished. The cumulative effect of a short interval between contractions is hypoxia with a risk of acidemia, respiratory acidosis, and metabolic acidosis.

If contractions are more frequent than every 2 minutes, or the interval between them is less than 1.5 minutes, fetal SaO_2 decreases to as low as 18%. Less than 30% is abnormal. When there are fewer contractions, fetal SaO_2 is 54% or higher. The normal fetal SaO_2 is between 30 and 70%. Maternal supplemental oxygen increases fetal SaO_2 7 to 11% within 3 minutes (McNamara & Johnson, 1995; Johnson, Johnson, McNamara,

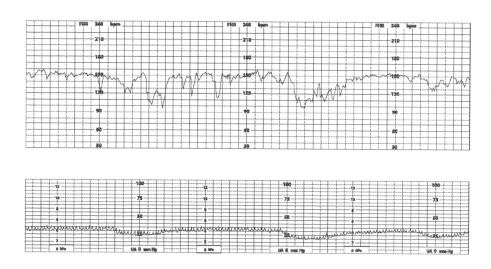

Figure 9.9: Uterine reversal pattern. There are three contractions in this image. During and between these contractions there are variable decelerations of the fetal heart rate.

Montague, Jongsma, & Aumeerally, 1994; Johnson, van Oudgaarden, Montagne, & McNamara, 1994). Therefore, it is best for fetal health if at least 1 1/2 minutes elapses between contractions.

UTERINE HYPERSTIMULATION

Under normal conditions, hyperstimulation is unlikely during labor since plasma concentrations of oxytocin do not fluctuate (Thornton, Davison, & Baylis, 1990). Hyperstimulation is likely to occur when uterine stimulants are administered, including Dinoprostone E₂ (Prepidil® or Cervidil®), prostaglandin E₁ (misoprostol or Cytotec®), and oxytocin (Pitocin® or Syntocinon®).

To avoid hyperstimulation when exogenous prostaglandins or oxytocin are administered, these medications should be discontinued once the patient is contracting and dilating. Oxytocin should be discontinued when the patient is in the active phase of labor and dilating. Discontinuing oxytocin does not significantly lengthen labor. Physicians found that there were fewer instances of hyperstimulation in the group whose oxytocin was discontinued at the beginning of the active phase of labor (4.8%) than in women who received oxytocin up until the time of delivery (6.9%) (Ustunyurt et al., 2007).

Hyperstimulation may also occur as a natural phenomenon when the patient has uterine fibroids. The presence of fibroids was related to an increased frequency of contractions (six or more in 10 minutes) during labor (Sheiner et al., 2004).

COCAINE AND UTERINE HYPERSTIMULATION

Cocaine use may precede uterine hyperstimulation and decreased uterine relaxation due to the increase of calcium from intracellular stores (Fomin, Singh, Brown, Natarajan, & Hurd,

1999). Cocaine use has also been associated with miscarriage, placental abruption, spontaneous uterine rupture (not related to a history of cesarean section or vaginal birth after cesarean), and preterm labor (Ferraro, Ferraro, & Massard, 1997). Placental abruption has occurred within 1 to 5 hours, and as late as 18 hours, after cocaine use (Flowers, Clark, & Westney, 1991; Cohen, Green, & Crombleholme, 1991).

Women who use cocaine have decreased prostacyclin production, which is needed to relax blood vessels. These women also have high levels of norepinephrine (Wang, Dombrowski, & Hurd, 1996; Smith, Dombrowski, Leach, & Hurd, 1995; Ferraro et al., 1997; Zhao & Sun, 2004; Mastrogiannis, Luckenbau, & O'Brien, 2003; Wang, Gauvin et al., 1996). As a result of these physiological changes, women who use cocaine will have an increased heart rate and blood pressure, and decreased uterine and placental perfusion with uterine artery vasoconstriction (Chao, 1996; George, Smith, & Curet, 1995; Sutliff, Gayheart-Walsten, Snyder, Roberts, & Johnson, 1999). Cocaine administration to pregnant rats was associated with a 27% reduction in uterine blood flow and a 30% reduction of blood flow to the placenta (Patel, Laungani, Grose, & Dow-Edwards, 1999).

URINE TOXICOLOGY

If a toxicology screen is ordered, the patient should be informed of the purpose of the test and should consent to the test. A toxicology screen may detect the presence of many substances including ethanol, methanol, acetone, isopropanol, acetaminophen, amphetamines, barbiturates, benzodiazepines, cocaine, codeine, hydromorphone, glutethimide, meperidine, meprobamate, methadone, morphine, pentazocine, phencyclidine, phenothiazine, propoxyphene, amitriptyline, nortriptyline, doxepin, imipramine, and desipramine.

THROMBIN AND HYPERSTIMULATION

Labor occurs because there has been a change in the maternal–fetal interface between the decidua and placenta. This change is mediated by plasminogen activators and inhibitors. This same plasminogen activator/inhibitor system plays a role in hemorrhage-mediated physiological events related to placental abruption. Thrombin is a protease, which is an active enzyme found in the blood (Elovitz, Saunders, Ascher-Landsberg, & Phillippe, 2000). Thrombin promotes the production of enzymes by the decidua. These enzymes stimulate the migration of neutrophils that infiltrate the decidua and they are related to an increase in the number of contractions (Norwitz et al., 2007). Thrombin also stimulates the uterus to contract because of the activation of protease-activated receptors (PARs) in the uterus (Allen, O'Brien, Friel, Smith, & Morrison, 2007). Thrombin can stimulate contractions even when there is no cervical dilatation (Elovitz, Ascher-Landsberg, Saunders, & Phillippe, 2000; Elovitz, Saunders, Ascher-Landsberg, & Phillippe, 2000; Pan, Goharkhay, Felix, & Wing, 2003). The presence of uterine irritability or tachysystole may be due to the effect of thrombin related to bleeding from a placental abruption.

HISTAMINE, BRADYKININ, AND HYPERSTIMULATION

It is believed that cytokines, prostaglandins, leukotrienes, thromboxane, and histamine are released in response to exposure to amniotic fluid (Clark, Hankins, Dudley, Dildy, & Porter, 1995). Histamine increases spontaneous contractions in uterine tissue from term pregnant nonlaboring women. The massive release of histamine associated with an amniotic fluid embolism appears to be related to tachysystole (Bytautiene, Vedernikov, Saade, Romero, & Garfield, 2003).

Bradykinin is also released into the maternal blood stream during an amniotic fluid embolism (Schoening, 2006). Bradykinin acts on the uterus to increase the strength of contractions (Brown, Leite, Engler, Discher, & Strauss III, 2006). Robillard and colleagues (2005) demonstrated a sudden and massive consumption of plasma bradykinin-generating capacity that occurred simultaneously with clinical and biologic signs suggestive of an amniotic fluid embolism. Symptoms of amniotic fluid embolism may include seizures, followed by hypotension, tachysystole, and coagulopathy. When these patients are intubated, it is difficult to inflate their lungs.

TACHYSYSTOLE

Tachysystole is the waveform recorded by the electronic fetal monitor when there is uterine hyperstimulation. Tachysystole means there are five or more contractions in 10 minutes. Nurses must act to decrease uterine activity when they see tachysystole. If you observe tachysystole and/or an abnormal fetal heart rate pattern, try to determine its cause after you discontinue the uterine stimulant. If a medication such as a prostaglandin vaginal insert is in use, remove it. If oxytocin is infusing, decrease or discontinue it. The goal is to obtain a maximum of four contractions in 10 minutes during labor.

If there are five or more contractions in 10 minutes, then significant fetal oxygen desaturation will occur (Simpson & James, 2008). If there are five or more contractions in 10 minutes, the interval between contractions is usually less than 1 1/2 minutes (see Figure 9.10). In addition to discontinuing the uterine stimulant, supplemental oxygen should be administered to the laboring patient if there is an abnormal fetal heart rate pattern. The administration of 10 L/minute of oxygen via a tight-fitting, nonrebreather face mask substantially and significantly increases fetal oxygen saturation (Haydon et al., 2006).

> **Documentation example:** Tachysystole. Oxytocin discontinued. Fetal heart rate 150 to 160, suspect fetal PVCs (or suspect fetal arrhythmia). Patient turned to right side, intravenous bolus of lactated Ringer's solution infusing. Physician notified that oxytocin was discontinued and informed of suspected fetal arrhythmia.

In the fetal heart rate in Figure 9.10, there is evidence of a fetal arrhythmia. The image of upward and downward deflections is common with premature ventricular contractions (PVCs) of the fetus. PVCs have been reported as an adverse reaction to oxytocin in the fetus and infant. Small amounts of infused oxytocin probably reach the fetus (*Physicians' Desk Reference*, 1995).

Fetal brain oxygen decreases when the frequency or strength of contractions increases. Fetal cerebral oxygen was found to be at its lowest level when the peak-to-peak time between contractions was less than 2.3 minutes (Peebles et al., 1994). A fetal defense mechanism is the redistribution of blood from the limbs to the vital organs (Fu & Olofsson, 2007). The fetal vital organs are the brain, the heart, and the adrenal glands. In animal studies, brief periods of hypoxia disrupted nerve function and caused the death of brain cells (Tomimatsu, Peña, & Longo, 2007). To increase brain oxygen, the fetus automatically responds by dilating the middle cerebral artery, and blood flow to the fetal brain increases (Li, Gudmundsson, & Olofsson, 2006; Tomimatsu et al., 2007).

If there is hypoxia, there may also be carbon-dioxide retention (hypercarbia or hypercapnia) in the fetal blood stream (Tomimatsu et al., 2007). If there is a high level of carbon dioxide, oxygen will be released from hemoglobin for use by the tissues. If the delivery of oxygen to the fetus does not increase between contractions, the fetus will eventually deplete oxygen in its bloodstream and in its red blood cells, and may decompensate or even die.

The risk of fetal acidemia increases when the number of contractions in a 10-minute period increases. Recently, the intrauterine pressure catheter (IUPC) recordings taken during the last hour of the first stage of labor and the entire length of the second stage of labor (33 to 37 minutes), as well as the umbilical venous and arterial blood gases of 1,433 neonates, were evaluated to determine the relationship between neonatal acidemia and the frequency and strength of uterine contrac-

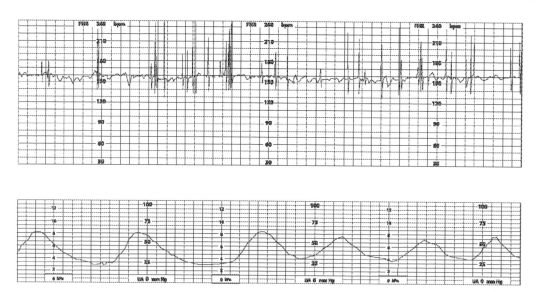

Figure 9.10: Tachysystole as a result of hyperstimulation due to oxytocin (16 mU/minute). Tachysystole due to an overdose of oxytocin significantly increases the risk of fetal acidemia.

tions. Seventy-seven newborns had an umbilical arterial pH of 7.11 or less, and the remaining neonates were nonacidemic. A computer program was used to analyze uterine activity. An inverse relationship was found between the number of contractions in a 10-minute period and the umbilical artery pH. The mothers of nonacidemic newborns had significantly fewer contractions during the last hour of the first stage of labor and during the second stage of labor than mothers with acidemic fetuses (4.3 versus 5.7, and 4.4 versus 6.4, respectively). The goal to prevent fetal acidemia is no more than four contractions every 10 minutes (Bakker, Kurver, Kuik, & van Geijn, 2007).

Acidemia is also related to contraction intensity, that is, 175 to 347 Montevideo units (MVUs) during the first stage of labor, and 309 to 575 MVUs during the second stage of labor, were related to acidemia (Bakker et al., 2007). Based on this information, oxygen delivery to the fetus is enhanced when there are four or fewer contractions every 10 minutes. In addition, it appears that exceeding 175 MVUs during the first stage of labor, and 300 MVUs during the second stage of labor, increases the risk of acidemia.

AUGMENTATION WITH EXOGENOUS OXYTOCIN

If the uterine power is weak, then hypotonic contractions are probably present. If there are hypotonic contractions, the cervix may not change or the fetus may not descend. Weak contractions produce functional dystocia. Functional dystocia may be due to the lack of an increase in prostaglandin $F_{2\alpha}$. When membranes rupture spontaneously women have more prostaglandin $F_{2\alpha}$ in their plasma than when membranes are ruptured by a health care provider (Fuchs, Goeschen, Husslein, Rasmussen, & Fuchs, 1983).

Weak contractions may be mild, or mild to moderate, and may be irregular in their timing. The midwife or physician should be informed of your assessment and he or she may decide to order the infusion of oxytocin. The infusion of oxytocin to augment hypotonic contractions is called "augmentation."

The World Health Organization recommends amniotomy and oxytocin administration until there are three or four contractions every 10 minutes, or until the pain perceived is too intense (Nordstrom & Waldenstrom, 2002). If there are more than four contractions every 10 minutes or if the pain is too intense, the oxytocin infusion should be decreased or discontinued.

The only adverse effect of exogenous oxytocin on the fetus is dose-related hyperstimulation (Clark et al., 2007). If there are abnormal fetal heart rate patterns or tachysystole, or both, the oxytocin should be discontinued. You should document the fetal heart rate pattern and uterine activity you observed before and after the oxytocin infusion was discontinued.

Even if the oxytocin order calls for a low-dose, a high-dose, active management of labor, or "Pit to distress," the nurse needs to follow a conservative protocol and decrease or discontinue the oxytocin infusion to protect the fetus (Clark et al., 2007; Freeman & Nageotte, 2007). The best plan is to discontinue the infusion to allow the uterus time to rest, and to allow the placenta and fetus time to receive oxygen. In addition, "Pit to distress" is not an acceptable order. If a provider writes "Pit to distress," notify your charge nurse or supervisor. Nursing management will have to discuss the order with the person who wrote it. At all times, you must practice to prevent harm.

Exhibit 9.1: Bishop score or Bishop index.

Score	Dilatation (cm)	Effacement (%)	Station (cm)	Consistency	Position
0	Closed	0–25	−3	Firm	Posterior
1	1–2	25–50	−2	Medium	Mid
2	3–4	50–75	−1/0	Soft	Anterior
3	>5	75	+1/+2		

SCHEDULED, PREVENTIVE, OR ELECTIVE INDUCTION?

The indications for induction of labor may be a pregnancy that is *postdates* (past the estimated date of delivery), hypertension, or rupture of the membranes prior to the onset of contractions or intrauterine growth restriction (Peregrine, O'Brien, Omar, & Jauniaux, 2006). Induction may be elective because the obstetrician or perinatologist decides that a "preventive" induction is needed due to maternal risk factors (Nicholson et al., 2007). A preventive induction has also been called a "risk-guided, prostaglandin-assisted labor induction" or "active management of risk." Prostaglandins will be administered to ripen the cervix, followed by the infusion of oxytocin (Nicholson et al., 2008).

As pregnant women age, the number of inductions increases (Nicholson et al., 2008). In one study, 30% of women over 40 years of age were induced compared with 12.2% of women younger than 25, 16.7% of women 25 to 34 years of age, and 22.1% of women 34 to 39 years of age. Women over 40 also have an increased risk of cesarean section for failure to progress or an abnormal fetal heart rate pattern even though the use of oxytocin or the length of labor did not vary in each age group (Ecker, Chen, Cohen, Riley, & Lieberman, 2001).

IS THE CERVIX RIPE?

When a woman is admitted for induction, she usually has a closed or nearly closed, firm (unripe) cervix. In some parts of the United States, nurses will say, "The cervix is green." This does not mean it is the color green or that there is meconium staining of the cervix. It means that the cervix is unripe and hard, just as fruit is hard when it is unripe and soft when it is ripe.

The cervix needs to ripen (soften) in order to dilate. The physician or midwife will determine if the cervix is unripe or ripe by calculating a Bishop score (see Exhibit 9.1). An unripe cervix will have a Bishop score (Bishop index) of less than 6. If the cervix is unripe it will usually exceed 30 mm (3 cm) in length (Bartha, Romero-Carmona, Martinez-del-Fresno, & Comino-Delgado, 2005).

The degree of dilatation is the factor in the Bishop score that best predicts the success of an elective induction (Bremme & Nilsson, 1984). The consistency of the cervix and parity are also related to a successful induction. The highest rate of spontaneous vaginal delivery is found in multiparous women who have a favorable (ripe) cervix.

Clinical example: A secundigravida presented at 0600 for induction due to pregnancy-induced hypertension. Her cervix was dilated 2 cm, was 50% effaced, with a fetus at a −2 station. The cervix was firm and posterior. What was the Bishop score? If you calculated a score of 3 you are right. Therefore, her cervix was unripe.

MECHANICAL RIPENING OF THE CERVIX

If the cervix is nearly closed, firm and unripe, the obstetric provider may choose to mechanically dilate the cervix. Mechanical dilation requires the insertion of a medication or a device into the os (opening) of the cervix. Prostaglandin E_2 gel, a catheter with or without use of a saline infusion, and laminaria are often used for this purpose.

Laminaria are made of seaweed ("sea-grown plants") and they absorb water and expand. Laminaria may have viable spores present even after they are processed with ethylene oxide. Therefore, laminaria are not sterile and they increase the risk of infection. When laminaria enlarge, they push on the inside wall of the cervix to open the os. Laminaria are also called "laminaria tents." They are usually removed 12 hours after they were inserted by the obstetric provider.

Women who have an extraovular catheter inserted into their cervical os with a saline infusion are more dilated and effaced than women who receive laminaria or a prostaglandin gel. Therefore, many physicians choose not to use laminaria or gel and have changed their practice to include insertion of a catheter in the cervical os with or without the simultaneous infusion of normal saline (Guinn, Goepfert, Christine, Owen, & Hauth, 2000).

The use of an extraovular or extraamniotic balloon, inflated above the internal cervical os, is a nonpharmacologic, mechanical method of cervical ripening. Traction may be applied to the catheter and normal saline may be infused through the end of the catheter or into the catheter's port into the extraamniotic space (Sherman et al., 1996).

A Foley catheter is often used for this purpose. A Foley catheter is measured in French (F) units. 1F unit is 0.33 mm. For mechanical ripening, a 30F Foley catheter is placed inside the internal os, under the membranes and fetal presenting part. A 30F Foley catheter is almost 1 cm in diameter. After it is inserted, the balloon is filled with 50 mL of sterile water.

If a Foley catheter is used for mechanical ripening, women have an increased risk of fever, chorioamnionitis, and endomyometritis. Neonates have an increased risk of infection (Sanchez-Ramos, Heinemann, & Kaunitz, 2007; Williams, Wilson, Ganesh, White, & Apuzzio, 2007). In addition, a Foley catheter may be made of latex and absolutely must not be used if the woman has a latex hypersensitivity. Prior to this procedure, you must inform the physician that your patient has a latex allergy and provide a latex-free catheter.

After the extraovular catheter is in the cervix and the physician confirms placement, intravenous tubing is inserted into the end of the Foley catheter instead of inserting a urine collection bag, or the intravenous solution will be connected to the port on the catheter. Saline is infused by a pump at 40 to 60 mL per hour into the catheter. The saline infusion rate may vary depending on the physician's order.

An intravenous oxytocin infusion may also be ordered. The patient will experience pain with the insertion of the intracervical catheter. You may wish to hold her hand (if this is culturally accepted) and encourage her to use slow breathing. The patient may need intravenous sedation for placement of the extra-amniotic balloon. Some women also complain of feeling cramps after the insertion of the catheter, and some women will need an epidural early in their labor.

> **Documentation example:** Dr. Begentle discussed plan of care and patient consented. No known allergies. Cervix fingertip dilated and 2-cm long. 30F Foley catheter inserted by physician. Patient reports some cramping. Encouraged slow breathing during procedure. Normal saline infusing via pump into Foley at 40 mL/hour.

A latex-free catheter has been developed by Cook Medical specifically for mechanical ripening of the cervix. The Cook Cervical Ripening Balloon® has two balloons that are separately inflated. One is placed above the internal os and one is designed so that it is below the external os. It stays in place 12 hours before the balloons are deflated and the catheter is removed. When this device is used, labor averages 6.9 hours after removal of the cervical catheter (Atad, Hallak, Ben-David, Auslender, & Abramovici, 1997).

PHARMACOLOGIC CERVICAL RIPENING

Prostaglandin gel and intravenous oxytocin (Syntocinon®) are contraindicated for use if a woman has had a previous cesarean section (Dodd & Crowther, 2006). In some cases, however, these will be ordered and administered. Extreme caution and vigilance are required. Any abnormal finding should be reported immediately to the physician. The lowest possible dose of oxytocin should be used to ensure that hyperstimulation is avoided.

MISOPROSTOL (CYTOTEC®)

In women with an unscarred uterus, misoprostol can be used to ripen the cervix. Misoprostol should never be used, however, if the patient has a history of cesarean section due to the high risk of uterine rupture. Vaginal misoprostol is placed in the upper back part of the vagina (in the posterior fornix) (see Figure 9.11). Misoprostol may also be placed inside the cheek (buccal administration) where it slowly dissolves, or it may be swallowed (Fisher, Davies, & Mackenzie, 2001; Russell, O'Leary, Destafano, Deutsch, & Carlan, 2007).

In one study, oral doses as high as 200 micrograms hyperstimulated the uterus in more than half of the women participants. These women needed terbutaline to decrease the number of contractions (Adair et al., 1998). A better dosing regimen for oral misoprostol (Cytotec®) is 50 micrograms followed by 100 micrograms, if needed, every 4 hours for up to four doses.

This regimen was as effective as vaginal misoprostol (25 micrograms) given every 4 hours (Colon, Clawson, Taslimi, & Druzin, 2005). Oral misoprostol has no different beneficial or harmful effects compared with vaginal prostaglandins (Alfirevic, 2000).

Usually 25 micrograms will be inserted in the posterior fornix when there are no regular uterine contractions, and the fetus has a normal, reassuring fetal heart rate pattern. Since 25 micrograms is a quarter of a 100 microgram unscored tablet, it may be more easily inserted when it is in lubricant placed on the tip of the gloved finger. The use of lubricant results in a decreased perception of pain when the drug is inserted and has no adverse effect on cervical ripening (Rivas & Anasti, 2005). Intravaginal Cytotec® has also been administered as a sustained-release hydrogel with a retrieval system that is removed 24 hours after it is inserted. Misoprostol acid has an average half-life of less than 1 hour (Powers, Wing, Carr, Ewert, & Di Spirito, 2008).

Prior to drug use, maternal vital signs should be assessed and recorded, and the fetal heart rate and maternal uterine activity should be monitored to confirm a well fetus and the lack of regular contractions. If there are contractions, there is an increased risk of uterine hyperstimulation. You should consult your hospital protocol for further guidance.

DINOPROSTONE (CERVIDIL®)

When a dinoprostone insert (Cervidil®) was inserted into the posterior fornix, women began labor an average of 5 1/2 hours later. Women who have received Cervidil® should remain in the hospital and the fetal heart rate and maternal uterine activity should be assessed while the Cervidil® is in place. Cervidil® contains 10 mg of prostaglandin E_2 and releases 0.3 mg every hour. It is contraindicated in patients who are hypersensitive to the drug, where there is evidence of an abnormal fetal heart rate pattern ("fetal distress"), if there is unexplained vaginal bleeding, if there is evidence of or a strong suspicion of marked cephalopelvic disproportion, if oxytocic drugs are contraindicated, in patients already receiving an oxytocin infusion, or in a multiparous woman with six or more prior term pregnancies (Cervidil, 2001). Prostaglandins such as dinoprostone (prostaglandin E_2) can also cause bronchospasms and should be avoided if a woman has a history of asthma or currently has asthma. Misoprostol (prostaglandin E_1) appears to be safer for women who have asthma because there is less risk of bronchospasm.

INDUCTION INCREASES THE RISK OF A CESAREAN SECTION

Induction of labor increases the risk of a cesarean section (Herbst, Doyle, & Ramin, 2005) and nulliparous women with a term fetus in particular have an increased risk of a cesarean section when they are induced (Cammu, Martens, Ruyssinck, & Amy, 2002; Coonrod, Drachman, Hobson, & Manriquez, 2008). The risk of cesarean section is highest in older women, women of African American descent, and women

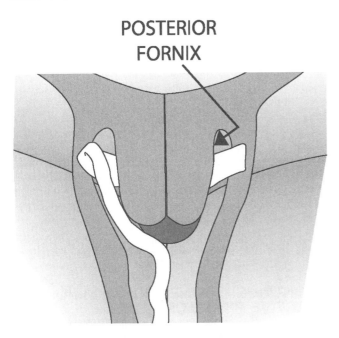

Figure 9.11: The location of the posterior fornix where a prostaglandin insert or part of a prostaglandin tablet might be placed. In this example, Cervidil® would be placed as illustrated. It is removed by pulling on the attached tape.

who have more education. If the fetal weight is very low or very high, there is an increased risk of a cesarean section (Coonrod et al., 2008). Before you infuse oxytocin for induction, be sure that the patient is aware of the plan of care and that her midwife or physician has obtained her informed consent.

The benefits and potential risks of an elective, repeat cesarean section compared with a planned induction of labor for women with a prior cesarean section are unclear (Dodd & Crowther, 2006). The use of prostaglandins and oxytocin, however, are known to increase the risk of uterine rupture. Women with a history of prior cesarean section should be carefully monitored during induction. Informed consent should be obtained by the patient's midwife or physician prior to her admission to labor and delivery and you should confirm her understanding of the procedure. A vaginal examination should be done within 24 hours or less. If she is contracting, you should withhold prostaglandins and oxytocin and discuss the plan of care with the physician.

Clinical example: The patient was frightened. When the nurse asked her what was wrong, she said the doctor just informed her that she was going to be seduced. The nurse calmly explained that the doctor said "induced." She asked the physician to return to the patient, explain the plan of care, and obtain informed consent.

Documentation example: Patient admitted for a planned induction due to pregnancy-induced hyperten-

sion. She has a history of one prior cesarean section and one vaginal birth after cesarean. Patient reports that physician discussed risks and benefits of induction at the office yesterday. Cervix was 1 cm/50%/−2. Occasional contractions, fetal heart rate 140s with accelerations, no decelerations. Fetal movement palpated. Orders received for oxytocin infusion. IV started with 18 gauge in left hand on first attempt. Oxytocin infusing at 1 mU/minute.

BEFORE OXYTOCIN IS INFUSED

Exogenous oxytocin (Pitocin® or Syntocinon®) are similar to the naturally occurring hormone oxytocin, except that a preservative has been added to the solution. Before you infuse oxytocin, you should confirm that your patient has never had an allergic reaction to the medication in the past. Contraindications for the infusion of oxytocin include "significant cephalopelvic disproportion, unfavorable fetal positions or presentations that are undeliverable without conversion prior to delivery, that is, transverse lie, hypertonic uterine patterns, hypersensitivity to the drug, prolonged use in uterine inertia or severe toxemia (preeclampsia), or where vaginal delivery is not indicated, such as a cord presentation or prolapse, total placenta previa, and vasa previa" (*Physicians' Desk Reference*, 1995). Simply put, a vaginal delivery must be possible if oxytocin will be administered for induction or augmentation.

Before administering oxytocin, you should confirm that there is a written or computer-entered order for the medication. Apply the electronic fetal monitor. Start a primary intravenous line with a large-bore catheter (such as one that is 18 gauge). Infuse crystalloid at the ordered rate. Initiate and monitor intake and output. Determine the status of the patient's cervix, the fetal station, and the status of the membranes.

If the patient was examined in the physician's or midwife's office the day prior to induction, the dilatation, effacement, and station are recorded, and she is not contracting on a regular basis, she does not need a vaginal examination prior to starting the oxytocin infusion. If she is contracting every 5 to 10 minutes or less, assess her cervix and the fetal station prior to infusing oxytocin. The examination will establish the baseline dilatation and descent at the onset of the induction.

Amniotomy may be used by the midwife or physician to induce labor (Atkinson, 2001; Rogers et al., 1997). In that case, he or she will determine the dilatation, effacement, and station. You should record in your notes the dilatation, effacement, and station along with the color, amount, and odor of the amniotic fluid after amniotomy.

You should also monitor and record your assessment of contractions and the fetal heart rate during the 20 or more minutes prior to the infusion. Confirm fetal well-being. There should be accelerations with no decelerations. Document your assessments. If there is an abnormal fetal heart rate pattern or the patient is already in labor, do not administer the oxytocin until a midwife or a physician evaluate your patient because the plan of care may change.

THE OXYTOCIN MIXTURE

Oxytocin should be administered using an infusion pump to avoid a bolus of oxytocin. The dose for augmentation is generally half of the dose used for induction. Drs. Edward Hayes and Louis Weinstein (2008) suggest 10 units of oxytocin diluted in 1000 mL of normal saline. If the initial ordered infusion rate is 1 mU/minute, an infusion of 6 mL/hour will deliver that dose. Some hospitals buy the oxytocin premixed in an isotonic solution such as 20 U of oxytocin in 1000 mL of normal saline or 5% dextrose in water. With that dilution, 1 mU/minute will be delivered with an infusion of 3 mL/hour. In cases where fluid restriction is required, a low-dose protocol will restrict the intravenous infusion. Adding more oxytocin to less solution will also restrict the fluid intake. In that case, the mL/hour needed to deliver the ordered dose must be recalculated. Follow your hospital's policies and procedures related to the administration of oxytocin.

You should wait 45 minutes to increase the dose, if you can, because that is the time it takes for the medication to reach a steady state (Hayes & Weinstein, 2008). When a steady state is reached, the amount of the drug infused is equal to the amount of the drug that has been metabolized. A measurable response to oxytocin is usually apparent within the first few hours after the infusion is initiated (Gibb, 1993). Patience here is very important. If contractions are increasing in frequency and strength, then the oxytocin is working and there is no need to increase the dose. You should simply maintain the dose. If contractions weaken or space out, however, you should increase the dose. Changing the infusion rate and oxytocin dose to obtain the proper frequency and strength of contractions is called "titration."

> **Documentation example:** IV started in right hand with second attempt. Labs drawn and lactated Ringer's solution infusing at 125 mL/hour. Patient reports she feels no contractions. Occasional contraction recorded by electronic fetal monitor, but not palpable. Fetal heart rate 120 to 130 with accelerations, no decelerations. Oxytocin started at 2 mU/minute. Ampicillin 2 grams IVPB over 30 minutes due to GBS positive status.

ANAPHYLAXIS: A RARE ADVERSE RESPONSE

A rare but potentially fatal adverse reaction when exogenous oxytocin is administered is anaphylaxis. Women who have anaphylaxis are not allergic to oxytocin itself, but are hypersensitive to chlorobutanol, the preservative in the oxytocin solution. Chlorobutanol is used as a hypnotic, a sedative, and a local anesthetic. It is a chloroform derivative (*Physicians' Desk Reference*, 1995). It has bacteriostatic properties and is widely used as a preservative for injectables such as oxytocin (Hofmann, Goerz, & Plewig, 1986).

Anaphylaxis is a type-I allergic response (Hofman, Goerz, & Plewig, 1986). The histamine reaction may also cause uterine hyperstimulation. After less than 1 minute of the oxytocin infusion, the patient may sit up, grab her neck with both hands and say, "I can't breathe," or she may begin coughing. Immediately discontinue the oxytocin infusion and note the time.

Recognize, vocalize, and mobilize. Anaphylaxis may be delayed from the time the infusion was initiated. Therefore, it is critical that you stay in the room for a few minutes after you begin the infusion. Start the infusion at the lowest possible dose until you see how the patient responds. If she has a type-I anaphylactic response, call for help. Assess your patient's lung sounds and apical heart rate, feel her pulse. If you can write down the findings at the time, you should do so. If the fetal monitor becomes detached, do not try to reapply it until she is evaluated by the physician. The patient is your priority at that moment. That is why the physician, who can manage complications, should be available at all times (*Physicians' Desk Reference*, 1995). You may need to administer a steroid, epinephrine, or order a breathing treatment to open her airway.

DISCONTINUE THE INFUSION DURING THE ACTIVE PHASE OF LABOR

When there are four contractions in a 10-minute period there is no need to increase the oxytocin dose. Maintain, decrease, or discontinue the oxytocin infusion once the patient has reached the active phase of labor.

Researchers found that there is no significant decrease in the duration of labor if the oxytocin is discontinued during the active phase of labor. It was also found that discontinuing the infusion at 5 cm of dilatation with three to five contractions in each 10-minute period was sufficient for a woman to continue her labor and deliver vaginally without any increased risk of a cesarean section. The oxytocin was discontinued during the active phase of labor because researchers were concerned that the duration and concentration of oxytocin administered during induction over a long period of time would desensitize oxytocin receptors in the uterus to both exogenous and endogenous oxytocin (Daniel-Spiegel, Weiner, Ben-Shlomo, & Shalev, 2004).

DISCONTINUE THE INFUSION IN THE CASE OF TACHYSYSTOLE

An infusion at 4 to 6 mU/minute corresponds to the natural level of oxytocin during the entire first stage of labor. Higher doses of oxytocin result in higher rates of uterine hyperstimulation (Hayes & Weinstein, 2008). Any time you infuse more than 6 mU/minute you increase the risk of adverse events, including uterine hyperstimulation.

You should discontinue the oxytocin infusion if there is evidence of tachysystole. Labor should not be prolonged, and there should be no increase in the number of operative interventions. The number of cesarean sections actually decreases and the 1-minute Apgar scores were higher when an oxytocin checklist was used (Clark et al., 2007). In their study, oxytocin was discontinued when there were five or more contractions in 10 minutes for two consecutive 10-minute periods.

The response of the uterus and the fetus is far more important than the dose of oxytocin (Freeman & Nageotte, 2007). Your nursing duty is to monitor the fetus and contractions and then decrease or discontinue the oxytocin infusion if there is evidence of fetal hypoxia or uterine hyperstimulation, or both. Consult your hospital's policies and procedures for more guidance.

MONITORING THE FETUS AND CONTRACTIONS

Intravenous oxytocin is a powerful and dangerous drug. The manufacturer recommends that "all patients receiving intravenous infusions of oxytocin must be under continuous observation by trained personnel with a thorough knowledge of the drug and qualified to identify complications. A physician qualified to manage any complications should be immediately available." The manufacturer also advises that "overstimulation of the uterus by improper administration can be hazardous to both mother and fetus" (*Physicians' Desk Reference*, 1995).

While oxytocin is infusing, you should assess and record the fetal heart rate and uterine activity every 15 minutes during the first stage of labor, and every 5 minutes during the second stage of labor. Once the oxytocin infusion is discontinued, you may be able to resume a low-risk protocol for monitoring contractions and the fetal heart rate, especially if there is a normal fetal heart rate pattern and two to four contractions every 10 minutes.

Any abnormal finding should be reported immediately to the midwife or physician. If there are signs of fetal hypoxia, such as a decrease in baseline variability, the lack of accelerations, or variable, late, or prolonged decelerations, the oxytocin infusion should be discontinued. To increase maternal cardiac output and blood flow, and oxygen delivery to the uterus, position your patient in a nonsupine position, that is, on her side or upright. Place a tight-fitting face mask on her and administer 10 L/minute. A nonrebreather mask delivers slightly more oxygen than a simple mask. You should know which types of oxygen mask are available in your hospital's labor rooms. Notify the obstetric provider of your assessments, interventions, and the current fetal status.

Documentation example: Patient presents to labor and delivery for a scheduled induction due to postdates and hypertension. Cervix FT/thick/high. Fetal heart rate 120 to 130, with accelerations and no decelerations. Occasional mild contraction for 30 to 40 seconds. Dr. Pittuday explained plan of care. Patient verbally consented to the procedure. AROM, clear, large amount, normal odor. Oxytocin infusing IVPB via pump at 1 mU/minute.

Documentation example: 5 cm/100%/0 with contractions every 2 minutes. Oxytocin infusion discontinued. Fetal heart rate 120 to 130 bpm with accelerations, no decelerations. Patient to tub to soak in warm water.

INTRAUTERINE RESUSCITATION

If the fetus has an abnormal heart rate, discontinue the oxytocin infusion, position your patient on her side, and apply oxygen with a tight-fitting face mask. Maternal hyperoxygenation with 10 L/minute helps increase the blood oxygen level of the hypoxic or borderline hypoxic fetus (Dildy & Clark, 2007).

If the mother has abnormal vital signs, abnormal uterine activity, or an abnormal resting tone (above 25 mm Hg and/or firm to palpation between contractions), discontinue the oxytocin infusion until your patient is evaluated by the midwife or physician. Notify the obstetric provider of your assessments and actions. Document your assessment of the fetal heart rate, uterine activity, other findings, your actions, and the response of the mother, her uterus, and the fetus to your actions.

WHEN INDUCTION FAILS TO ACCOMPLISH DELIVERY

It has been shown that nulliparous women at 36 or more weeks of gestation who dilate 2 cm or less per hour and who are less than 100% effaced will have an increased risk of a cesarean section. They also have a decreased risk for vaginal delivery if the latent phase of labor lasts 13 or more hours or they fail to progress to the active phase of labor. If the latent phase lasts more than 12 hours, the induction is deemed a failure, and 36.8% of the women have a vaginal delivery whereas 29.4% develop chorioamnionitis or endometritis (Rouse, 2007). Therefore, if you admit a nulliparous woman at 0700 and she is still dilated less than 4 cm 12 hours later, a cesarean section may be the most reasonable plan, especially if she has an elevated temperature or fever, and if chorioamnionitis has been diagnosed. You should always keep the midwife or physician informed of her labor progress and any abnormal findings.

CONCLUSIONS

Power generated by uterine contractions is a prerequisite for vaginal delivery. Uterine smooth-muscle cells are responsive to uterotonic substances such as norepinephrine, thrombin, adenosine triphosphate, histamine, and bradykinin that are produced by the woman's body.

Nurses are responsible for palpating uterine activity to identify the frequency, duration, and strength of contractions, and they determine if the resting tone is firm or soft. They document their findings, report abnormal uterine activity, and act to decrease uterine tachysystole if a uterine stimulant is the cause.

Uterine preparation for labor involves three phases prior to the onset of coordinated contractions that change the cervix. The third phase, stimulation, is a naturally occurring process. In contrast, hyperstimulation is a response to elevated levels of norepinephrine, thrombin, histamine, bradykinin, or adenosine triphosphate. Hyperstimulation is also associated with the presence of fibroids or exogenous stimulants such as prostaglandins, oxytocin, or cocaine.

Based on the available evidence, a maximum of four contractions every 10 minutes should provide an adequate interval between contractions to replenish cerebral and arteriolar oxygen in the fetus. Therefore, a rate of five or more contractions in 10 minutes that persists is evidence of tachysystole, which increases the risk of fetal hypoxia and acidemia. Nurses must remove uterine stimulants in order to decrease tachysystole and/or if they observe an abnormal fetal heart rate pattern.

If uterine hyperstimulation occurs in the absence of a uterine stimulant, nurses should assess the patient for signs of a placental abruption, such as uterine tenderness or bleeding, an abnormal fetal heart rate pattern, or maternal restlessness or pain. Nurses must communicate their concerns and assessments with the midwife or physician. When necessary, they should act to increase fetal oxygenation.

REVIEW QUESTIONS

True/False: Decide if the statements are true or false.

1. The processes leading to contractions are downregulation, activation, and stimulation.

2. Dilatation of the cervix requires the synchronous contraction of uterine smooth-muscle cells.

3. Uterine irritability is the same as uterine hyperstimulation.

4. Fetal brain oxygenation should be stable when the contraction interval is 1 1/2 minutes.

5. The force of uterine contractions depends on the levels of oxytocin and magnesium.

6. Catecholamines bind with uterine beta-receptors to increase the number of contractions.

7. Thrombin increases uterine activity by binding with receptors in the chorion.

8. Uterine rupture at the site of a prior uterine scar is more common when prostaglandins rather than oxytocin are used to ripen the cervix.

9. Six uterine contractions in a 10-minute period is an example of tachysystole.

10. If there are more than five contractions in 10 minutes with a normal fetal heart rate pattern, the oxytocin infusion should continue at the current infusion rate.

References

Adair, C. D., Weeks, J. W., Barrilleaux, P. S., Philibert, L., Edwards, M. S., & Lewis, D. F. (1998). Labor induction with oral versus vaginal misoprostol: A randomized, double-blind trial. *American Journal of Obstetrics and Gynecology, 178*(1, Part 2), S93.

Alfirevic, Z. (2000). Oral misoprostol for induction of labour. *Cochrane Database of Systematic Reviews*, Issue 4:CD001338.

Allen, N. M., O'Brien, M., Friel, A. M., Smith, T. J., & Morrison, J. J. (2007). Expression and function of protease-activated receptor 4 in human myometrium. *American Journal of Obstetrics & Gynecology, 196*(2), 161–163.

Allix, S., Reyes-Gomez, E., Aubin-Houzelstein, G., Noël, D., Tiret, L., Panthier, J. J., & Bernex, F. (2008). Uterine contractions depend on KIT-positive interstitial cells in the mouse: Genetic and pharmacological evidence [Abstract]. *Biology and Reproduction*. Retrieved July 7, 2008 from http://www.ncbi.nlm.nih.gov.libproxy.unm.edu/pubmed/1840468?ordin alpos=1&itool=Ent

Allman, A. C., & Steer, P. J. (1993). Monitoring uterine activity. *British Journal of Hospital Medicine, 49*(9), 649–653.

American College of Obstetricians and Gynecologists. (2005). Intrapartum fetal heart rate monitoring. *ACOG Practice Bulletin Clinical Management Guidelines for Obstetrician-Gynecologists*. Number 70.

Arrabal, P. P., & Nagey, D. A. (1996). Is manual palpation of uterine contractions accurate? *American Journal of Obstetrics and Gynecology, 174*(1, Part 1), 217–219.

Arthur, P., Taggart, M. J., & Mitchell, B. F. (2007). Oxytocin and parturition: A role of increased myometrial calcium and calcium sensitization. *Frontiers in Bioscience, 12*, 619–633.

Ascher, B. H. (1978). Maternal anxiety in pregnancy and fetal homeostasis. *Journal of Obstetric, Gynecologic, and Neonatal Nursing, 7*(3), 18–21.

Astle, S., Newton, R., Thornton, S., Vatish, M., & Slater, D. M. (2007). Expression and regulation of prostaglandin E synthase isoforms in human myometrium with labour. *Molecular Human Reproduction, 13*(1), 69–75.

Atad, J., Hallak, M., Ben-David, Y., Auslender, R., & Abramovici, H. (1997). Ripening and dilation of the unfavorable cervix for induction of labor by a double balloon device: Experience with 250 cases. *British Journal of Obstetrics and Gynaecology, 104*(Part 1), 29–32.

Atkinson, M. W. (2001). Misoprostol for third trimester labor induction: A survey of labor induction methods [Abstract]. *American Journal of Obstetrics and Gynecology, 184*(1), S125.

Bakker, P. C. A. M., Kurver, P. H. J., Kuik, D. J., & van Geijn, H. P. (2007). Elevated uterine activity increases the risk of fetal acidosis at birth. *American Journal of Obstetrics and Gynecology, 196*(4), 313–315, 313.e1–6.

Bakker, P. C. A. M., & van Geijn, H. P. (2008). Uterine activity: Implications for the condition of the fetus. *Journal of Perinatal Medicine, 36*, 30–37.

Bakker, W. W., & Faas, M. M. (2007). The incidence of pregnancy-induced hypertension and smoking: An alternative explanation [Letter to the editor]. *American Journal of Obstetrics and Gynecology, 197*(5), 556.

Bartha, J. L., Romero-Carmona, R., Martinez-del-Fresno, P., & Comino-Delgado, R. (2005). Bishop score and transvaginal ultrasound for preinduction of cervical assessment: A randomized clinical trial. *Obstetrical & Gynecological Survey, 60*(8), 507–508.

Blanks, A. M., Zhao, Z.-H., Shmygol, A., Bru-Mercier, G., Astle, S., & Thornton, S. (2007). Characterization of the molecular and electrophysiological properties of the T-type calcium channel in human myometrium. *Journal of Physiology, 581*, 915–926.

Bremme, K., & Nilsson, B. (1984). Prediction of time to delivery from start of contractions in induced labor: A life table analysis approach. *International Journal of Gynaecology and Obstetrics, 22*, 225–229.

Brown, A. G., Leite, R. S., Engler, A. J., Discher, D. E., & Strauss III, J. F. (2006). A hemoglobin fragment found in cervicovaginal fluid from women in labor potentiates the action of agents that promote contraction of smooth muscle cells. *Peptides, 27*, 1794–1800.

Bugg, G. J., Crocker, I., Baker, P. N., Johnston, T. A., & Taggart, M. J. (2005). The effect of superoxide free radicals on human myometrial contractility in vitro [Letter to the editor]. *European Journal of Obstetrics & Gynecology and Reproductive Biology, 125*, 139–145.

Bursztyn, L., Eytan, O., Jaffa, A. J., & Elad, D. (2007). Modeling myometrial smooth muscle contraction. *Annals of the New York Academy of Science, 1101*, 110–138.

Bytautiene, E., Vedernikov, Y. P., Saade, G. R., Romero, R., & Garfield, R. E. (2003). Effect of histamine on phasic and tonic contractions of isolated uterine tissue from pregnant women. *American Journal of Obstetrics and Gynecology, 188*(3), 774–778.

Caldeyro-Barcia, R., & Poseiro, J. J. (1960). Physiology of the uterine contraction. *Clinical Obstetrics and Gynecology, 3*(2), 388–408.

Cammu, H., Martens, G., Ruyssinck, G., & Amy, J.-J. (2002). Outcome after elective labor induction in nulliparous women: A matched cohort study. *American Journal of Obstetrics and Gynecology, 186*, 240–244.

Cervidil. (2001). Brand of dinoprostone vaginal insert. St. Louis, MO: Forest Pharmaceuticals, Inc.

Chalmers, B., Mangiaterra, V., & Porter, R. (2001). WHO principles of perinatal care: The essential antenatal, perinatal, and postpartum care course. *Birth, 28*(3), 202–207.

Chao, C. R. (1996). Cardiovascular effects of cocaine during pregnancy. *Seminars in Perinatology, 20*(2), 107–114.

Choi, S. J., Oh, S. Y., Kim, J. H., & Roh, C. R. (2007). Changes of nuclear factor kappa B (NF-?B), cyclooxygenase-2 (COX-2) and matrix metalloproteinase-9 (MMP-9) in human myometrium before and during term labor. *European Journal of Obstetrics, Gynecology, and Reproductive Biology, 132*, 182–188.

Clark, S., Belfort, M., Saade, G., Hankins, G., Miller, D., Frye, D., & Meyers, J. (2007). Implementation of a conservative checklist-based protocol for oxytocin administration: Maternal and newborn outcomes. *American Journal of Obstetrics and Gynecology, 197*, 480.e1–480.e5.

Clark, S. L., Hankins, G. D., Dudley, D. A., Dildy, G. A., & Porter, T. F. (1995). Amniotic fluid embolism: Analysis of the national registry. *American Journal of Obstetrics and Gynecology, 172*, 1159–1167.

Cohen, H. R., Green, J. R., & Crombleholme, W. R. (1991). Peripartum cocaine use: Estimating risk of adverse pregnancy outcome. *International Journal of Gynaecology and Obstetrics, 35*(1), 51–54.

Collins, P. L., Idriss, E., & Moore, J. J. (1995). Fetal membranes inhibit prostaglandin but not oxytocin-induced uterine contractions. *American Journal of Obstetrics and Gynecology, 172*, 1216–1223.

Colon, I., Clawson, K., Taslimi, M., & Druzen, M. (2005). Prospective randomized clinical trial of inpatient cervical ripening with stepwise oral misoprostol versus vaginal misoprostol [Abstract]. *American Journal of Obstetrics and Gynecology*, S15.

Condon, J. C., Jeyasuria, P., Faust, J. M., & Mendelson, C. R. (2004). Surfactant protein secreted by the maturing mouse fetal lung acts as a hormone that signals the initiation of parturition. *Proceedings of the National Academy of Science, 101*, 4978–4983.

Coonrod, D. V., Drachman, D., Hobson, P., & Manriquez, M. (2008). Nulliparous term singleton vertex cesarean delivery rates: Institutional and individual level predictors. *American Journal of Obstetrics and Gynecology, 198*, 694.e1–694.e11.

Csonka, D., Zupkó, I., Minorics, R., Márki, A., Csík, G., & Falkay, G. (2007). The effects of α-methyldopa on myometrial noradrenaline release and myometrial contractility in the rat. *Acta Obstetricia et Gynecologica, 86*, 986–994.

Daniel-Spiegel, E., Weiner, Z., Ben-Shlomo, I., & Shalev, E. (2004). For how long should oxytocin be continued during induction of labor? *British Journal of Obstetrics and Gynaecology, 111*, 331–334.

Dawood, M. Y. (1989). Evolving concepts of oxytocin for induction of labor. *American Journal of Perinatology, 6*(2), 167–172.

Dawood, M. Y., Wang, C. F., Gupta, R., & Fuchs, F. (1978). Fetal contribution to oxytocin in human labor. *Obstetrics & Gynecology, 52*(2), 205–209.

Dawood, M. Y., Ylikorkala, O., Trivedi, D., & Fuchs, F. (1979). Oxytocin in maternal circulation and amniotic fluid during pregnancy. *Journal of Clinical Endocrinology and Metabolism, 49*(3), 429–434.

Dildy, G. A. III, & Clark, S. L. (2007). Effects of maternal oxygen administration on fetal pulse oximetry measured by fetal pulse oximetry [Letter to the editor]. *American Journal of Obstetrics and Gynecology, 196*(4), e.13.

Dodd, J. M., & Crowther, C. A. (2006). Elective repeat caesarean section versus induction of labour for women with a previous caesarean birth [Review]. *Cochrane Database of Systematic Reviews*, Issue 4. Art. No.: CD004906. doi: 10.1002/14651858.CD004906.pub2

East, C. E., Dunster, K. R., & Colditz, P. B. (1998). Fetal oxygen saturation and uterine contractions during labor. *American Journal of Perinatology, 15*(6), 345–349.

Ecker, J., Chen, K., Cohen, A., Riley, L., & Lieberman, E. (2001). Increased risk for cesarean section delivery after a trial of labor with advancing maternal age: Cesarean indications and role of induction [Abstract]. *American Journal of Obstetrics and Gynecology, 184*(1), S183.

Egarter, C., Husslein, P. W., & Rayburn, W. F. (1990). Uterine stimulation after low-dose prostaglandin E$_2$ therapy: Tocolytic treatment in 181 cases. *American Journal of Obstetrics and Gynecology, 163*(3), 794–796.

Elovitz, M., Ascher-Landsberg, J., Saunders, T., & Phillippe, M. (2000). The mechanism underlying the stimulatory effects of thrombin on myometrial smooth muscle. *American Journal of Obstetrics & Gynecology, 183*, 674–681.

Elovitz, M., Saunders, T., Ascher-Landsberg, J., & Phillippe, M. (2000). Effects of thrombin on myometrial contractions in vitro and in vivo. *American Journal of Obstetrics and Gynecology, 183*, 799–804.

Feltovich, H., Ji, H., Carroll, C., Janowski, J., Bonney, E., & Chien, E. (2005). EP4 receptor activation produces quantifiable decrease in cervical collagen content [Abstract]. *American Journal of Obstetrics and Gynecology*, S15.

Ferraro, F., Ferraro, R., & Massard, A. (1997). Consequences of cocaine addiction during pregnancy on the development of the child. *Archives in Pediatrics, 4*(7), 677–682.

Field, T., Diego, M., Hernandez-Reif, M., Figueiredo, B., Schanberg, S., & Kuhn, C. (2007). Sleep disturbances in depressed pregnant women and their newborns. *Infant Behavioral Development, 30*, 127–133.

Fisher, S., Davies, G., & Mackenzie, P. (2001). Oral versus vaginal misoprostol for induction of labour: A double-blind, placebo-controlled randomized trial [Abstract]. *American Journal of Obstetrics and Gynecology, 184*(1), S117.

Flowers, D., Clark, J. F., & Westney, L. S. (1991). Cocaine intoxication associated with abruption placentae. *Journal of the National Medical Association, 83*(3), 912–915.

Fomin, V. P., Singh, D. M., Brown, H. L., Natarajan, V., & Hurd, W. W. (1999). Effect of cocaine on intracellular calcium regulation in myometrium from pregnant women. *Journal for the Society of Gynecologic Investigation, 6*(3), 147–152.

Freeman, R. K., & Nageotte, M. (2007). A protocol for use of oxytocin [Editorial]. *American Journal of Obstetrics and Gynecology, 197*, 445–446.

Fu, J., & Olofsson, P. (2007). Intracerebral regional distribution of blood flow in response to uterine contractions in growth-restricted human fetuses. *Early Human Development, 83*, 607–612.

Fuchs, A. R., Fuchs, F., Husslein, P., & Soloff, M.S. (1984). Oxytocin receptors in the human uterus during pregnancy and parturition. *American Journal of Obstetrics and Gynecology, 150*(6), 734–741.

Fuchs, A. R., Goeschen, K., Husslein, P., Rasmussen, A. B., & Fuchs, F. (1983). Oxytocin and initiation of human parturition: III. Plasma concentrations of oxytocin and 13, 14-dihydro-15-keto-prostaglandin F2 alpha in spontaneous and oxytocin-induced labor at term [Abstract]. *American Journal of Obstetrics and Gynecology, 147*(5), 497–502.

Garfield, R. E., Maner, W. L., MacKay, L. B., Schlembach, D., & Saade, G. R. (2005). Comparing uterine electromyography activity of antepartum patients versus term labor patients. *American Journal of Obstetrics and Gynecology, 193*, 23–29.

George, K., Smith, J. F., & Curet, L. B. (1995). Doppler velocimetry and fetal heart rate pattern observations in acute cocaine intoxication: A case report. *Journal of Reproductive Medicine, 40*(1), 65–67.

Gibb, D. M. (1993). Measurement of uterine activity in labour-clinical aspects. *British Journal of Obstetrics and Gynaecology, 100*(10), 970–971.

Graham, E. M. (2007). Elevated uterine activity increases the risk of fetal acidosis at birth [Letter to the editor]. *American Journal of Obstetrics and Gynecology, 197*(4), 441.

Grammatopoulos, D. K. (2007). The role of CRH receptors and their agonists in myometrial contractility and quiescence during pregnancy and labour. *Frontiers in Bioscience, 12*, 561–571.

Grobman, W. A., Gilbert, S., Landon, M. B., Spong, C. Y., Leveno, K. J., & Rouse, D. J. (2007). Outcomes of induction of labor after one prior cesarean [Abstract]. *Obstetrics & Gynecology, 109*(2, Part 1), 262–269.

Guinn, D. A., Goepfert, A. R., Christine, M., Owen, J., & Hauth, J. C. (2000). Extra-amniotic saline, laminaria, or prostaglandin E$_2$ gel for labor induction with unfavorable cervix: A randomized controlled trial. *Obstetrics & Gynecology, 96*(1), 106–112.

Gyselaers, W., Vansteelant, L., Spitz, B., Odendaal, H. J., & Van Assche, F. A. (1991). Do biphasic uterine contractions imply poor uterine function? *European Journal of Obstetrics, Gynecology, & Reproductive Biology, 42*(2), 111–114.

Haydon, M. L., Gorenberg, D. M., Nageotte, M. P., Ghamsary, M., Rumney, P. J., & Patillo, C. (2006). The effect of maternal oxygen administration on fetal pulse oximetry during labor in fetuses with nonreassuring fetal heart rate patterns. *American Journal of Obstetrics and Gynecology, 195*, 735–738.

Hayes, E. J., & Weinstein, L. (2008). Improving patient safety and uniformity of care by a standardized regimen for the use of oxytocin. *American Journal of Obstetrics and Gynecology, 198*, 622.e1–622.e7.

Herbst, M., Doyle, N., & Ramin, S. (2005). Cervical ripening for labor induction at term: A cost-analysis [Abstract]. *American Journal of Obstetrics and Gynecology*, S186.

Hinton, A., Grigsby, P., Pitzer, B., Brockman, D., & Myatt, L. (2005a). Localization of contractile prostaglandin E2 receptors in rat cervical tissue [Abstract]. *American Journal of Obstetrics and Gynecology*, S131.

Hinton, A., Grigsby, P., Pitzer, B., Brockman, D., & Myatt, L. (2005b). Localization of relaxatory prostaglandin E2 receptors in rat cervical tissue [Abstract]. *American Journal of Obstetrics and Gynecology*, S131.

Hofmann, H., Goerz, G., & Plewig, G. (1986). Short communications: Anaphylactic shock from chlorobutanol-preserved oxytocin. *Contact Dermatitis, 15*, 241–260.

Johnson, N., Johnson, V. A., McNamara, H., Montague, I. A., Jongsma, H. W., & Aumeerally, Z. (1994). Fetal pulse oximetry: A new method of monitoring the fetus. *Australia New Zealand Journal of Obstetrics and Gynaecology, 34*(4), 428–432.

Johnson, N., van Oudgaarden, E., Montagne, I., & McNamara, H. (1994). The effect of oxytocin-induced hyperstimulation on fetal oxygen. *British Journal of Obstetrics and Gynaecology, 101*(9), 805–807.

Justus, K., Arora, C., Sandhu, M., & Hobel, C. (2005). The effect of smoking on the time course release of catecholamines and corticotrophin releasing (CRH) hormone [Abstract]. *American Journal of Obstetrics and Gynecology,* S21.

Kavanagh, J., Kelly, A. J., & Thomas, J. (2005). Breast stimulation for cervical ripening and induction of labour. *Cochrane Database of Systematic Reviews,* Issue 3.

Khan-Dawood, F. S., & Dawood, M.Y. (1984). Oxytocin content of human fetal pituitary glands. *American Journal of Obstetrics & Gynecology, 148*(4), 420–423.

Kim, C. J., Han, Y. M., Kim, J.-S., Kim. S. K., Tarca, A. L. & Draghici (2007). First evidence that the human amnion is functionally heterogeneous: A study of the amnion transcriptome [Abstract]. *American Journal of Obstetrics and Gynecology,* S93.

Lawson, Y., Dombrowski, M. P., Carter, S., & Hagglund, K. H. (2003). Does external tocodynamometry increase maternal perception of uterine contractions. *American Journal of Obstetrics and Gynecology, 189,* 1396–1397.

Leman, H., Marque, C., & Gondry, J. (1999). Use of the electrohysterogram signal for characterization of contractions during pregnancy. *IEEE Transactions on Biomedical Engineering, 46*(10), 1222–1229.

Lenke, R. L., & Nemes, J. M. (1984). Use of nipple stimulation to obtain contraction stress test. *Obstetrics & Gynecology, 63,* 345–348.

Li, H., Gudmundsson, S., & Olofsson, P. (2006). Acute centralization of blood flow in compromised human fetuses evoked by uterine contractions. *Early Human Development, 82,* 747–752.

Lindgren, L. (1973). The influence of uterine motility upon cervical dilatation in labor. *American Journal of Obstetrics and Gynecology, 117*(4), 530–536.

Makino, S., Zaragoza, D. B., Mitchell, M. F., Yonemoto, H., & Olson, D. M. (2007). Decidual activation: Abundance and localization of prostaglandin F_{2a} receptor (FP) mRNA and protein and uterine activation proteins in human deciduas at preterm birth and term birth. *Placenta, 28,* 557–565.

Mastrogiannis, D. S., Luckenbau, A., & O'Brien, W. F. (2003). Cocaine decreases urinary prostacyclin release in pregnancy: Correlation with uterine and umbilical Doppler velocimetry. *Journal of Maternal, Fetal, and Neonatal Medicine, 14*(6), 383–388.

Maul, H., Maner, W. L., Olson, G., Saade, G. R., & Garfield, R. E. (2004). Non-invasive transabdominal uterine electromyography correlates with the strength of intrauterine pressure and is predictive of labor and delivery. *Journal of Maternal, Fetal, and Neonatal Medicine, 15,* 297–301.

McNamara, H., & Johnson, N. (1995). The effect of uterine contractions on fetal oxygen saturation. *British Journal of Obstetrics and Gynaecology, 102*(8), 644–647.

Meniru, G. I., Brister, E., Neumanaitis-Keller, J., Gill, P., Krew, M., & Hopkins, M. P. (2002). Spontaneous prolonged hypertonic uterine contractions (essential uterine hypertonus) and a possible infective etiology. *Archives in Gynecology and Obstetrics, 266,* 238–240.

Muleba, N., Havelock, J., Casey, B., Keller, P., Word, R., & Rainey, W. (2004). Gene expression in the human pregnant uterus before and during parturition [Abstract]. *American Journal of Obstetrics and Gynecology, 191*(6), S17.

Nicholson, J., Caughey, A., Parry, S., Rosen, S., Evans, A., & Macones, G. (2007). Prospective randomized trial of the active management of risk in pregnancy at term: Improved birth outcomes from prostaglandin-assisted preventive labor induction [Abstract]. *American Journal of Obstetrics and Gynecology,* S37.

Nicholson, J. M., Parry, S., Caughey, A. B., Rosen, S., Keen, A., & Macones, G. A. (2008). The impact of the active management of risk in pregnancy at term on birth outcomes: A randomized clinical trial. *American Journal of Obstetrics and Gynecology, 198,* 511.e1–511.e15.

Nordstrom, L., & Waldenstrom U. (2002). *Management in normal birth: State of the art guidelines.* Stockholm: Swedish Health Association.

Norwitz, E. R., Snegovskikh, V., Schatz, F., Foyouzi, N., Rahman, M., & Buchwalder, L. (2007). Progestin inhibits and thrombin stimulates the plasminogen activator/inhibitor system in term decidual stromal cells: Implications for parturition. *American Journal of Obstetrics and Gynecology, 196,* 382.e1–382.e8.

O'Brien, W. F. (1995). The role of prostaglandins in labor and delivery. *Clinical Perinatology, 22*(4), 973–984.

Oh, S.-Y., Park, I.-S., Kim, C. J., Romero, R., & Shim, S.-S. (2005). Progesterone receptor isoforms (A/B) ratio of human fetal membrane increases during term parturition [Abstract]. *American Journal of Obstetrics and Gynecology,* S185.

Oppenheimer, L. W., Bland, E. S., Dabrowski, A., Holmes, P., McDonald, O., & Wen, S. W. (2002). Uterine contraction pattern as a predictor of the mode of delivery. *Journal of Perinatology, 22,* 149–153.

Pan, V. L., Goharkhay, N., Felix, J. C., & Wing, D. A. (2003). FGL2 prothrombinase messenger RNA expression in gravid and nongravid human myometrium. *American Journal of Obstetrics and Gynecology, 188*(4), 1057–1062.

Patel, T. G., Laungani, R. G., Grose, E. A., & Dow-Edwards, D. L. (1999). Cocaine decreases uteroplacental blood flow in the rat. *Neurotoxicology and Teratology, 21*(5), 559–565.

Pavan, B., Buzzi, M., Ginanni-Corradini, F., Ferretti, M. E., Vesce, F., & Biondi, C. (2000). Influence of oxytocin on prostaglandin E_2, intracellular calcium, and cyclic adenosine monophosphate in human amnion-derived (WISH) cells. *American Journal of Obstetrics and* Gynecology, *183*(1), 76–82.

Peebles, D. M., Spencer, J. A., Edwards, A. D., Wyatt, J. S., Reynolds, E. O., & Cope, M. (1994). Relation between frequency of uterine contractions and human fetal cerebral oxygen saturation studied during labour by near infrared spectroscopy. *British Journal of Obstetrics and Gynaecology, 101*(1), 44–48.

Peregrine, E., O'Brien, P., Omar, R., & Jauniaux, E. (2006). Clinical and ultrasound parameters to predict the risk of cesarean delivery after induction of labor. *Obstetrics & Gynecology, 107*(2, Part 1), 227–233.

Physicians' desk reference. (1995). Oxytocin. Montvale, NJ: Medical Economics Company, Inc.

Powers, B. L., Wing, D. A., Carr, D., Ewert, K., & Di Spirito, M. (2008). Pharmacokinetic profiles of controlled-release hydrogel polymer vaginal inserts containing misoprostol [Abstract]. *Journal of Clinical Pharmacology, 48*(1), 26–34.

Rihana, S., Lefrançois, E., & Marque, C. (2007). A two dimension model of the uterine electrical wave propagation. *Conference Proceedings IEEE Engineering Medical Biology Society*, 1108-1112. Retrieved July 7, 2008 from http://www.ncbi.nlm.nih.gov.libproxy.unm.edu/pubmed/18002156?ordi nalpos=2 &itool=Ent.

Rivas, J., & Anasti, J. N. (2005). The effects of vaginal lubricants on insertional pain and efficacy of misoprostol for cervical ripening. *Obstetrics & Gynecology, 105*(4), 425.

Robillard, J., Gauvin, F., Molinaro, G., Leduc, L., Adam, A., & Rivard, G. (2005). The syndrome of amniotic fluid embolism: A potential contribution of bradykinin. *American Journal of Obstetrics and Gynecology, 194*, 1508–1512.

Rogers, R., Gilson, G. J., Miller, A. C., Izquierdo, L. E., Curet, L. B., & Qualls, C. R. (1997). Active management of labor: Does it make a difference? *American Journal of Obstetrics and Gynecology, 177*, 599–605.

Rouse, D. (2007). When should labor induction be discontinued in the latent phase? [Abstract]. *American Journal of Obstetrics and Gynecology, 197*(6), S103.

Ruddock, N., Shi, S.-Q., Jain, S., Moore, G., Hankins, G. D. V., Romero, R., & Garfield, R. (2007). Progesterone (P4), but not 17alpha hydroxyprogesterone caproate (17P), inhibits human myometrial contractions [Abstract]. *American Journal of Obstetrics and Gynecology, 56*.

Russell, Z., O'Leary, T., Destefano, K., Deutsch, A., & Carlan, S. (2007). Buccal versus vaginal misoprostol administration for cervical ripening [Abstract]. *American Journal of Obstetrics and Gynecology, S37*.

Sanchez-Ramos, L., Heinemann, J., & Kaunitz, A. (2007). Infectious complications of pre-induction cervical ripening with the intracervical foley catheter balloon: A systematic review with meta-analysis [Abstract]. *American Journal of Obstetrics and Gynecology, 197*(6), S103.

Schellpfeffer, M. A., Hoyle, D., & Johnson, J. W. (1985). Antepartal uterine hypercontractility secondary to nipple stimulation. *Obstetrics & Gynecology, 65*(4), 588–591.

Schoening, A. M. (2006). Amniotic fluid embolism: Historical perspectives and new possibilities. *American Journal of Maternal Child Nursing, 31*(2), 78–83.

Shafik, A., El-Sibai, O., & Shafik, I. (2004). Identification of c-kit-positive cells in the uterus. *International Journal of Gynecology and Obstetrics, 87*, 254–255.

Sheiner, E., Biderman-Madar, T., Katz, M., Levy, A., Hadar, A., & Mazor, M. (2004). Higher rates of tachysystole among patients with clinically apparent uterine leiomyomas. *American Journal of Obstetrics and Gynecology, 191*(3), 945–948.

Sheiner, E., Levy, A., Ofir, K., Hadar, A., Shoham-Vardi, I., & Hallak, M. (2004). Changes in fetal heart rate and uterine patterns associated with uterine rupture. *Journal of Reproductive Medicine, 49*(5), 373–378.

Sherman, D. J., Frenkel, E., Tovbin, J., Arieli, S., Caspi, E., & Bukovsky, I. (1996). Ripening of the unfavorable cervix with extraamniotic catheter balloon: Clinical experience and review. *Obstetrical and Gynecological Survey, 51*(10), 621–627.

Shmygol, A., Gullam, J., Blanks, A., & Thornton, S. (2006). Multiple mechanisms involved in oxytocin-induced modulation of myometrial contractility. *Acta Pharmacologica Sinica, 27*(7), 827–832.

Sieprath, P. J., Koninckx, P. R., & Van Assche, F. A. (1986). Essential prolonged and hypertonic contractions. *European Journal of Obstetrics, Gynecology, and Reproductive Biology, 21*, 49–52.

Simpson, K. R., & James, D. C. (2008). Effects of oxytocin-induced uterine hyperstimulation during labor on fetal oxygen status and fetal heart rate patterns. *American Journal of Obstetrics and Gynecology, 199*(1), 34.e1–34.e5.

Smith, G., Cordeaux, Y., White, I., Charnock-Jones, S., Pasupathy, D., & Missfelder-Lobos, H. (2007). Maternal age and uterine function: A biological basis for rising rates of cesarean delivery [Abstract]. *American Journal of Obstetrics and Gynecology, S100*.

Smith, R. (2007). Mechanisms of disease: Parturition. *New England Journal of Medicine, 356*(3), 271–283.

Smith, Y. R., Dombrowski, M. P., Leach, K. C., & Hurd, W. W. (1995). Decrease in myometrial beta-adrenergic receptors with prenatal cocaine use. *Obstetrics & Gynecology, 85*(3), 357–360.

Sutliff, R. L., Gayheart-Walsten, P. A., Snyder, D. L., Roberts, J., & Johnson, M. D. (1999). Cardiovascular effects of actue and chronic cocaine administration in pregnant and nonpregnant rabbits. *Toxicology and Applied Pharmacology, 158*, 278–287.

Thornton, S., Davison, J. M., & Baylis, P. H. (1990). Effect of human pregnancy on metabolic clearance of oxytocin. *American Journal of Physiology, Regulatory, Integrative and Comparative Physiology, 259*, R21–R24.

Tomimatsu, T., Peña, J. P., & Longo, L. D. (2007). Fetal cerebral oxygenation: The role of maternal hyperoxia with supplemental CO_2 in sheep. *American Journal of Obstetrics and Gynecology, 196*(4), 359–361.

Ustunyurt, E., Ugur, M., Ustunyurt, B. O., Iskender, T. C., Ozkan, O., & Mollamahmutoglu, L. (2007). Prospective randomized study of oxytocin discontinuation after the active stage of labor is established. *Journal of Obstetric Gynaecologic Research, 33*(6), 799–803.

Vedernikov, Y. P., Betancourt, A., Wentz, M. J., Saade, G. R, & Garfield, R. E. (2006). Adaptation to pregnancy leads to attenuated RAT uterine artery smooth muscle sensitivity to oxytocin. *American Journal of Obstetrics and Gynecology, 194*, 252–260.

Wang, F. L., Dombrowski, M. P., & Hurd, W. W. (1996). Obstetrics: Cocaine and beta-adrenergic receptor function in pregnant myometrium. *American Journal of Obstetrics and Gynecology, 175*(6), 1651–1652.

Wang, F. L., Gauvin, J. M., Dombrowski, M. P., Smith, Y. R., Christopher, K. A., & Hurd, W. W. (1996). Cocaine downregulates beta-adrenergic receptors in pregnant sheep myometrium. *Reproductive Toxicology, 10*(2), 119–123.

Williams, S., Wilson, S., Ganesh, S., White, P., & Apuzzio, J. (2007). Risk of febrile morbidity with addition of intracervical foley for induction of labor [Abstract]. *American Journal of Obstetrics and Gynecology,* S105.

Witcher, P. M., & Harvey, C. J. (2006). Modifying labor routines for the woman with cardiac disease. *Journal of Perinatal and Neonatal Nursing, 20*(4), 303–310.

Woodcock, N. A., Taylor, C. W., & Thornton, S. (2006). Prostaglandin $F_2\alpha$ increases the sensitivity of the contractile proteins to Ca^{2+} in human myometrium. *American Journal of Obstetrics and Gynecology, 195*, 1404–1406.

Yamaguchi, E. T., Cardoso, M. M. S. C., & Torres, M. L. A. (2007). Oxytocin in cesarean sections. What is the best way to use it? *Revista Brasileira de Anestesiologia, 57*(3), 324–330.

Yasuda, K., Nakamoto, T., Yasuhara, M., Okada, H., Nakajima, T., & Kanzaki, H. (2007). Role of protein kinase Cβ in rhythmic contractions of human pregnant myometrium. *Reproduction, 133*, 797–806.

Zhao, Y., & Sun, L. (2004). Perinatal cocaine exposure reduces myocardial norepinephrine transporter function in the neonatal rat. *Neurotoxicology and Teratology, 26*(3), 443–450.

Ziganshin, A. U., Zefirova, J. T., Zefirova, T. P., Ziganshina, L. E., Hoyle, C. H. V., & Burnstock, G. (2005). Potentiation of uterine effects of prostaglandin F2a by adenosine 5'-triphosphate. *Obstetrics & Gynecology, 105*(6), 1429–1436.

10

Psyche, Spirituality, and the Cultural Dimensions of Care

He who knows the road can ride at full trot.

—*Italian Proverb*

The last "P" that is essential for labor and delivery nurses to understand is the patient's psyche. *Psyche* means the "self, soul, or mind." The patient's psyche is a product of her previous experiences, emotional readiness, culture and ethnicity, support systems, coping ability, and self-confidence (VandeVusse, 1999). This chapter explores the psyche of the pregnant woman, her spirituality, and her culture, and how they might affect her experiences during pregnancy, labor, and birth.

THE MEANING OF BEING PREGNANT

Becoming pregnant may define some women's purpose in life (Wesley, 2007). In such cases, pregnancy enriches the self. Other women perceive pregnancy as part of their spiritual growth, as something good for their soul and a gift from God. Other women may think of pregnancy as a time they can "eat for two."

The meaning of pregnancy may also be negative or positive (Simkin, 1996). In any case, each woman will create her own meaning for the pregnancy. Some women may consider the pregnancy unwanted. They may not feel joy or they will be concerned about the financial burden created by the pregnancy, the labor, and the addition of a child to the household.

THE FIRST HOSPITAL EXPERIENCE

Pregnancy begins a journey that ends with labor and birth. Women having their first baby are facing the unknown and are often scared, even when they have attended childbirth preparation classes. Admission to the hospital and the labor room has been referred to as "the point of no return" (Low & Moffat, 2006).

Women who are in labor and planning to have a vaginal delivery may be as fearful as women who have been admitted for a scheduled cesarean section. Even women who have an elective cesarean section feel fearful (Keogh, Hughes, Ellery, Daniel, & Holdcroft, 2005). Some women are frightened because they have listened to unpleasant birth stories from their friends or family members. Some women believe the events of others may now happen during their labors. And then there are the women who seem to have no fear because they learned everything about labor and delivery from watching programs about birth on television.

Your role is to build trust and diminish fear. Listen to your patient's expressions of fear. She is more likely to report fear during the labor than during the pregnancy (Alehagen, Wijma & Wijma, 2006). Laboring women may be subjected to new procedures such as intravenous infusion, amniotomy, epidural anesthesia, use of forceps or a vacuum extractor, or even a cesarean section.

When women present to the hospital after many months of anticipation, it is important for nurses to assess their emotional readiness for the tasks of labor and birth. Does she have a support system? Who is her coach? Is she able to cope? Is she confident or fearful? It is important to speak confidently to your patient and her family members. Do not tell her, "Hi, I'm new!" or "This is my first month here" or "I've never done this before." It is critical that your patient and her family have confidence in you. As labor progresses, your patient may have an overwhelming fear of the actual delivery, even the fear of dying. She may become silent and it will be up to you to acknowledge her fear. You might say, "Many women are scared the first time they have a baby. I will be with you the whole time. We'll do this together."

In fact, you may be the first caregiver she encounters. The nurse–patient relationship is a valued and honored relationship. Nurses establish a trusting relationship with the patient and her family. To begin this relationship, greet them and tell them your name. If you cannot communicate in the language they understand, locate a translator using the translator service that your hospital provides. Document the name of the translator in the medical record. Let your patient and the family know you will be with them to support and help them.

When your patient tells you about her previous birth experience, do not say "Oh, that happens a lot." Give her the time to tell her story and listen. Listening allows her to validate her thoughts and gives meaning to the life-changing event of birth (Callister, 2003). When your patient is in pain do not say, "Relax." It is better to encourage her to look toward a focal point and breathe rhythmically (which you might need to help her do if she did not attend childbirth preparation classes). Breathing this way does not relieve the pain, but it may help her to manage the contraction. Remind her to get through "one contraction at a time." It is best if she does not see the clock.

Tell the patient and her family the hours that you will be working and caring for them. Ask them to feel free to call you at any time. Encourage them to ask for you by name if you are out of the room. Demonstrate the use of the call light. This is an important first step in reducing anxiety and stress in your patient. This interaction should take place before other nursing assessments. Place your hands on the patient if it is culturally accepted. A compassionate first touch can build trust between you and your patient.

Nurses are both teachers and patient advocates. You should assess your patient's learning needs and provide information based on her readiness to learn. Your interactions with your patient become part of her birth story. Simkin (1992) wrote that some women remember the events surrounding birth and how they felt for at least 20 years.

In anticipation of the day of delivery, some women lose sleep. Your patient may be fatigued. Fatigue diminishes the ability to cope with the pain of labor. Fear, anxiety, loneliness, stress, anger, exhaustion, discouragement, and feelings of hopelessness all diminish the ability to cope with pain (Simkin & Ancheta, 2005). Women who are depressed may also feel lonely or angry, exhausted and discouraged, or hopeless. These feelings may be accepted as normal during pregnancy (Records & Rice, 2007). Your role is to discover how your

patient is coping. For example, does she have a history of depression?

Provide your patient with a safe environment. Act to decrease her stress and promote comfort and rest. Bolster her courage and inspire hope so that she can confidently participate in the childbirth process.

When women think they are in labor, they are often anxious. Anxious women contract but may not dilate. Listen to the cadence of her words and look at her face to determine if she is anxious. She may be anxious because this is her first labor or because she lacks social support or the financial resources to be a parent. She may be homeless. She may be very prepared for childbirth or not prepared at all.

Once you determine if your patient is anxious and/or fearful, assess her pain and how she copes with pain. Is she doubled over, crying, complaining the pain is deep and constant, yet is only 1-centimeter dilated? This is not normal and requires you to summon the physician to the bedside to evaluate her. She may have a placental abruption. Is she stoic and nonverbal, but tenses her arms and legs during contractions? Palpate contractions and monitor the fetus. Document your assessments.

> **Documentation example**: Patient crying and thrashing in bed. No vaginal bleeding. Fingertip dilated. States she is due in 1 month. No prenatal care. Dr. Beritethere called at her office. Reports she will arrive in 5 to 10 minutes.

DEPRESSION DURING PREGNANCY

Pregnant women have depression as often as women who are not pregnant. As many as 14.5% experience an episode of depression during pregnancy (Records & Rice, 2007). Labor and delivery nurses should perform a psychosocial patient interview as part of the initial patient assessment. Your patient may share her history of depression and discuss her current medications. Include this information in the nursing admission database and inform the incoming nurse of her history of depression and medication when care is transferred. During the patient interview and physical assessment, you may be able to identify symptoms of depression (see Exhibit 10.1). Adverse maternal and infant outcomes occur when depression worsens (Marcus, Flynn, Blow, & Barry, 2003). Therefore, it is important that nurses read the prenatal record to determine a woman's history of depression. Ask her when she last took her antidepressant and document the medication and the time she took it.

If your patient has a flat affect, share your assessment with the midwife or physician because routine monitoring for depression symptoms may not have occurred during prenatal care. Women with a history of depression and women who are currently receiving psychotherapy or drug therapy for depression are more likely to be assessed and monitored during pregnancy. A study of 3,472 women found that several factors were strongly predictive of depressive symptoms dur-

---

> ### Exhibit 10.1: Some signs and symptoms related to depression.
>
> - Feeling sad or blue
> - Losing all interest in things such as work
> - Fatigue and confusion
> - Mood swings and irritability
> - Tearfulness
> - Sleep disturbances
> - Appetite changes

ing pregnancy. These factors are: previous episodes of major depressive illness, poor self-rated health, and the use of tobacco and alcohol. Depression is also more common in women who are unemployed or unmarried, and in women who smoke and drink alcohol (Marcus, Flynn, Blow, & Barry, 2003).

> **Clinical example:** A pregnant woman in her 32nd week of pregnancy walked into the labor and delivery unit and stopped at the nurses' station. With a calm demeanor and quiet voice she said, "I just swallowed a whole bottle of Tylenol." This woman was depressed. She was immediately treated for the overdose after seeing the triage physician.

It is critical that the diagnosis of depression or anxiety be addressed by nurses and caregivers prior to the patient's discharge from the hospital. Postpartum women with increasing depressive symptoms are at greater risk of developing clinical depression (Skouteris, Wetheim, Rallis, Milgrom & Paxton, 2008).

CHEMICAL DEPENDENCE DURING PREGNANCY

Another area that needs to be explored during the psychosocial patient interview is the abuse of tobacco, alcohol, or other drugs. Alcohol, cigarettes, and street drugs such as cocaine, marijuana, and heroin may, directly or indirectly, harm the mother and the fetus. Women who are addicted to narcotics are at risk for hepatitis, human immunodeficiency virus (HIV), venereal disease, skin abscesses, glomerulonephritis, vasculitis, and bacterial endocarditis (Chan & Tang, 1995).

Pregnant women and their partners may both need treatment for drug dependency. Women who have a chemical dependency may live a chaotic lifestyle, be impoverished, or feel shame or guilt, and may even be malnourished due to lack of food. They need your nonjudgmental compassion when they are in labor. If a urine test is ordered to screen for drugs, the patient must consent to the test prior to the collection of urine. Let her know the test is to help the nurses and physicians know how to care for her and for her baby in the nursery. After she consents, you must be present when the urine is collected or you should obtain a sample by catheterizing her. Document her verbal consent or refusal in your notes.

> **Documentation example:** Discussed the need for a urine test to check for drugs. Mother said, "Okay, I will." Cath urine obtained and sent to lab.

> **Documentation example:** Discussed the need for a urine test to check for drugs. Mother refused. Dr. Ohno notified of maternal refusal for a urine toxicology test.

Women who are addicted to alcohol or opiates may be intoxicated or in withdrawal when they arrive at the hospital. Addiction is a disease. They may have cravings, compulsive use of these drugs (even when they are in the hospital), continued use despite harm or consequences, impaired control over their drug use, and chronicity (Christensen, 2008).

Adolescents 16 to 19 years of age who are chemically dependent and in a drug-treatment program with adults were mostly addicted to alcohol and marijuana. Adult women are more likely to be addicted to opiates and cocaine (Farrow, Watts, Krohn, & Olson, 1999).

Some women with a chemical dependency do not seek prenatal care. In a study from Pennsylvania and Georgia, 62% of women who received no prenatal care were addicted to cocaine (Spence, Williams, Digregorio, Kirby-McDonnel, & Polansky, 1991). Even if a woman receives prenatal care, her provider may fail to use a standardized screening tool to assess her alcohol use during pregnancy (Davis & Carr, 2008). Therefore, the full extent of her alcohol use may be undetected. Occasionally, a woman who is drunk will present to labor and delivery. She will need assistance to stabilize her gait and to get into bed. She may slur her words. If her baby has fetal alcohol syndrome, there may be facial anomalies, intrauterine growth restriction (IUGR), and cognitive impairment (Christensen, 2008). Women with an addiction to alcohol are usually cigarette smokers as well. Smoking cigarettes increases the risk of IUGR.

> **Clinical example:** A patient arrived in active labor. She had no prenatal care and she appeared to be about 26 weeks pregnant. She delivered within 1 hour. Her newborn was a full-term, 3 pound 6 ounce baby. The pediatrician was present for the birth. He asked her if she smoked. She said she smoked a pack a day (20 cigarettes). He asked her what other drugs she used. She looked at her boyfriend. He asked again and she said, "I did crack last night."

In this example, and based on her history, she did not use cocaine (crack) just last night. Addiction implies chronicity. She had been using cocaine for 1 year. Her boyfriend was walking quickly around her room. She asked him after the delivery to go across the street and buy her a hamburger. He came back to the room 1 hour later with nothing in his hands. She asked him, "Where's my burger?" His response was, "I couldn't find the place."

The partner was also addicted to cocaine. When addiction is detected, a social services professional should be contacted because an evaluation is needed to determine if it is safe for the neonate to go home with the mother.

Clinical example: A pregnant woman near term was brought into the labor unit by the ambulance crew who picked her up at a known "crack" house. She was intoxicated on cocaine. She admitted to having sex in exchange for the cocaine. Upon arrival, she was screaming and in pain. This was her second child. Her mascara was smeared and her hair was in disarray. The labor nurse managed to assist the patient into a hospital gown and into the bed. The midwife assessed the patient and found her to be ready to deliver. As the baby was delivering, she tried to leave the bed. With forceful commands, the midwife was able to redirect the woman's attention and the baby was safely delivered. Within 30 minutes of the delivery, the woman was walking in the hall barefoot and asking the other nurses if there was any food anywhere on the unit. The woman was assisted back to her room and a sandwich was located for her to eat.

As a labor and delivery nurse, you cannot treat addiction. Your priority will be to assess the patient's most recent drug use, her vital signs, her contractions (women addicted to cocaine may have tachysystole), signs and symptoms of placental abruption, the estimated fetal weight, and the psychosocial factors that influence the patient's behavior. If she has had prenatal care, read the prenatal record to identify drug use. You might ask her, "Do you smoke cigarettes?" You might also ask her, "When is the last time you smoked a cigarette?" If your patient is an adolescent, you might ask, "When is the last time you drank alcohol?" You could also ask, "When is the last time you used marijuana?" You can ask the same questions of your adult patients, but add a question about heroin and cocaine use.

Clinical example: A woman who has two children presented to labor and delivery. She smelled of alcohol, could not walk a straight line, and slurred her words. After the nurse assisted her into bed, she asked if the woman had been drinking. The woman's response was, "I don't know what everyone's problem is. All I had was two shots of tequila and a couple of beers." The nurse documented this as a quote in the nursing notes, then notified her charge nurse and a social services representative. Prior to discharge, a social worker met with the patient and the baby was placed in foster care. Her other two children were also in foster care.

CHEMICAL WITHDRAWAL DURING LABOR

Withdrawal may occur during labor. Never administer nalbuphine hydrochloride (Nubain®) or butorphanol to women who are addicted to opiates because this will put them into withdrawal. If your patient is a heroin addict (opioid addict), she may complain of back pain, leg pain, sweating, headache, and nausea when she is experiencing withdrawal. During labor, women addicted to opiates will need frequent doses of narcotics such as morphine, fentanyl, or meperidine (Demerol® or Pethidine®). If there are no contraindications and she can sit still, she may be able to receive neuraxial analgesia or anesthesia.

Women who are addicted to opiates have a much greater risk for preterm delivery and IUGR. Their husbands or male partners may also be addicted to narcotics or may be in jail. They may be poor and refuse to attend therapy. At least 85% of the women who are addicted to opiates are also cigarette smokers. These women are also more likely to have a sexually transmitted disease and it is more likely that their babies will go through withdrawal (Chan & Tang, 1995).

Women with a history of heroin addiction and who are in a treatment program may be taking methadone or a drug such as buprenorphine (Buprenex, Subutex, or Suboxone), a partial opiate agonist. Buprenex is injectable; Subutex and Suboxone are sublingual. Consult your formulary or hospital pharmacist if you have questions about these drugs. You should not begin buprenorphine during labor as the initial dose can trigger withdrawal. If the patient is able to wean off of methadone during the pregnancy, there should be an improved neonatal outcome (Christensen, 2008).

Women who have a chemical dependency are often users of more than one drug. This is known as polydrug use. These women may smoke cigarettes, use benzodiazepines such as Valium, and even smoke, inject, or snort cocaine. They may also use amphetamines.

Clinical example: The patient was a known amphetamine user and cigarette smoker. She presented in labor at 35 weeks of gestation. During labor she asked to smoke a cigarette. She was allowed to step outside (Labor and Delivery is on the first floor). She returned to bed and the fetal heart rate was tachycardic. The woman admitted to smoking amphetamines.

Women should be discouraged from smoking during labor. Nicotine triggers the release of catecholamines and may be related to tachycardia. Amphetamine use also causes fetal tachycardia. In this clinical example, the woman smoked amphetamines in the car with her friend and did not smoke a cigarette.

Even if you determine that your patient has a chemical dependency, the fetal heart rate or fetal heart rate pattern may be normal. You job is to assess her vital signs, her contractions, the fetal heart rate, and her uterine activity, and to communicate abnormal findings to the obstetric care provider. When you give report to the nurse who will assume care of the patient, you will need to discuss your patient's chemical dependency so that a social services representative can be contacted.

SPIRITUALITY

There are 19 major world religions, subdivided into 270 large groups and many smaller ones. There are 34,000 separate Christian religious groups that have been identified in the world (Barrett, Kurian, & Johnson, 2001). Therefore, it is possible that you will not be familiar with the religious beliefs of your patient. If the patient or her family members listen to music, place icons in the room or juniper seeds around the laboring woman's neck, or perform other unfamiliar rituals, this is obviously something they need for this part of the pregnancy journey.

Spiritually focused interventions may reduce maternal anxiety and increase confidence (Breen, Price, & Lake, 2007). Labor and delivery nurses do not have to understand or accept religious aspects or teachings that differ from their own religion or beliefs. On the contrary, nurses must be tolerant of their patients' spiritual needs and beliefs, and provide deliberate, safe care. Tolerance is different from acceptance. Tolerance is evidenced by a quiet respect for the patient and her family's right to practice religious and cultural beliefs and customs of their choosing. Obviously, you must also follow hospital protocol. There should be no use of electrical or gas cooking equipment in the room. If there is no contraindication to eating after delivery, however, the woman's family members may offer her special foods they have prepared.

Occasionally, a woman seeks a blessing from a spiritual leader during labor or after the birth of her child. Most hospitals have a chaplain or pastoral care provider for this purpose and your patient may also call in a religious leader for this purpose. Ask your charge nurse or supervisor to contact a pastoral care provider if it is requested. Your should familiarize yourself with the patient services that he or she provides.

CONFIDENCE AND CONTROL

Part of the psyche that is important to having the strength to labor and to push a child out of the womb is related to confidence and self-control. When labor and delivery nurses and/or a doula provide support, they help the patient gain both confidence and control (Association of Women's Health, Obstetric and Neonatal Nurses, 2000). The labor support you provide will vary based on your patient's cultural childbirth practices and rituals. Regardless of the woman's ethnic identity, your responsibility is to provide individualized, safe care to enhance labor using the labor support interventions that your patient accepts.

THE BIRTH PLAN

Women provide a birth plan to satisfy their need to control what happens to them during labor and birth. Satisfaction with their birthing experience is enhanced when expectations are met. The birth plan should be thought of as a "wish list." A birth plan is a way of expressing preferences and communicating with care providers. Take time to read the birth plan and discuss it with your patient and her partner or family. Discuss any requests that you cannot meet in the hospital

---

> **Exhibit 10.2: Examples of statements from birth plans.**
>
> - Please keep the room quiet. I want to be the only one screaming.
> - I do not want any procedures that rhyme with "otomy or ectomy."
> - Please keep me covered at all times. I do not want anyone to see me poop.
> - I do not want any monitoring of my baby during labor. What possibly could go wrong?
> - Do not offer me any pain medication. Pain is good and I want to feel my body on fire.

setting with the patient and the provider. Some birth plan statements will make you smile (see Exhibit 10.2).

SOME WISHES WILL BE UNFULFILLED

Rouse, Owen, Savage, and Hauth (2001) found that 18% of nulliparous women and 5% of parous women who began spontaneous labor nevertheless needed to be augmented with oxytocin. These women had an arrest of dilatation for 2 or more hours during the active phase and they all eventually had to have a cesarean section. If there is a birth plan, there may be a desire to avoid interventions such as augmentation and cesarean section. Demonstrate empathy when you explain changes in the plan that may contradict your patient's wishes. The obstetric care provider should also explain the rationale for any change in the plan of care.

You may be the labor and delivery nurse for a patient who is a Jehovah's Witness and who has refused a blood transfusion in her birthing plan. A policy or procedure for meeting the needs of Jehovah's Witness patients has been developed in some hospitals. The program involves options for infusion of nonblood substances in the case of hemorrhage. Ask your charge nurse or supervisor if your hospital has a similar policy or procedure.

There are also programs in some hospitals and birthing centers that provide an additional support person called a doula. *Doula* is a Greek word meaning "woman caregiver." The effect of support from a doula is a shorter labor (Campbell, Lake, Falk, & Backstrand, 2006). If your hospital has a doula program or doula group, and your patient would benefit from this program, contact your charge nurse or supervisor to help you obtain this additional support.

If you are unfamiliar or uncomfortable performing a procedure or using obstetric technology, ask a more experienced nurse for help. It is wise to say, "I don't know. Can you help?" Do not perform tasks or give medications for which you have not received education and training.

CULTURAL ASSESSMENT

Labor and delivery nurses must provide support, build confidence, and promote self-control within the context of the patient's culture and expectations. Allowing for cultural variations in the health care setting is a key principle of perinatal care endorsed by the World Health Organization (WHO) (Chalmers, Mangiaterra, & Porter, 2001).

A careful cultural assessment takes a long time which may not be possible during labor. A quick assessment of cultural needs should be done when an in-depth patient interview is not possible (see Exhibit 10.3).

INTERPRETER SERVICES

If your patient does not speak English, you should find a translator or use a translation service. It is important to avoid using a family member, especially when questions to ascertain domestic violence are asked. Some hospitals use a telephone translation program or may have a list of credentialed individuals within the hospital who you can contact. Ask your charge nurse or supervisor how you can obtain language translation for your patient. You should also determine if consent forms are available in other languages and document the name of the translator in the medical records.

CULTURE AFFECTS EXPECTATIONS

The psyche is created within a culture. Foods, the use of touch, and the role of males and females during labor and birth are part of that culture. Hot or cold foods may be unacceptable depending on the climate. The presence of a male as a care provider, such as a male nurse or male physician, may be unacceptable. Greetings with handshakes, a hug, or a smiling face may be either welcome or unwanted, depending on the acceptance of direct physical or eye contact within the patient's culture.

Clinical example: A male nurse who was trained in Kenya and who was present for the labor of his wife at a hospital in the United States said this about his wife's labor experience: "I expected them to help her ambulate, walk around and come back, check the fetal heart rate, make sure everything is fine, walk again, and let the baby descend naturally." In his experience in Kenya as a community nurse who provided primary care and monitored babies using a fetoscope, he could not understand why in the United States there was a need to put women in a bed and strap on the fetal monitor. His wife said "I didn't want an epidural. I wanted to do it the natural way. In Kenya we don't even know about epidurals. I didn't want to have an epidural."

After all, this is their labor and birth experience. In order to meet their expectations, you should ask during the psychosocial interview what they would like to see happen during labor and birth, and then provide them with information as to why the plan of care may have to change.

TRANSCULTURAL NURSING CARE

Transcultural nursing care reflects an understanding of another person's culture, language, verbal and nonverbal communication, and food preferences. Transcultural nursing ensures patient privacy and protects a woman's modesty. It is nursing that is tolerant of birth ceremonies or observances, health practices, and beliefs about illness and wellness.

First Nation and Native American Cultures

First Nation is a term of ethnicity, often used to refer to persons who inhabited lands in North America prior to the arrival of immigrants from Europe. In the United States, these people are called Native Americans. Native American women may demonstrate firm restraint when they experience labor pain. Because the woman may not freely offer complaints of pain or discomfort, you will need to be alert to indirect signs of her pain. Does she walk and pause every minute or two? If so, she may be contracting every 1 to 2 minutes, and may even be completely dilated. What is her pulse and blood pressure? Are they elevated? What is her body language?

Traditional Native American women may request that certain blood, urine, or the placenta and umbilical cord be returned after the birth (Abramo, 2001). The placenta will be buried at a site on the family's land. For example, the placenta may be buried near the weaving loom. A traditional Native American may also request that ceremonies be performed by a tribal member or healer, especially if there is a fetal demise. Tribal elders will be involved, and there may be a procession of tribe members who elevate and chant as they leave with the mother and her deceased infant. The infant will be wrapped in special fabrics during a ceremony that may be held in the postpartal room.

Amish Culture

Amish women in labor may not verbally express pain. The Amish woman and her husband may be uncomfortable with technology used in the hospital setting. If she is a low-risk patient, avoid the use of the fetal monitor. If she can drink fluids, postpone starting an intravenous line. Her husband may not show outward affection toward her or the newborn after delivery. The laboring woman also may prefer eating food grown by her family instead of hospital food (Lipson, Dibble, & Minarik, 1996).

Mexican Culture

Women of Mexican descent who are in labor may be very vocal and loud and they may repeat their words during painful contractions (Darby, 2007). You may hear "Aye, aye, aye" during strong contractions. Multiple female family members may attend to the woman as her labor coaches. Hospital policy of restricting visitors during labor and birth may not be popular with the family (Lipson, Dibble, & Minarik, 1996). She may avoid cold foods in cold weather and avoid warm foods in warm weather.

Arab Culture

Women who speak Arabic as their native language generally have been raised in an Arab culture. Traditional Arab women may be quiet, and their husbands may make the decisions related to labor and birth. Modesty and privacy are extremely important to them. Ask permission before exposing your patient's body. Some women wax their body hair, so it is important not to act surprised by the absence of pubic hair.

Arab women may also have greater fear of a cesarean section than a vaginal delivery. A cesarean section may be perceived as mutilation (Lipson, Dibble, & Minarik, 1996). If your patient is financially dependent on her husband, he may refuse the cesarean section and threaten to divorce her if she consents to the surgery. In Arab cultures, foods are considered either hot or cold, and the general rule is to avoid cold foods in warm seasons and hot foods in cold seasons (Abramo, 2001).

Iranian Culture

Women from Iran speak Farsi. Iranian fathers very are involved in the labor process, and female family members act as support persons. Reaction to pain may vary from moaning to more vocal expressions of pain. If you cannot understand what she is saying, but her body language reflects severe pain and you palpate regular, moderate to strong contractions, ask an English-speaking family member or translator what she is saying. If he or she says "I can't tell you because it is bad words," check her immediately! She may be completely dilated. Iranian women may request warm fluids to drink and they may wish to avoid ice cold-water. Above all, do not serve pork (Lipson, Dibble, & Minarik, 1996).

ASIAN CULTURES

Women from Asia will have one of several Asian cultures. This section explores the childbirth and food preferences of traditional Chinese, Japanese, Vietnamese, Hmong, and Korean women.

Chinese

Traditional Chinese parents may not be joyous with the birth of an infant girl due to social constraints on childbearing. Laboring women may be nonverbal and demonstrate restraint during contractions to avoid being considered weak. They may have beads of sweat on their forehead as a sign they are 10-cm dilated. During the second stage, hold her hand if she accepts this. If she squeezes it, she is probably pushing. Occasionally, the Chinese husband will count in Chinese during pushing. Do not discourage this supportive behavior. Hot foods should be avoided in cold seasons and cold foods should be avoided during warm seasons (Abramo, 2001).

Japanese

Japanese women may not voice their discomfort during labor and birth, because this is viewed as weakness. Japanese women will, however, express their needs. They are modest and may prefer a female birth attendant. The father of the baby will be expected to be present for the birth. Japanese women may request tea instead of water or juice (Lipson, Dibble, & Minarik, 1996).

Vietnamese

Vietnamese women in labor are often stoic and do not vocalize their need for pain medication. Hot and cold balance is very important during labor. These women will drink only warm or hot liquids during labor. The labor coach will most often be a female family member instead of her husband (Abramo, 2001; Lipson, Dibble, & Minarik, 1996).

Hmong

Childbearing women of Hmong families may have had many pregnancies and may delay seeking prenatal care because they are embarrassed by physical examination. They are often quiet during their labor. They will voice extreme discomfort during vaginal examinations (Levine, Anderson, & McCullough, 2004). They may refuse a cesarean section and request warm water or diluted tea during labor (Lipson, Dibble, & Minarik, 1996).

Koreans

Korean women in labor may be quiet and stoic, and may avoid vocalizing pain or a need for pain medication. The birth of a female infant may not be embraced with enthusiasm. They will be modest and perineal cleanliness is very important. They avoid cold liquids and may request lukewarm water to drink (Lipson, Dibble, & Minarik, 1996).

SOUTH EAST ASIAN CULTURE
Filipinos

Filipino families may attend to the laboring woman with great care and attention. Often, the laboring woman will request her mother be in attendance at the delivery instead of her husband. Filipino women are modest and they may desire a female birth attendant. They will often vocalize their requests during labor and delivery and may even scream during labor. They prefer drinking fluids at room temperature or slightly warmer than room temperature (Lipson, Dibble, & Minarik, 1996).

Indians

Traditional women from India will act subservient to their husbands and will not make their own decisions. Male infants are more highly valued than female infants. Women from India in labor may quietly accept pain, but may permit pain relief measures when offered. Women from India are modest and will prefer being draped and covered during procedures and during childbirth.

Pakistanis

Traditional Pakistani women may not make their own decisions regarding labor and birth, leaving decisions to a male family member. The father of the baby may stay at the hospital for her protection, but will not attend the birth. These women refrain from taking in hot foods during cold seasons and cold foods during warm seasons (Abramo, 2001).

Afghans

Afghan women in labor will often have a female birth-support person. They prefer female nurses and female medical providers. The father of the baby may not be present for the delivery, but will be nearby. The birth of a male infant may be preferred over the birth of a female infant (Lipson, Dibble, & Minarik, 1996). Afghans believe food can produce hot or cold, or be neutral in the body. Food is well appreciated and even has special meaning. For example, stepping on a piece of dropped bread is considered sinful.

CARIBBEAN CULTURES

Laboring women from islands such as the West Indies may be quiet and nonverbal during labor and birth. They may feel too ashamed to cry out in pain. They may be embarrassed with exposure of their body and prefer a female caregiver. The woman's husband or partner may or may not be present for the labor and birth. Women from the Caribbean may drink fluids with ice, unless they are ill (Lipson, Dibble, & Minarik, 1996).

PACIFIC ISLANDS CULTURE

Pacific Islanders may be found in Hawaii, American Samoa, Guam, and the Commonwealth of the Northern Mariana Islands. Pacific Island women may not vocally express labor pain. They may be accompanied by multiple female family members who will attend the birth. Their husband may or may not attend the birth (Abrano, 2001).

LATIN AMERICAN CULTURES

In some of Latin America, including the regions of Central and South America, and the Caribbean islands of Cuba, the Dominican Republic, Puerto Rico, and Haiti, Spanish is the most common language spoken (with French being spoken in Haiti and Portuguese in Brazil). Laboring women from Latin America may not participate during labor due to their fear of birth, and they may respond to pain by screaming. Men are not usually involved in the labor and birth process. These women may request that liquids be served without ice (Lipson, Dibble, & Minarik, 1996).

Cubans

The mother of the laboring Cuban woman may be the dominant decision maker during this time. The husband may not be present and may not take an active role. The laboring Cuban woman will vocalize her pain. She may request cold liquids to drink (Lipson, Dibble, & Minarik, 1996).

Puerto Ricans

Puerto Rican women in labor prefer to have family members present, with the father of the baby accepting a supportive role. Outward expressions of pain are socially accepted and encouraged. The laboring woman may be modest. Hygiene is very important. She may request cold liquids to drink during labor (Lipson, Dibble, & Minarik, 1996).

Haitians

Behavior during labor may vary from stoic to screaming and cursing. The husband will not participate in the labor, as the traditional belief is that labor is best handled by women. Female family members will give support to the laboring woman but may not coach her. Haitian women believe hot and cold food imbalances affect wellness. Pregnant Haitian women may avoid eating tomatoes and white beans due to the belief that they may cause hemorrhage (Lipson, Dibble, & Minarik, 1996).

CENTRAL AMERICAN CULTURES

Central America includes the countries of Belize, Costa Rica, El Salvador, Guatemala, Honduras, Nicaragua, and Panama. Family members and husbands are supportive of laboring woman in these countries. The woman may loudly express her labor pain. She may avoid cold foods in cold weather and avoid hot food in hot weather. Liquids should be served at room temperature (Lipson, Dibble, & Minarik, 1996).

RUSSIAN CULTURE

Women from Russia, also known as the Russian Federation, receive strong support from family members. The husband may be the decision maker during labor if he has the stronger personality. In that case, the laboring woman's behavior may be passive. He may not attend the delivery. She will request no ice in her drinks and may desire hot tea (Lipson, Dibble, & Minarik, 1996).

WHEN THINGS GO WRONG

An adverse outcome or the birth of an anomalous infant may threaten a woman's psyche. Parents will need emotional support and may suffer from chronic sorrow due to the birth of an anomalous baby or a stillborn. Adverse outcomes in labor and delivery require completion of a report such as an occurrence report or an incident report. Adverse outcomes that trigger the need to write a report include stillbirth, neonatal death, meconium aspiration syndrome, an acidemic pH, a 5-minute Apgar score of 5 or less, neonatal trauma, neonatal seizures, maternal seizures, hemorrhage, hysterectomy, and maternal death. Of course, if there is an unplanned removal of a body part or injury during an operative procedure, or an incorrect surgical sponge or instrument count, these events are also considered adverse outcomes. A medication error is also an adverse outcome, especially if the mother or her baby is affected. You should be familiar with your hospital's policies, procedures, and protocol regarding adverse outcomes.

Most current resuscitation guidelines suggest that clinicians consider withdrawing resuscitation if there are no signs of life after 10 minutes of adequate resuscitation. Harrington, Redman, Moulden, and Greenwood (2007) identified seven studies that evaluated the outcomes of infants who had an Apgar score of 0 at 10 minutes. Ninety-four percent of the infants died or were severely handicapped. The rest were mildly or moderately handicapped. The outcome of three infants was not reported. The birth of an infant who has an Apgar score of 0 at 10 minutes will usually require a report of an adverse outcome, unless the birth of a stillborn was anticipated.

THE ANOMALOUS BABY

Providing emotional support is essential when a woman is expecting to deliver a baby who needs surgery or intensive care. Active listening is helpful for the patient, the family, and the caregiver.

> **Clinical example of a conversation with a labor and delivery nurse**: Yesterday I had a patient who knew that her baby had gastroschisis. She came in on Wednesday at 38 weeks for induction. We tried prostaglandin gel, but she made no progress. She came back 2 days later for oxytocin. After 6 hours her cervix still had not changed. Her contractions were mostly every 2 minutes, but difficult to record due to her size. I sat there and palpated most of them. The tracing was fine. We were all discouraged. She just wanted a cesarean section. I didn't think that was a good idea and asked the physician to reassess her. After the amniotomy and with oxytocin, she started to really labor. We didn't want to use an intrauterine pressure catheter due to the gastroschisis. So, I just continued to palpate the contractions. She eventually delivered with the neonatal team there.

SATISFACTION WITH THE BIRTHING EXPERIENCE

Satisfaction is a complex and multidimensional phenomenon (Hodnett, 2002). Satisfaction with the birthing experience will be context specific and influenced by the woman's culture, the birthing environment, and expectations based on previous experiences (Bricker & Lavender, 2002). As a labor and delivery nurse, you are in a position to influence the birthing environment and to meet the patient's expectations.

Your support and the relationship you create with your patient will influence her satisfaction with the childbirth expe-

---

> **Exhibit 10.4: Actions to express patient satisfaction messages (modified from Leebov, 2008).**
>
> 1. Provide nursing care with compassion.
> 2. Make sure caring comes across.
> 3. Pay quality attention.
> 4. Reduce patient anxiety.
> 5. Make nursing your personal calling.

rience. Personal expectations, the amount of support from caregivers, the quality of the caregiver–patient relationship, and the woman's involvement in the decisions related to childbirth are the four most important variables women consider when they evaluate their birthing experience. Pain and pain relief do not seem to play a major role in rating satisfaction with the childbirth experience unless the patient's expectations related to pain relief were unmet (Hodnett, 2002).

"Customer service" is a term you would use if you worked in a service-oriented environment. As a nurse, you are probably more familiar with the term "patient satisfaction." Some hospitals mail surveys to their patients and ask them to rate their hospital stay, including room cleanliness, the quality of food, and the nursing care they received. Hospitals also support learning events and activities that encourage caregivers to acquire skills that improve patient satisfaction scores on these surveys. Some of these skills include greeting all patients and visitors with a smile and/or asking all patients and visitors if there is anything else that you can do for them. Nurses may feel that these customer-service strategies are superficial or staged. Nurses also may feel insulted that they have to be taught how to care about patients (Leebov, 2008). By changing some of the words and phrases used to reach patient-satisfaction goals, Leebov (2008) found that nurses were more accepting of the customer-service messages. The messages are based on key nursing actions (see Exhibit 10.4).

CONCLUSIONS

Nurses who conduct a psychosocial assessment will be better able to appreciate their patient's unique needs. Women may be fearful or chemically dependent. They may be depressed or unable to cope with labor pain. Women come from many different cultures, and nurses will interact with a diverse population during their careers. Tolerance of differences enhances the childbirth experience. The support nurses and doulas provide and the quality of the nurse–patient relationship can shorten labor, improve patient satisfaction, and create positive long-term memories.

Labor and delivery nurses must communicate effectively, advocate for their patients, and use the chain of command. They must assess their patients' needs, understand the phases and stages of labor, and act to diminish pain. Labor nurses should assist their patients in finding a position of comfort during labor. They must understand the relationship between the passenger, the placenta, the umbilical cord, and the passageway. They must estimate fetal weight, assess the fetal presentation, and monitor the fetal station. They determine dilatation and effacement. They understand the powers of labor, and act when there are abnormal powers or an abnormal fetal heart rate. They are aware of the psyche, spirituality, and culture of their patients, and they create a plan of care that reflects the patient's needs and desired outcomes. Labor and delivery nurses who have an evidence-based practice recognize learning is a lifelong process.

REVIEW QUESTIONS

True/False: Decide if the statements are true or false.

1. Women who deliver their babies vaginally are more fearful than women who have a cesarean section.
2. Birth plans are a communication tool and a wish list.
3. Nalbuphine hydrochloride (Nubain®) is contraindicated if the patient is an opiate addict.
4. Some signs of depression are appetite changes, mood swings, and insomnia.
5. Spiritually focused interventions may help to reduce maternal anxiety and increase confidence in the caregivers.
6. An in-depth cultural needs assessment is required to provide transcultural care.
7. Cuban women in labor prefer their mothers to make decisions for them.
8. Pacific Islanders prefer a limit on the number of family members and visitors present during labor.
9. Vietnamese women in labor prefer their husbands as their labor coach.
10. An intrauterine pressure catheter should be avoided if the fetus has gastroschisis.

References

Abramo, L. (2001). *Transcultural competencies for healthcare providers.* Agoura Hills, CA: Author.

Alehagen, S., Wijma, B., & Wijma, K. (2006). Fear of childbirth before, during, and after childbirth. *Acta Obstetricia et Gynecologica, 85,* 56–62.

Association of Women's Health, Obstetric, and Neonatal Nurses. (2000). Issue: Professional nursing support of laboring women. Washington, D.C.: Author.

Barrett, D. B., Kurian, G. T. & Johnson, T. M. (Eds.). (2001). *World Christian encyclopedia: A comparative survey of churches and religions in the modern world, AD 1900–2000. New York:* Oxford University Press.

Breen, G. V., Price, S., & Lake, M. (2007). Spirituality and high-risk pregnancy: Another aspect of patient care. *AWHONN Lifelines, 10*(6), 467–473

Bricker, L., & Lavender, T. (2002). Parenteral opioids for labor pain relief: A systematic review. *American Journal of Obstetrics and Gynecology, 186,* S94–S109.

Callister, L. C. (2003). Making meaning: Women's birth narratives. *Journal of Obstetric, Gynecologic, and Neonatal Nursing, 33*(4), 508–518.

Campbell, D. A., Lake, M. F., Falk, M., & Backstrand, J. R. (2006). A randomized control trial of continuous support in labor by a lay doula. *Journal of Obstetric, Gynecologic, and Neonatal Nursing, 35*(4), 456—464.

Chalmers, B., Mangiaterra, V., & Porter, R. (2001). WHO principles of perinatal care: The essential antenatal, perinatal, and postpartum care course. *Birth, 28*(3), 202–207.

Chan, K. S., & Tang, L. C. H. (1995). Narcotic addiction in pregnancy. *Hong Kong Medical Journal, 1*(3), 201–206.

Christensen, C. (2008). Management of chemical dependence in pregnancy. *Clinical Obstetrics and Gynecology, 51*(2), 445–455.

Darby, S. B. (2007). Pre- and perinatal care of Hispanic families: Implications for nurses. *Nursing for Women's Health, 11*(2), 162–169.

Davis, P. M., & Carr, T. L. (2008). Needs assessment and current practice of alcohol risk assessment of pregnant women and women of childbearing age by primary health care professionals. *Canadian Journal of Clinical Pharmacology, 15*(2), e214–e222.

Debby, A., Rotmensch, S., Girtler, O., Celentano, C., Geva, D., Sadan, O., & Golan, A. (1999). Clinical significance of the unengaged fetal head in laboring nulliparous women. *American Journal of Obstetrics and Gynecology, 180*(1, Part 2), S130.

Farrow, J., Watts, D., Krohn, M., & Olson, H. (1999). Pregnant adolescents in chemical dependency treatment: Description and outcomes. *Journal of Substance Abuse Treatment, 16*(2), 157–161.

Harrington, D. J., Redman, C. W., Moulden, M., & Greenwood, C. E. (2007). Long-term outcome in surviving infants with Apgar zero at 10 minutes: A systematic review of the literature and hospital-based cohort. *American Journal of Obstetrics and Gynecology, 196,* 463.e1–463.e5.

Hodnett, E. D. (2002). Pain and women's satisfaction with the experience of childbirth: A systematic review. *American Journal of Obstetrics and Gynecology, 164*(5), S160–S172.

Keogh, E., Hughes, S., Ellery, D., Daniel, C., & Holdcroft, A. (2005). Psychosocial influences on women's experience of planned elective cesarean section. *Psychosomatic Medicine,* *68,* 167–174.

Leebov, W. (2008). Beyond customer service. *American Nurse Today, 3*(1), 21–23.

Levine, M., Anderson, L., & McCullough, N. (2004). Hmong birthing: Bridging the cultural gap in a rural community in northern California. *AWHONN Lifelines 8*(2), 147–149.

Lipson, J. G., Dibble, S. L., & Minarik, P. A. (1996). *Culture & nursing care.* San Francisco: USCF Nursing Press.

Low, L. K., & Moffat, A., (2006). Every labor is unique. *American Journal of Maternal Child Nursing, 31*(5), 307–312.

Marcus, S. M., Flynn, H. A., Blow, F. C., & Barry, K. L. (2003). Depressive symptoms among pregnant women screened in obstetrics settings. *Journal of Women's Health, 12*(4), 373–380.

Records, K., & Rice, M. (2007). Psychosocial correlates of depression symptoms during the third trimester of pregnancy. *Journal of Obstetric, Gynecologic, and Neonatal Nursing, 36*(3), 231–242.

Rouse, D. J., Owen, J., Savage, K. G., & Hauth, J. C. (2001). Active phase labor arrest: Revisting the 2-hour minimum (2001). *Obstetric Gynecology, 98*(4), 550–554.

Simkin, P. (1992). Just another day in a woman's life?: Part 2. Nature and consistency of women's long term memories of their first birth experiences. *Birth: Issues in Perinatal Care, 19,* 64–81.

Simkin, P., (1996). The experience of maternity in woman's life. *Journal of Obstetric, Gynecologic, and Neonatal Nursing, 25,* 247–252.

Simkin, P., & Ancheta, R. (2005). *The labor progress handbook* (2nd ed.). Oxford, England: Blackwell Publishing.

Skouteris, H., Wetheim, E. H., Rallis, S., Milgrom, J., & Paxton, S. J. (2008). Depression and anxiety through pregnancy and the early postpartum: An examination of prospective relationships. *Journal of Affective Disorders,* doi:10.1016/j.jad.2008.06.002

Spence, M. R., Williams, R., Digregorio, G. J., Kirby-McDonnel, A., & Polansky, M. (1991). The relationship between recent cocaine use and pregnancy outcome. *Obstetrics & Gynecology, 78,* 326–327.

VandeVusse, L. (1999). The essential forces of labor revisited: 13 Ps reported in womens' stories. *American Journal of Maternal Child Nursing, 24*(4), 176–184.

Wesley, Y., (2007). Why women want children: Defining the meaning of desire and the construction of an index. *Journal of National Black Nurses' Association, 18*(1), 14–20.

Glossary

Abortion: Another name for miscarriage or a spontaneous abortion (SAB), however, it can be an elective procedure (EAB), previously referred to as a therapeutic abortion (TAB).

Abruption (abruptio placentae): The premature separation of part or all of the placenta from the uterine wall. Thrombin causes the uterus to contract frequently when there is bleeding inside the uterus.

Acceleration: An independent event, not attached to a deceleration. A transitory increase above the fetal heart rate baseline. An acceleration lasts 10 or more seconds and increases 10 or more beats per minute above the baseline. It is distinct from the cycles of (long-term) variability in the baseline.

Accreta: Deeper than normal invasion of the placenta (trophoblast) into the uterine wall.

Acidemia: pH lower than an acceptable level in the blood. Associated with acidosis.

Acidosis: A pathophysiologic state with an abnormally elevated cardon dioxide concentration (respiratory acidosis) or an abnormally elevated lactic acid concentration (metabolic acidosis) or both (mixed acidosis).

Adequate labor progress: Close to a 1-centimeter change in dilatation every hour with less than five contractions every 10 minutes during the active phase of labor. Adequate labor progress is accompanied by fetal descent. Dystocia is the opposite of adequate labor progress. Contractions can be effective yet there is dystocia due to the size or fit of the fetus in the pelvis (mechanical dystocia).

Advocacy: Acceptance of others as they are, supporting their choices, helping them explore their feelings, options, and possible consequences of their decisions. Speaking and acting on their behalf.

Amniocentesis: Removal of amniotic fluid through the abdomen and uterus. The fluid is analyzed for various factors and to detect genetic diseases and analyze chromosomes of the fetus.

Amnion: The thin, avascular, tough inner membranous layer of the sac around the fetus.

Amnion bands: After rupture of the membranes, bands of the membrane that wrap around fetal body parts and can lead to structural malformations or amputations.

Amniotic fluid: Also known as liquor. Mostly fetal urine around the fetus that cushions the umbilical cord and lubricates the fetus to aid in fetal descent. There should be approximately 1000 mL (500–1500 mL) of fluid at term with an amniotic fluid index of 8 to 25 cm.

Amniotic fluid index: An ultrasound calculation adding up the diameter of fluid from each of the four uterine quadrants. An amniotic fluid index of over 25 cm is polyhydramnios, less than 8 cm is oligohydramnios. Some physicians use less than 5 cm as a sign of oligohydramnios.

Amniotomy: Artificial rupture of the membranes with a device such as a hook that looks a little like a crochet hook.

Anembryonic: Empty sac.

Aneuploidy: Chromosome number is not a multiple of 23, usually caused by random errors.

Anhydramnios: Severe oligohydramnios or an amniotic fluid index less than the 2.5nd percentile.

Anoxia: Total lack of oxygen delivery with a rise in carbon dioxide. Reflects complete failure of maternal perfusion and/or placental oxygen uptake and/or oxygen transfer from the placenta to the fetus.

Anterior lip: Approximately 0.5 centimeter of cervix is left between the 11 o'clock and 1 o'clock positions. Some believe it is formed by uneven pressure by the presenting part on the cervix or the anterior cervix being caught between the fetal head and pubic arch (Simkin & Ancheta, 2005). Once this retracts, the woman will be dilated 10 centimeters.

Apgar score: Named after the anesthesiologist who invented it, Dr. Virginia Apgar. The clinical tool used to score the newborn's heart rate, respiratory effort, muscle tone, skin color, and response to stimuli. Each of these five factors receives a score of 0, 1, or 2 points. It is customary to calculate the Apgar score at 1 and 5 minutes but calculations can continue to be assessed every 5 minutes until a score of 7 is reached.

Ascending infection: Microorganisms move up into the uterus and infect the membranes or crossed the membranes into the amniotic fluid.

Asphyxia: Impaired gas exchange resulting in hypoxemia, hypercapnia, anaerobic metabolism and metabolic acidosis.

Asynclitism: The fetal head is angled with one of the parietal bones, not the vertex, presenting at the pelvic inlet. This is expected as the fetal head passes through the pelvic inlet but if it persists it can keep the fetus from rotating and descending.

Attitude: The relation of the different parts of the fetus to one another. Usually, there is an attitude of flexion with the arms folded in front of the chest, the head flexed toward the chest, and the legs flexed in front of the abdomen.

Augmentation of labor: The stimulation of contractions during labor by the administration of intravenous oxytocin.

Auscultation: The act of listening for sounds within the body. Healthcare providers can hear fetal heart sounds when they use a fetoscope or stethoscope. Sounds produced by any other device, such as a hand-held Doppler, are not the sounds of the fetal heart. They are sounds produced when the Doppler shift was analyzed by the device.

B

Base excess: A nonrespiratory reflection of acid–base status. Reported in millimoles per liter (mmol/L) of base.

Baseline: The fetal heart rate over a period of time, not including accelerations or decelerations. The baseline may be documented as a range or an average.

Beat-to-beat variability: The difference between consecutive sets of heartbeats in milliseconds or the R-to-R interval time on the electrocardiogram. When the computer calculates the fetal heart rate, the beats per minute rates will change if there is beat-to-beat variability. This creates a bumpy looking baseline, sometimes with little lines as long as 9 to 10 beats per minute. This bumpy appearance and/or short lines are called short-term variability. The presence of short-term variability requires beat-to-beat variability.

Bicarbonate (HCO$_3$): An alkaline, basic substance in the blood.

Birth: The fetus is expelled from the uterus and emerges from the mother's body.

Bleeding: The active loss of blood. This is blood alone, not blood mixed with cervical mucus. Bleeding may occur when there is placenta previa, a placental abruption, or a ruptured vasa previa. Estimate blood loss (1 mL weighs about 1 gram). Weigh the linen protector (Chux) and subtract the weight of a dry Chux to obtain the estimated blood loss.

Bloody show: Blood mixed with mucus. When the cervix begins to dilate, capillaries may rupture and bleed. The blood is mixed with cervical mucus. This is not bleeding. Bleeding will be thin, watery, and bright red. Bloody show is often seen early in labor but not during active labor when the cervix is dilated 4 or more centimeters.

Bradycardia: An abnormally slow heart rate. In general, a fetal heart rate below 100 to 110 bpm that is sustained for 10 or more minutes.

Braxton-Hicks contractions: Painless, intermittent, usually irregular contractions without dilation.

Breech: Buttocks first. The fetus is usually sitting in the pelvis. If you feel the buttocks and no feet (because the legs are straight with the fetal feet near the fetal head, that is a frank breech. If the legs are flexed and the buttocks and feet are presenting, that is a complete breech. A footling breech can be single (one foot presents) or double (two feet present).

Brow presentation: The head of the fetus is extended back so that the forehead is the presenting part.

C

Caput Succedaneum: Localized edema or swelling of the fetal scalp that develops during labor due to pressure of the cervix against the fetal head.

Cardiac output: Amount of blood pumped by the left ventricle into the aorta each minute.

Cephalic: Head first.

Cephalhematoma (also spelled cephalohematoma): Blood between the skull bone and the periosteum on the fetal head. A cephalhematoma usually forms on the parietal bone that was against the maternal sacral prominence.

Cephalopelvic disproportion: When the size of the fetal head is greater than the size of the midpelvis or pelvic inlet.

Chimera: Two or more genetically distinct cells that originated in different zygotes emerging in the same zygote; also known as mosaicism.

Chlamydia: A sexually transmitted disease related to infertility. It may be symptomless in the woman.

Chorangioma: Benign, nontrophoblastic mass of capillaries in the placenta. If large, there can be high output fetal congestive heart failure and polyhydramnios. Associated with placenta previa, cutaneous hemangiomas, and preterm delivery.

Chorangiosis: Hypervascular villi. Instead of 5 capillaries per villus, there are 10 in 3 or more random, noninfarcted placental areas.

Chorioamnionitis: Polymorphonuclear leukocytes (neutrophils) in the membranes and sometimes in the amniotic fluid. The infection may enter the uterus from the ascending route (vagina), through the abdomen after an amniocentesis, or be hematogenous (from the mother's blood).

Choriocarcinoma: A malignant growth of trophoblastic cells without the production of chorionic villi.

Chorion: The outermost layer of the two fetal membranes that surround the fetus.

Chorionicity: The number of chorions (related to the number of placentas with multiples).

Chorionic plate: The base from which the villous trees are suspended in the maternal blood in the intervillous space.

Chorionic villi: The two-cell layer extension or "fingers" that hold the fetal capillaries and the site of oxygen and carbon dioxide transfer (to and from the fetal and maternal blood).

Chorionic villus sampling: A test done early in the pregnancy to detect abnormalities and genetic diseases.

Chronic hypertension: High blood pressure that existed prior to the pregnancy.

Chux: Also known as a linen saver, linen protector, blue pad, yellow pad, or pink pad. This is placed under the woman in labor to absorb any amniotic fluid that may leak after rupture of the membranes.

Complete: 10-centimeters dilatation. "Fully" is an alternative word for "complete."

Compound presentation: The fetal hand, arm, foot, or leg is presenting with the fetal head or buttocks.

Contraction Stress Test (CST): An antenatal test used to evaluate placental function and fetal oxygenation during contractions. A spontaneous CST is obtained when there are three or more contractions in a 10-minute period. Otherwise, nipple stimulation or an infusion of oxytocin can be used to create contractions. The desired test result is a reactive (see NST) negative test. A negative test could be a flat line that may be related to fetal neurologic impairment. Therefore, it is very important that there are no decelerations, at least two "reactive" accelerations in 20 minutes of monitoring, and (long-term) variability prior to her discharge.

Cord prolapse: Presentation of the umbilical cord in front of the fetus. The cord prolapse may be occult and only suspected or overt and palpated in front of the presenting part.

Cotyledon: Fifteen to 20 septa divide the maternal surface of the placenta creating cotyledons. Cotyledons are not separate functional units.

Crowning: The fetal head is showing at the vaginal opening and staying there with every contraction, that is, it does not retract between contractions. Delivery usually occurs within minutes of crowning.

Culture: Accepted patterns of physical, cognitive, affective, and social behaviors of the individuals in a society or organization. The totality of ideas, beliefs, values, and knowledge of a group who share historical experiences.

D

Decidua: Gestational endometrium.

DeLee catheter: A clear plastic catheter attached to a mucus trap used for suctioning the newborn.

Descent: The way the baby adapts itself and passes down and through the maternal pelvis (see Figure G.1).

Dichorionic: Two chorions and two placentas

Dichorionic, diamnionic: Two chorions, two placentas, two amniotic sacs and fraternal twins. The placentas may be separate or fused (see Figure G.2).

Dilatation: The size of the opening. In the case of the cervix, it is estimated in centimeters.

Dilation: The act of expanding an opening, such as the cervix.

Domestic abuse: Physical, psychological, sexual, economic, or verbal behaviors within an intimate relationship to gain or maintain control over another person.

Duration: From beginning to end.

Dystocia (dysfunctional labor): A slow or difficult labor and/or delivery. From the Greek word *dystokos* meaning difficult birth. The opposite of adequate labor progress (eutocia). It may be evident as a cessation of labor progress (failure to progress) during the active phase of labor or an arrest of

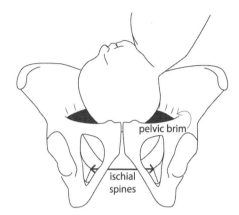

Flexion and descent
Figure G.1

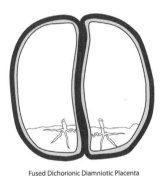

Fused Dichorionic Diamniotic Placenta

Figure G.2

dilation, that is, no change in dilatation for more than 2 hours with or without at least 200 Montevideo Units (when an intrauterine pressure catheter is in place) or an arrest of descent at 10-centimeters dilatation (no change for 1 or more hours). Dystocia is the most common reason for a cesarean section. It is related to a failed induction with no dilatation or a persistent OP position until delivery. Dystocia is also related to cephalopelvic disproportion with failure of the fetal head to descend into the pelvis at 10 cm dilatation. Protraction and arrest disorders (dystocia) are more common in women who are 35 years old or older.

E

Early deceleration: A fetal vagal response from increased intracranial pressure, may be related to cephalopelvic disproportion. The nadir of the deceleration is usually 18 or fewer seconds after the contraction peak.

Effacement: The thinness of the cervix. The cervix is "taking up" and merging with the lower uterine segment. Most clinicians estimate it as a percentage.

Effective contractions: Contractions that last 30 to 90 seconds with a mild to moderate quality or strength until the second stage of labor when they become strong to palpation. They are usually associated with a change in the cervix (effacement and/or dilatation) and descent of the fetus. Effective contractions may not be associated with adequate labor progress when there is cephalopelvic or fetopelvic disproportion (dystocia).

Endometrium: Mucous membrane lining the uterus in the nonpregnant woman.

En face: Eye contact with the newborn. Face-to-face interaction between mother and child.

Engagement: The largest diameter of the head (biparietal diameter) has passed the pelvic inlet and the tip of the skull is at the level of the ischial spines. If the fetus is not vertex, engagement occurs when the chin or sacrum are below the maternal pelvic inlet at the level of the ischial spines.

Episiotomy: A small incision made on the lower edge of the vaginal opening usually after crowning has occurred. The surgical enlargement of the vaginal opening before delivery first described by Sir Fielding Ould in Dublin who recommended an incision from the posterior vaginal fourchette toward the anus in women undergoing a very difficult delivery (median episiotomy) (Mueller-Heubach, 2007).

Erb's palsy: Brachial plexus palsy with weakness of the affected arm and often diminished or no use of the arm and hand on the affected side.

Ethnic group: A group that shares a common language, race, and religion.

Ethnocentrism: A tendency to judge people using one's own group as the standard.

Evaluation: Obtaining evidence as part of the feedback process that demonstrates whether or not actions had an effect.

Expected date of confinement (EDC): Forty weeks after the first day of the last menstrual period (LMP). EDC is also known as the expected date of delivery (EDD).

F

Face presentation: The fetal head is hyperextended with the chin or mentum presenting (see Figure G.3).

Failed induction: Labor induction of nulliparous women at 36 or more weeks of gestation and at *least 12 hours after*

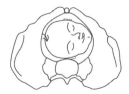

LMT

Figure G.3

ruptured membranes and the active phase of labor has not yet begun. After more than a 12-hour latent phase only 36.8% of the women had a vaginal delivery (Rouse, 2007).

False labor: Regular contractions without dilation.

Fetal death: Death of the fetus prior to complete expulsion or extraction from the uterus, irrespective of the duration of pregnancy. The death is indicated by the fact that after such expulsion or extraction the baby does not breathe or show any evidence of life such as beating of the heart, pulsation of the umbilical cord, or definite movement of voluntary muscles. A reportable fetal death is usually when the baby weighs 500 grams or more.

Fetal distress: Significant fetal oxygen deprivation with a fetal heart rate pattern suggestive of hypoxia, metabolic acidosis, and/or asphyxia severe enough to cause neurologic impairment. It is best to not use this term unless your work has a lexicon or glossary of terms and everyone knows what you mean when you say "fetal distress."

Fetal inflammatory response syndrome (FIRS): A fetal response to exposure to pathogens such as bacteria related to maternal urinary tract infection or intrauterine infection such as chorioamnionitis. Funisitis is a marker for FIRS.

Fetal intolerance: Evidence of oxygen deprivation during contractions.

Fetal intolerance of labor prior to 5-centimeters: An abnormal or nonreassuring fetal heart rate pattern (related to oxygen deprivation). Late decelerations, severe variable decelerations, absent or minimal (long-term) variability, a lack of accelerations, a falling baseline, or bradycardia near 60 bpm are examples of an abnormal, nonreassuring pattern. If the laboring woman is less than 5-centimeters dilated actions to increase fetal oxygenation should be undertaken. A cesarean section is needed if the fetal heart rate pattern does not return to a normal, reassuring pattern.

Fetal intolerance of labor with poor labor progress: A nonreassuring fetal heart rate pattern with a protracted or arrested labor (dystocia).

Fontanel: Also spelled fontanelle, a soft spot such as the membrane-covered space on the incompletely ossified skull of a fetus or infant.

Fourchette: From the French word for "little fork" or used to describe a dessert fork. The fourchette is a fold of tissue that joins the labia minora at the back of the vaginal orifice. Above the fourchette is the vestibule. Below the fourchette is the perineum. The fourchette may be torn if there is sudden stretching of the vulval orifice. An episiotomy is a cut through the fourchette and the perineum.

Fully: Ten centimeters.

Fundal pressure during the second stage of labor: A dangerous practice previously thought to expedite the second stage of labor. Requires firm and steady pressure with an arm or hands on the fundus of the uterus prior to the birth of the baby. The procedure has been related to maternal and fetal harm, including uterine rupture, third- and fourth-degree lacerations, and impaction of the anterior (fetal) shoulder causing a shoulder dystocia and subsequent fetal injury such as Erb's palsy or even asphyxia from a delayed delivery (Mollberg, Hagberg, Bager, Lilja, & Ladfors, 2005; Phelan, Ouzounian, Gherman, Korst, & Goodwin, 1997; Simpson & Knox, 2001; Zetterström, Lopez, Anzen, Norman, Holmström, & Mellgren, 1999).

Fundus: Section of the top of the uterus where the spiral artery (maternal artery) density is the greatest; the preferential area for placental implantation.

Funisitis: Umbilical cord inflammation. Activated neutrophils migrate through the muscular layers of the cord vessels into the Wharton's jelly toward the bacterially infected amniotic fluid. This diagnosis will be made by a placental pathologist when macrophages or leukocytes invade the Wharton's jelly of the cord.

G

Gestational age: Number of weeks and days since a pregnant woman's last menstrual period began.

Gestational diabetes: Impaired glucose tolerance during pregnancy.

Grandmultiparity: Parity of 5 to 7 or more. Grand multiparity increases risks for obstetric complications such as a spontaneous uterine rupture, premature rupture of the membranes, and precipitous labor.

Gravida (G): The number of pregnancies.

H

HELLP syndrome: Hemolysis, elevated liver enzymes, and a low platelet count. A complication of severe preeclampsia.

Hemorrhage: Severe bleeding. A loss of 500 mL or more of blood after vaginal delivery is considered a postpartum hemorrhage.

High risk: A condition or conditions that increase the risk of injury to the mother or her fetus.

Hydramnios: Also known as polyhydramnios. More than 2 liters of amniotic fluid. Associated with maternal diabetes mellitus, Rh sensitization, and twin-to-twin transfusion in which the recipient twin has polycythemia. An amniotic fluid index of 25 or more.

Hypercarbia: The same as hypercapnia, meaning carbon dioxide retention. If a fetus has a very high level of carbon dioxide in its blood at the time it is born, it will be limp, blue, and not breathing.

Hyperemesis gravidarum: Intractable nausea and vomiting, weight loss, electrolyte and fluid disturbances, acetonuria, and ketonuria. Hyperemesis occurs in approximately 2% of all pregnancies and typically during the first trimester or early in the second trimester. It usually resolves by 15 to 16 weeks of gestation.

Hyperoxygenation: The maternal partial pressure of oxygen is greater than 100 mm Hg. This is achieved in labor only when a tight-fitting oxygen mask is applied to the woman at 6 or more liters/minute. However, to maximize fetal oxygenation, 10 liters/minute should be the flow rate with a nonrebreather mask.

Hyperstimulation: An overstimulated uterus. There may be more than four contractions in a 10-minute period and/or an interval between contractions of less than 1 minute. Hyperstimulation increases the risk of fetal hypoxemia.

Hypotension: A 30% or greater reduction from the baseline blood pressure usually with a systolic blood pressure less than 90 mm Hg.

Hypoxemia: Deficient oxygen in the blood, a low partial pressure of arterial oxygen.

Hypoxia: Low oxygen delivery to the cells or tissues. Hypoxia can be chronic or acute.

I

Increta: Abnormally deep invasion of the villi that penetrates and goes through the uterus. Placenta increta can result in a uterine rupture and hysterectomy.

Induction of labor: The deliberate initiation of contractions prior to the onset of labor.

Intensity: When an intrauterine pressure catheter is in the uterus and accurately recording the peak pressure and the baseline resting tone, intensity can be calculated. It is the peak pressure minus the resting tone. Active pressure is another term that means intensity.

Intervention: An act to prevent harm from occurring to a person or to improve the mental, emotional, or physical function of a person.

Interconception: The time between pregnancies.

Intrauterine growth restriction (IUGR): Estimated fetal weight less than the 10th percentile for that gestational age.

Intrauterine resuscitation: Actions taken by a health care provider to ameliorate fetal hypoxia. Intrauterine resuscitation actions include: discontinuation of a uterine stimulant, lateral positioning, administration of a tocolytic or intravenous fluid to decrease uterine activity, the application of oxygen with a tight-fitting face mask.

Introitus: Entrance to the vagina.

Ischemia: Decreased blood flow to tissue and organs.

L

Laceration(s): A tear of tissue such as the vulva, vagina, cervix, perineum or into the rectum.

Late deceleration: A vagal response of the fetus due to hypoxia. The nadir (lowest point) of the deceleration is usually more than 18 seconds after the contraction peak.

Leadership: Approach to managing conflict and relationships, building teams, implementing solutions, and responding to everyday work situations to achieve one or more particular goals.

Lie: The relationship of the maternal spine to the fetal spine, usually longitudinal. A transverse lie occurs when the fetal spine is at a right angle to the maternal spine. It may be an oblique lie, at an angle to the maternal spine. It could also be an unstable lie in a woman who has had many babies and who has weak uterine muscles.

Live birth: The complete expulsion or extraction of the infant from its mother, irrespective of the duration of pregnancy.

After expulsion or extraction, the infant breathes or shows evidence of life such as beating of the heart, pulsation of the umbilical cord, or definite movement of voluntary muscles, whether or not the umbilical cord has been cut or the placenta is attached.

Long-term variability (LTV): Also known as variability. The up and down oscillations of the fetal heart rate baseline of at least two or more cycles per minute. Documented based on the bandwidth or amplitude. Less than two cycles or a flat baseline is absent LTV.

Low risk: Little to no risk of injury to the mother or fetus.

M

Macrosomia: A weight greater than the 90th percentile for that gestational age. These babies are large for their gestational age (LGA).

McRoberts' maneuver: The maternal legs are flexed at the knees and hips, abducted, and pulled back toward the maternal chest.

Mean arterial pressure (MAP): The average pressure inside the arteries, closer to the diastolic pressure than the systolic pressure. MAP is the product of cardiac output times total peripheral vascular resistance. Calculated as the diastolic pressure plus (systolic pressure minus diastolic pressure) divided by 3. Normal MAP is between 77 and 97. An MAP of 120 mm Hg or higher increases the chance of stroke.

Meconium: Bile-stained contents from the fetal intestine.

Midpelvis: The imaginary line between the narrowest bony points connecting the ischial spines, which typically exceeds 12 cm.

Molding (also spelled moulding) of the head: Alteration in the shape of the fetal head to reduce the skull diameter up to 4 millimeters (in normal labor). Usually physiological and harmless but if excessive can result in brain compression trauma, and even permanent injury.

Monochorionic: One chorion and one placenta. There can be one or two amniotic sacs (see Figure G.4).

Monochorionic, monoamnionic: One chorion and one placenta, one amniotic sac for both twins. Except in the case of a chimera in which one baby can be male and the other female, the twins are usually identical. The concerns are entanglement of the umbilical cords and twin-to-twin transfusion.

Montevideo Units (MVUs): A calculation of uterine intensity or active pressure over a 10-minute period. An intrauterine pressure catheter records the contraction pressures. The resting tone in mm Hg is subtracted from the peak pressure in mm Hg and added for each contraction in the 10-minute period. An alternative method to calculate MVUs is to calculate the average peak in mm Hg and subtract the average resting tone in mm Hg and multiply that value by the number of contractions in the 10-minute period.

Morbidity: An illness or complication.

Mortality: Death.

Mosaicism: Two or more cell lines that are genetically distinct found in one zygote.

MSAFP: Maternal serum alpha-fetoprotein, a marker to screen for neural tube (spine) defects, such as, spina bifida or anencephaly. These may be prevented by ingestion of 400 micrograms of folic acid a day prior to and during the pregnancy.

Mucous plug: Thick mucus that collected in the cervical opening. A barrier against bacterial invasion and ascending infection.

Müller-Hillis maneuver: An assessment to determine whether or not the unengaged fetal head can enter the pelvic inlet. While the physician pushes gently on the fundus and grasps (through the abdomen) the fetal brow and suboccipital region, someone else assesses the change in station. This is done during the peak of a contraction. If the fetus descends, additional space in the pelvis exists. After this is done, there should also be an evaluation of flexion, rotation, synclitism, caput, and molding. If the fetus does not descend with this maneuver, fetopelvic disproportion is probable.

Multiparous: Has delivered more than one baby. However, instead of saying multigravida for a woman in labor who has delivered one baby, you may hear her called multiparous or a "multip."

N

Nadir: The bottom.

Neutrophil: A granular leukocyte or white blood cell.

Nonstress test (NST): A noninvasive test of fetal oxygenation when a woman is not in labor and not contracting on a regular basis. The ultrasound transducer and tocotransducer are applied to the maternal abdomen. A reactive NST requires two accelerations within 20 minutes. The accelerations need to be 15 beats per minute or more above their base for 15 or more seconds at their base. In some cases, the fetal heart rate tracing may have gaps in it during the 20 minutes. If the accelerations are 10 to 15 bpm high and/or 10 to 15 seconds in duration the test result is reassuring but not reactive. An acceleration that is 10 bpm high or more that is 10 seconds or more at its base is associated

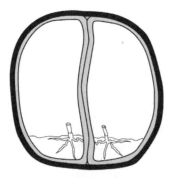

Monochorionic Diamniotic Placenta

Figure G.4

with a normal scalp blood pH. If there are no accelerations, the NST is categorized as nonreactive and the obstetric provider should be notified. Consult your hospital policy and procedure for guidance.

Nucleated red blood cells (nRBCs): Immature red blood cells produced when there is hypoxia. The production of nRBCs is stimulated by erythropoietin, also called hematopoietin or hemopoietin. This is a hormone produced by the liver in the fetus and kidneys in the adult.

O

Offset: The return to baseline from the bottom or nadir of the deceleration.

Oligohydramnios: Abnormally low amniotic fluid volume. An amniotic fluid index less than or equal to 5 cm may not reflect actual fluid volume but has been used in the past as a criterion for oligohydramnios (Johnson, Chauhan, Ennen, Niederhauser, & Magann, 2007).

Oliguria: Abnormally low urine production.

Ominous fetal heart rate pattern: A fetal heart rate pattern associated with metabolic acidosis. Severe variable decelerations, bradycardia with no recovery, absence of variability, and absence of accelerations with or without decelerations are examples of an ominous fetal heart rate pattern.

Onset: The beginning. The start of the drop in the fetal heart rate during a deceleration is the deceleration onset.

Oxycardiotocography: Maternal and fetal monitoring. Use of the pulse oximeter for the electronic fetal monitor in conjunction with fetal heart rate and uterine activity monitoring.

P

Parity: The number of pregnancies that have progressed to 20 or more weeks of gestation resulting in the birth of one or more infants who weighed 400 grams or more (Bai, Wong, Bauman, & Mohsin, 2002; Beebe, 2005). Parity is not based on the number of babies delivered. For example, a nulliparous woman who delivered a baby at 23 weeks of gestation would be a gravida 1 para 1 (G_1P_1). If she has twins at 36 weeks, she would be a gravida 1, para 1. If there is a stillborn, that adds to the count of parity. To help understand the number of births of preterm and term infants, miscarriages or elective abortions, and living children, a system has been devised for parity (P) followed by the letter T-P-A-L. $G_5P_{3-1-0-2}$ means the woman has been pregnant five times, had three infants at term (T), one who was preterm (P), no miscarriages or abortions (A), and two living children (L).

Partial pressure of oxygen (PO₂): The concentration or tension of a gas, such as oxygen, in the plasma, unbound to red blood cells or hemoglobin. PCO_2 is the partial pressure of carbon dioxide exerted in the plasma. Partial pressure is measured in mm Hg.

Pelvic inlet: The level of the brim of the pelvis.

Pelvic outlet: The lower pelvis. The pelvic outlet is surrounded by the pubic arch, the sacrum and coccyx, and the ischium.

Percreta: Abnormally deep invasion of the placenta in which all or part of the villi penetrate the entire thickness of the uterine wall. Placenta percreta can weaken the uterus resulting in a uterine rupture.

Periconception: The time immediately before conception through the period of organogenesis of the fetus.

pH: Denotes hydrogen ions using a logarithmic scale with a pH of 1 being the most acidic and 14 being the most basic or alkaline.

Phagiocephaly: If synostotic: abnormal suture development requiring surgical correction. If deformational: due to external molding forces imposed on a malleable cranium that can be prevented or improved with noninvasive interventions such as positioning.

Placenta previa: A placenta lying partly or completely over the opening of the cervix or the cervical os.

Polycythemia: Increased red blood cell count associated with an increased hemoglobin concentration in the blood.

Position: The location of the occiput or sacrum or mentum in relation to the maternal left or right side and the anterior or posterior part of the pelvis. For example, the ROA position means the fetal occiput is on the maternal right side near the top of the pelvis (see Figure G.5).

Precipitous labor and birth: Rapid labor. Closed cervix to completely or fully dilated in less than 3 hours with delivery soon thereafter.

Preconception: The woman's health status shortly before pregnancy.

Preconception care: Visit to a midwife or physician prior to becoming pregnant to achieve the healthiest possible outcome for the woman and her baby.

Preeclampsia: A disease related to primipaternity. Abnormal implantation of the trophoblast and abnormal placental development result in vasospasm with high blood pressure, swelling, and proteinuria.

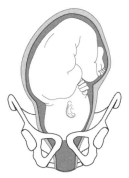

Right Occiput Anterior (ROA)

Figure G.5

Premature rupture of the membranes (PROM): A break in the amnion/chorion prior to the onset of labor. Some consider it PROM if labor does not begin for 12 or more hours.

Preterm premature rupture of the membranes (PPROM): A break in the amnion/chorion prior to the onset of preterm labor.

Presentation: The part of the fetus occupying the lower part of the uterus that presents at the cervical opening. At term, at least 96% of fetuses have a cephalic presentation and 3% are breech. The remaining 1% will have an arm, shoulder, or back presenting above the cervix.

Primigravida: Pregnant for the first time.

Primipaternity: Pregnancy resulting from exposure to semen/sperm from a new partner.

Prolonged labor: Labor lasting more than 20 hours.

Prolonged rupture of the membranes: PROM lasting 18 or more hours.

Pulmonary embolism: A blood clot to the lungs that blocks circulation.

R

Rales: Wet, crackling noises heard by auscultation of the lung fields during inspiration.

Rhonchi: Long, continuous extra sounds suggesting airway obstruction (wheezing).

Retroplacental hemorrhage: Bleeding behind the placenta.

Rim: Less than 1 cm of cervix is left until complete dilatation or 10 cm. There is no such concept as an "anterior rim" (see anterior lip).

Round ligament: The ligament attached to the uterus on either side in front of and below the fallopian tube and passing through the inguinal canal to the labia majora.

Rubella: German measles. A viral infection related to blindness, cardiac defects, and other problems in the exposed fetus.

Rubra: Dark red. Lochia rubra is mostly dark-red blood that is expelled by the uterus following a vaginal delivery. Over the 3 days after delivery the color and quantity will lighten.

Ruptured uterus: A tear through all layers of the uterus.

S

Secundigravida (Also spelled secundagravida): Pregnant with her second baby.

Shoulder dystocia: Birth of the fetal head with impaction of the fetal shoulder(s) and body.

Shoulder presentation: The fetus is in a transverse lie and the scapula is presenting over the cervical os. The fetal shoulder is trying to come out first. A cesarean section is the only exit route for this fetus.

Shunting: Passing of blood from the right side to the left side of the fetal heart without gas exchange in the lungs.

Sinciput: The top of the fetal head that is neither flexed or extended with the anterior fontanel as the presenting part. The fetus has a military attitude.

SpO$_2$: The percentage of saturation of hemoglobin with oxygen. Oxyhemoglobin is measured with a device such as a pulse oximeter versus a blood test of arteriolar oxygen saturation (SaO$_2$).

Spotting: A spot or spots of blood, often described based on their size. Spotting may consist of multiple bright red (or dark brown) spots, on underwear, tissue, or a peri-pad.

Station: If the fetus is vertex, it is where the tip of the fetal skull is above, at, or below the level of the ischial spines of the pelvis. When the tip of the skull (not the caput) is at the level of the ischial spines, the station is 0 (zero). When the fetus is crowning, the station is usually +5. A floating or ballotable fetus has a −3 or higher station. A dipping fetal station is −1 and −2.

Suprapubic pressure: The application of manual pressure to dislodge the impacted anterior shoulder. The pressure is applied just above the pubic bone on the lower abdomen.

Synclitism: How parallel the fetal head is with the maternal pelvis.

T

Tachysystole: *See* hyperstimulation.

Transverse lie: The fetal spine is perpendicular to the maternal spine. The fetus is oriented from one side of the mother to the other side.

Turtle sign: A sign of shoulder dystocia. The fetal head delivers then pulls tightly back against the perineum.

Twin-to-twin transfusion syndrome: Unbalanced intertwin blood flow through placental vascular anastomoses in a monochorionic twin pregnancy.

U

Uterine atony: Loss of uterine tone resulting in hemorrhage.

V

Velamentous insertion of the cord: Insertion of the umbilical cord vessels on the membranes where they are more susceptible to compression and are not protected by Wharton's jelly.

Vertex presentation: The highest point, acme, apex, peak or top of the head of a cephalic presentation that is felt with the gloved fingers during a vaginal examination.

Viable: A fetus that can live outside the womb, usually near 23 to 24 weeks of gestation providing adequate health care services were received. At 23 to 24 weeks of gestation there is a high rate of morbidity and mortality due to extreme prematurity.

Z

Zygosity: In the case of twins, the number of zygotes. One zygote is monozygosity, and two are dizygosity.

References

Johnson, J. M., Chauhan, S. P., Ennen, C. S., Niederhauser, A., & Mangann, E. F. (2007). Comparison of 3 criteria of oligohydramnios in identifying peripartum complications: A secondary analysis. *American Journal of Obstetrics & Gynecology, 197*, e1-e8.

Mollberg, M., Hagberg, H., Bager, B., Lilja, H., & Ladfors, L. (2005). Risk factors for obstetric brachial plexus palsy among neonates delivered by vacuum extraction. *Obstetrics & Gynecology, 106*, 913–918.

Mueller-Heubach, E. (2007). The pursuit of evidence. *American Journal of Obstetrics & Gynecology, 196*(4), 366–372.

Phelan, J. P., Ouzounian, J. G., Gherman, R. B., Korst, L. M., & Goodwin, T. M. (1997). Shoulder dystocia and permanent Erb's palsy: The role of fundal pressure? [Abstract]. *American Journal of Obstetrics & Gynecology*, S138.

Rouse, D. (2007). When should labor induction be discontinued in the latent phase? [Abstract]. *American Journal of Obstetrics & Gynecology, 197*(6), S103.

Simkin, P., & Ancheta, R. (2005). *The labor progress handbook* (2nd ed.). Oxford, England: Blackwell Publishing.

Simpson, K. R., & Knox, G. E. (2001). Fundal pressure during the second stage of labor: Clinical perspectives and risk management issues. *American Journal of Maternal/Child Nursing, 26*(2), 64–71.

Zetterstr§m, J., Lopez, A., Anzen, B., Norman, M., Holström, B., & Mellgren, A. (1999). Anal sphincter tears at vaginal delivery: Risk factors and clinical outcome of primary repair. *American Journal of Obstetrics & Gynecology, 94*(1), 21–28.

Abbreviations

A

A	arterial
AB	abortion
Abd	abdomen
ABG	arterial blood gas
ABX	antibiotics
AC	almost complete (almost 10 cm)
Accels	accelerations
ACTH	adrenocorticotropic hormone
ADB	Admission database
Adm	admission
AFE	amniotic fluid embolism
AFI	amniotic fluid index
AFP	alpha-fetoprotein
A/G	albumin/globulin ratio test
AGA	appropriate for gestational age
Alb	albuterol sulfate or albumin (consult your hospital list)
AMA	against medical advice or advanced maternal age
Amb	ambulate or ambulatory
AMFL	amniotic fluid
Amnio	amniocentesis
Amt	amount
ANA	antinuclear antibodies
Angio	angiocath (intravenous catheter)
AO	aorta
AP	apical pulse
A/P	attending physician present
A-P	anterior–posterior
ARDS	adult respiratory distress syndrome
ARM	artificial rupture of membranes
AROM	artificial rupture of membranes (also known as "pop the bag," "snag the bag," or "crack the sack")
ASA	aspirin (acetylsalicylic acid)
ASAP	as soon as possible
AST	antibody screening test
ATSO	admitted to the service of
A & W	alive and well

B

BBOW	bulging bag of water
BE	base excess
BF	black female
BID	twice a day
BL	baseline
BM	bowel movement
BOW	bag of water
BP	blood pressure
BPM	beats per minute
BPP	biophysical profile
BR	bathroom or breast
BTBV	beat-to-beat variability
BTL	bilateral tubal ligation or bottle
BUN	blood urea nitrogen

C

C	Celsius/centigrade
Ca	Calcium
CAN	cord around the neck (nuchal cord)
CBC	complete blood count
CBG	capillary blood gases or capillary blood glucose
cc	cubic centimeters
CVS	chorionic villus sampling
Chux	linen protector (also known as a "blue pad" or "yellow pad" or "soaker")
CL	clear
C/O	complaint of
CO	carbon monoxide
CO$_2$	carbon dioxide
COHb/ HbCO	carboxyhemoglobin
CPAP	continuous positive airway pressure
CPD	cephalopelvic disproportion (also known as fetopelvic disproportion)
CPK	creatine phosphokinase
CPR	cardiopulmonary resuscitation
C/S	cesarean section
CSE	continuous spinal epidural
CSF	cerebral spinal fluid

CST	contraction stress test		FBM	fetal breathing movements
CTSP	called to see patient		FBS	fasting blood sugar
Ctx or CTX	contractions (also abbreviated as UCs for "uterine contractions")		FD	fetal demise (also IUFD for "intrauterine fetal demise")
CVA	cerebral vascular accident		FDP	fibrinogen degradation products
CVP	central venous pressure		FE or Fe	iron
CWD	complies with dates		FECG	fetal electrocardiogram (assessed with a spiral electrode and transferred via a cable into the fetal monitor)
Cx or CX	cervix			

D

D_5LR	5% dextrose in lactated Ringer's solution		FF	fundus firm
Decel	deceleration		FFN	fetal fibrinonectin
DECG	direct electrocardiogram, obtained with a spiral electrode and transferred via a cable into the fetal monitor (see FECG)		FFP	fresh frozen plasma
			FHR	fetal heart rate (assessed with a Doppler device or fetal monitor)
Del	delivery		FIRS	fetal inflammatory response syndrome
DFM	decreased fetal movement		FHTs	fetal heart tones (auscultated with a fetoscope, pinard, or stethoscope)
DIC	disseminated intravascular coagulopathy or coagulation		FOB	father of the baby
Dig	digoxin		FOB NIP	father of the baby is not in the picture (uninvolved)
Dil	dilation, dilatation		FSE	fetal spiral electrode (also abbreviated as SE)
dL	deciliter		FT	fingertip
DM	diabetes mellitus		F/U	fundus at umbilicus
DNA	do not announce		Fully	10-cm dilated
DNI	do not intubate		FUO	fever of undetermined origin
DNR	do not resuscitate		Fx	fracture
DOB	date of birth			
DR	delivery room			
Drsg	dressing			
DTR	deep tendon reflexes			
Dx or DX	diagnosis			

G

			g	gauge
			g or gm	gram
			G	gravida

E

EBL	estimated blood loss		GA	gestational age
EBOW	evident bag of water		GBM	gross body movement(s)
ECG	electrocardiogram		GBS	group B streptococcus
Echo	echocardiogram		GETA	general endotracheal anesthesia
ECV	external cephalic version		GI	gastrointestinal
EDC	same as EDD, expected date of confinement or delivery		GTPAL	gravida, term, preterm, aborta, living children
			GTT	glucose tolerance test
EDH	epidural hematoma		gtt	drop(s)
EEG	electroencephalogram		GU	genitourinary
EF	ejection fraction		GYN	gynecology
Eff	effacement			

H

EFM	electronic fetal monitoring		h or hr	hour
EFW	estimated fetal weight		HA	headache
EGA	estimated gestational age		Hb or hgb	hemoglobin
Epis	episiotomy		HbA	adult hemoglobin
ETT	endotracheal tube		HbA_{1c}	glycosylated hemoglobin
Ext	external		HbF	fetal hemoglobin
			HBP	high blood pressure (also abbreviated as HTN for "hypertension")

F

F	fundus or fetal		HCT or hct	hematocrit
FA	fetus active			
FAS	fetal acoustic stimulator		HELLP	hemolysis, elevated liver enzymes, and low platelets

H & H	hemoglobin and hematocrit		Lb	pound
HL	heparin lock		LBP	low back pain
HOB	head of the bed		LBW	low birth weight
Hosp	hospital		LDR	labor-delivery-recovery room
H & P	history and physical		LDRP	labor-delivery-recovery-postpartum room
HPI	history of present illness		LFD	low forceps delivery
HR	high risk		LGA	large for gestational age
HS	at bedtime		LGE or lg	large
Ht	height		Liq	liquid
HX or Hx	history		LLQ	left lower quadrant
			LLT	left lateral tilt
I			LMA	left mentum anterior or laryngeal mask airway
I	intact (or iodine)		LMP	last menstrual period or left mentum posterior
IBOW	intact bag of water		LMW	low molecular weight
ICH	intracranial hemorrhage		LMT	left mentum transverse
ICN	intensive care nursery		LOA	left occiput anterior
ICU	intensive care unit		LOP	left occiput posterior
I & D	incision and drainage		LOT	left occiput transverse
IDDM	insulin-dependent diabetes mellitus		LPM	liters per minute
IDM	infant of a diabetic mother		LR	lactated Ringer's solution
IFSE	internal fetal spiral electrode		LSA	left sacrum anterior
IM	intramuscular injection		LSP	left sacrum posterior
Ind	induction		LST	left sacrum transverse
Inf	infection		LTV	long-term variability
Inj	injection		LUOQ	left upper outer quadrant
INT	intermittent therapy		LUQ	left upper quadrant
Irreg	irregular		Lytes	electrolytes
ITN	intrathecal			
IUC	intrauterine catheter		**M**	
IUFD	intrauterine fetal demise		M	mentum (chin)
IUGR	intrauterine growth restriction		MAP	mean arterial pressure
IUP	intrauterine pregnancy		Mat	maternal
IUPC	intrauterine pressure catheter		Max	maximum
IV	intravenous		MBU	mother–baby unit
IVF	in vitro fertilization or intravenous fluid		Mec	meconium
IVP	intravenous push		MED	medium
IVPB	intravenous piggyback		Memb	membranes
			MEq(s)	milliequivalent(s)
K			MET	medical emergency team
K	potassium		mg	milligram
K–B	Kleihauer–Betke test		Mg	magnesium
KCl	potassium chloride		$MgSO_4$	magnesium sulfate; MSO_4 is morphine sulfate.
Kg	kilogram		MHR	maternal heart rate
kPa	kilopascal unit (1 kPa = 7.5 mm Hg)		MI	myocardial infarction
			Midnoc	midnight (also abbreviated MN or noc for "night")
L			Min	minute or minimum
L or l	liter		ML	midline
Lab	laboratory		mL	milliliter(s)
Lac	laceration		MLE	midline episiotomy or midline extension
LAC	left antecubital vein		mm	millimeter
LAHF	low-amplitude high-frequency waves (uterine irritability)		mm Hg	millimeters of mercury
Lap	laparotomy or surgical lap sponges		mmol/L	millimoles per liter
LAT	left anterior thigh		MO	mineral oil
Lat	lateral		MOD	moderate

MOM	milk of magnesia		PP	postpartum
MPV	mean platelet volume		PPD	postpartum day
MSAF	meconium-stained amniotic fluid (also abbreviated MSF for meconium-stained fluid)		PPE	personal protective equipment
			PPH	postpartal or postpartum hemorrhage
MSAFP	maternal serum alpha fetoprotein		PPROM	preterm premature rupture of the membranes
mU	milliunits		PROM	premature rupture of the membranes (at term and before the onset of contractions)
mU/min	milliunits per minute			
MVU	Montevideo units		PRN	as needed
			PS	palpates soft
N			Pt	patient
N or n	number		PTB	preterm birth
NB	newborn		PTL	postpartal tubal ligation (also BTL for bilateral tubal ligation)
NBN	newborn nursery			
NIC	newborn intensive care		PTL	preterm labor
NICU	newborn intensive care unit		PVC	premature ventricular contraction
NIL	not in labor			
NKA	no known allergies		**Q**	
NKDA	no known drug allergy		q	every
NRBC (nRBC)	nucleated red blood cells		Q	blood flow
			QS	quantity sufficient
NST	nonstress test			
NSVD	normal spontaneous vaginal delivery		**R**	
NSY	nursery		R	rectal
N/V	nausea and vomiting		RAC	right antecubital vein
			RAT	right anterior thigh
O			RBCs	red blood cells
O$_2$	oxygen		R/CS	repeat cesarean section
OA	occiput anterior		RL	right lateral
OB	obstetrics		Reg	regular
OBRR	obstetrics recovery room		RMA	right mentum anterior
OBS	observation		RMP	right mentum posterior
OCT	oxytocin challenge test (see CST)		RMT	right mentum transverse
OP	occiput posterior		ROA	right occiput anterior
OR	operating room		ROM	rupture of the membranes
OT	occiput transverse		ROP	right occiput posterior
			ROT	right occiput transverse
P			RR	recovery room or respiratory rate
P	para, parity, probability, or partial pressure		RSA	right sacrum anterior
PaCO$_2$	partial pressure of carbon dioxide, also abbreviated PCO$_2$ or pCO$_2$		RSP	right sacrum posterior
			RST	right sacrum transverse
PAC	premature atrial contraction			
PACU	postanesthesia care unit		**S**	
PaO$_2$	partial pressure of oxygen, also abbreviated PO$_2$ or pO$_2$		S	sacrum (buttocks) or saturation as in SaO$_2$
			Sc	scapula (shoulder)
Pedi	pediatrician		SE	spiral electrode
PGE$_2$	prostaglandin E$_2$		SGA	small for gestational age
pH	acidity/alkalinity		SIDS	sudden infant death syndrome
PIH	pregnancy-induced hypertension		SIVP	slow intravenous push
Pit	Pitocin		SKB	single, keeping baby
PLTS	platelets		SM	small
POOC	premature onset of contractions		SNKB	single, not keeping baby
PNV	prenatal vitamins, prenatal visit, or postnatal visit		SO	significant other
			SOP	significant other person
PAS	postanesthesia score		SpO$_2$	oxygen saturation of hemoglobin (%)
Postop	postoperative			

Spont	spontaneous
SRM	spontaneous rupture of membranes (also SROM)
S/S	signs and symptoms
Sta	station
STAT	immediately
STD	sexually transmitted disease
STV	short-term variability
STV +	short-term variability present
STV 0	short-term variability absent
SVE	sterile vaginal examination
SVT	supraventricular tachycardia
SXN	suction

T

TAB	therapeutic abortion (also abbreviated EAB for "elective abortion")
ThAB	threatened abortion
THK	thick
T/L	tubal ligation
Toco	tocodynamometer or tocotransducer
TOL	trial of labor
TOLAC	trial of labor after cesarean (attempting a VBAC)
TTTS	Twin-to-twin transfusion syndrome
TX	treatment
Tymp	tympanic

U

UAC	umbilical artery catheter
UCs	uterine contractions
UMB	umbilical
US	ultrasound or unit secretary
UVC	umbilical venous catheter

V

Vag	vaginal
Var	variability
Var decels	variable decelerations
VAS	vibro-acoustic stimulation or visual analog scale (pain scale)
VBAC	vaginal birth after cesarean section
VE	vaginal examination
VO$_2$	oxygen consumption or delivery
VS or V/S	vital signs
VTX	vertex
VT	ventricular tachycardia
V-tach	ventricular tachycardia
VTX	vertex

W

WBC	white blood cells
WNL	within normal limits
WNWD	well-nourished and well-developed
Wt	weight

Y

YEL	yellow
YOB	year of birth (also abbreviated DOB for date of birth)

W

WF	White female
WHT	White

Abbreviations to Avoid in Documentation

BUD   big, ugly deceleration
CYA   cover your a—
FLK   funny looking kid
GOK   G-d only knows
PITA   pain in the a—
WNL   we never looked (others think this means
          "within normal limits" but the abbreviation can
          be misinterpreted and even misused, especially
          by nonmedical persons)

Orientation to Labor and Delivery

This is a list of suggested topics to cover during the orientation of a nurse who is new to the labor and delivery setting. It is not a competency list. Competency should be validated using a detailed skills checklist.

Week 1:
General hospital orientation

Week 2:
Tour the unit
Receive scrubs (if provided by the hospital) and locker assignment
Identify location of bulletin boards, mailbox
Initiate Orientation Skills Checklist
Identify learning objectives
Patient medical information privacy requirements (HIPPA)
Medical screening examination requirements (EMTALA)
Time clock, schedule (regular hours and call hours), overtime
Illness and absence policy, vacation and holiday policy
Pager and phone numbers of providers, call schedule
Yearly evaluation procedure and raises
Inservices and mandatory meetings policies
Location of information such as manuals on safety, evacuation, fire, patient care
Occurrence (incidence) reports location and procedure for completion
Delivery log book (if applicable)
Assignment sheet
Intradepartmental communication system
Telephone system
Preceptor role and orientee role
Clean utility room and location of linens
Location of other supplies for labor, delivery, and recovery
The blanket warmer:
   Never put bags of intravenous fluid in it because the temperature of the blanket warmer (120° F) usually exceeds manufacturer's guidelines (104° F).
Waste disposal and dirty utility room

Infection control requirements and location of personal protective equipment
Tour of Central Supply, Blood Bank, and Laboratory
Employee health procedures
Nursing attire in the operating room (cap, mask, shoe covers)
Dress code:
   No rings, bracelets, or watches on your dominant hand if it is used during a sterile procedure such as the abdominal scrub
   Earrings must be covered by the cap
   Neck chains should be placed inside scrubs
   Nails should be at a length to not perforate gloves
   No acrylic nails
Father's dressing room (operating-room attire: "bunny suit," hat, mask, shoe covers)
Assisting and observing patient care
Computer course (for documentation)

Week 3:
Read and discuss chapters 1, 2, and 3 of *Labor and Delivery Nursing: A Guide to Evidence-Based Practice*
Read policies, procedures, and protocols related to the topics in chapters 1, 2, and 3
Patient care with a preceptor

Week 4:
Read and discuss chapters 4 and 5
Read policies, procedures and protocols related to the topics in chapters 4 and 5
Patient care with a preceptor

Week 5:
Read and discuss chapters 6, 7, and 8
Read policies, procedures, and protocols related to the topics in chapters 6, 7, and 8
Patient care with a preceptor

Week 6:

Read and discuss chapters 8, 9, and 10

Read policies, procedures, and protocols related to the topics in chapters 8, 9, and 10

Patient care with a preceptor

Weeks 7 to 12:

Continue patient care with a preceptor

Read all other unit-specific policies, procedures, and protocols

Apply concepts you have learned by reading *Labor and Delivery Nursing: A Guide to Evidence-Based Practice*

Discuss the procedure for intrauterine fetal demise and/or stillbirth

Sample Orientation Skills Checklist

This is a list of other suggested topics that may be dated and signed by the preceptor. It is not a competency list. Competency should be validated using a detailed skills checklist.

Date Initiated:
Date Completed:
Date/Preceptor

Blood Bank
Laboratory
Nursery, NICU, Postpartum Units
Physical Layout of the Birthing Unit
Location of labor rooms
Location of other rooms:
   Nurse manager's office
   Clean utility room
   Dirty utility room
   Nurses changing room
   Staff bathroom(s)
   Schedule location
   Physicians changing room
   Supply room
   Call room
   Other:
      Linen storage
      Nurses lounge
      Nurses station
      Time clock
      Forms
      Whiteboard or patient screen on computer
      Waiting-room information
      Visitation rules
      Drug dispensing cabinet
      Refrigerator(s)
      Central monitor
      Charts
      Prenatal records
      Standing orders
      Exits
      Code cart

Precip Pack
Fire extinguishers/evacuation plan
Other:

Labor Room, LDR, or LDRP
Call light/emergency call
Newborn warmer equipment, medications
Kick buckets
Basins
Sutures
Yankauer suctions
Warm blankets/blanket warmer
Bathroom
Room lights
Emergency power
Use of the fetal monitor
   Leopold's maneuvers
   Application of ultrasound
   Application of tocotransducer
   Recognition of:
      Spontaneous accelerations
      Early decelerations
      Late decelerations
      Variable decelerations
Other:
Operation of labor/birthing bed
Operation of bedside table
Suction:
   Wall suction, replacement of canister
   Emergency suction equipment
Oxygen:
   Replacing the "Christmas tree"
   Location of replacement masks
   Nonrebreather vs. partial rebreather vs. simple mask
Precipitous Delivery Pack contents (example of a sample pack):
   2 Oschners
   1 Straight Mayo scissor
   4 Towels
   1 Baby blanket

1 Cord clamp
1 Straight needle holder
6 Towels

Birthing ball (also called a physio ball)
Medications: location and procedure to obtain
IV, amnioinfusion, blood tubing
Towels and washcloths
Labels for IV bags and tubing
Alligator clamps
Call light, emergency call light, intercom
Television
Room lighting
Computer system
Clock(s)
Delivery cart
Code (emergency) cart
Anesthesia cart
Sharps containers (location and procedure to replace them)

Antepartal Skills

(A detailed skills checklist for each procedure should be
used to confirm competency.)
Nonstress test
Contraction stress test (oxytocin challenge test)
Triage
Patient charges
Documentation

Labor and Delivery Skills

Sterile vaginal examination
Insertion of an intravenous catheter
Use of an intravenous infusion pump
Anesthesia pump (rules for use)
Amnioinfusion
Administration of magnesium sulfate
Spiral electrode application (if it is an approved nursing
skill)
IUPC insertion (if it is an approved nursing skill)
Set-up for vaginal delivery
Set-up of newborn warmer:
    If there is no meconium
    If there is meconium
Immediate care of the newborn:
    Airway & suctioning
    Temperature control
    Oxygen administration PRN
    Physical examination
    Apgar scores
    Documentation
Assist with a vacuum extraction
Assist with a forceps delivery
Patient charges
Documentation
Vaginal delivery

Recovery Skills

Fundal and lochia checks
Vital sign checks
Perineal care
Report to postpartum nurse

Operating-Room Skills

Preparation of surgical site
Preparation for cesarean section:
    Identification band verified
    Allergies noted
    Consent signed
    Preoperative orders reviewed
    Scrub nurse/tech notified
    Anesthesia personnel notified
    Neonatal care personnel notified
    Preoperative medications given
    Foley catheter inserted
    Patient transfer to OR table and legs secured
    Grounding pad applied to thigh and documented
    Cautery unit set to surgeon's preferences
    Confirm FHR checked prior to abdominal prep
    Surgeons' gowns
    Performs time-out
    Properly documents in the OR
    Opens packs using aseptic technique
    Adds instruments using aseptic technique
    Performs cricoid pressure when requested
    Properly labels and prepares specimens
    Addition of sterile supplies to back table
    Pouring sterile solutions into splash basins
    Sponge, needle, and instrument counts
    Neonatal warmer operable & equipped
    Newborn paperwork properly completed
    Assists with moving patient from table to bed
    Applies warm blankets to patient
    Safely transports patient to recovery room
    Gives report to recovery room nurse
Observed aseptic technique at all times
Limited conversation
Protected patient's modesty
Never left patient unattended
Other:

Labor Room Supplies

Exam gloves
Lubricant
Device for rupturing the membranes
Linen protector
Peri-pads
Sterile specimen container
Hair clipper (for abdomen prior to cesarean section)
Birthing bed pad
Bedpan
Warming devices

Culturette swabs
Endotracheal tubes (adult and neonatal)
Epidural cart/supplies
Spirometer, adult
Staple removal set
Spinal needles: 22 gauge, 27 gauge
Spiral electrode and cable
Compression stockings
Intrauterine pressure catheter and cable
Intravenous solutions
IV start kit or supplies
IV catheters
IV tubing
IV pumps
Amnioinfusion tubing
IV extension tubing
Microdrip tubing
Blood tubing
Additional IV pumps, IV poles
Foley catheter
Amniocentesis tray
Adult oxygen mask
Oxygen extension tubing
Graduated cylinder
Commode container hat
24-hour urine collection container
Clean-catch urine supplies
Red Robinson (straight) catheter
Perineal pads/linen protectors/Chux
Spiral electrode and cable
Stopcocks
Transducer belts
Shampoo
Hand lotion
Facial tissues
Disposable panties
Peri bottle (for cleansing after delivery)
Red bags
Vacuum cups: bell shaped, posterior
  (M or Mushroom) cups
Other:

Other Supplies

Physician preferences cards
Pudendal tray
Skin-prep tray
Betadine scrub/solution
OB Pack
Gown Pack
Gloves
Sutures
Lap sponges
Gauze (radio-opaque) 4 x 4s
Mayo stand cover
Drape sheet

Disposable speculum
1500 mL sterile water
1000 mL sterile water
1500 mL normal saline
Disposable "ice" pack
Suction canister
Suction tubing
Cautery unit and pad
Vacuum extractor and additional cups (bell and posterior
  (M/Mushroom) cups)
Forceps
Cord blood gas collection equipment and technique
Warm blankets
Specimen containers
Adhesion prevention supplies
Positioning wedge
Other:

Instruments That May Be Used During and After a Vaginal Delivery

2 Ring forceps
2 Towel clips
2 Hemostats
6 Allis clamps
2 Oschners
1 Needle holder
1 Tissue forcep with teeth
1 Curved Mayo scissor
1 Straight Mayo scissor
1 Instrument stringer
6 Towels
1 Small prep cup
1 Medicine cup
Also: sterile sutures, disposable scalpel and blade, needles
Mand syringes

Instruments That May Be Used to Repair a Laceration

4 Ring forceps
5 Allis clamps
1 Uterine dressing forcep
2 Heaney retractors
1 Large curved Mayo scissor
1 Short straight scissor
1 Large needle holder
1 Short needle holder
1 Heaney needle holder
1 Large tissue forcep with teeth
1 Short tissue forcep with teeth
1 Vaginal speculum
1 Instrument stringer
6 Towels

Instruments That May Be Used for a Dilatation and Curettage (D & C)

4 Ring forceps
1 Heaney scissor

1 Straight Mayo scissor
1 Needle holder
1 Vaginal speculum
1 Weighted vaginal speculum
2 Heaney retractors
1 Large curette
1 Instrument stringer
6 Towels

Instruments That May Be Used During a Cesarean Section

8 Curved hemostats
4 Allis clamps
4 Penningtons
2 Babcocks
1 Curved Kocher
4 Oschners
2 Heaneys
2 Ring forceps
2 Needle holders
6 Tissue forceps: 2 with teeth, 1 smooth, 2 Adson-Brown, 1 Russian
5 Scissors: 1 straight Mayo, 1 short, curved Mayo, 1 long Mayo, 1 Bandage, 1 Metzenbaum
1 #3 knife handle with #21 blade
1 #4 knife handle with #10 blade
3 Retractors: 1 bladder blade, 1 large Richardson-Eastman, 1 small Richardson-Eastman
1 Instrument rack with 2 parts

Instruments for a Hysterectomy

4 Ring forceps
4 Kochers
4 Rochester-Peons
4 Straight Heaney-Ballentines
4 Curved Heaney-Ballentines
4 Long Allis clamps
2 Collier hemostats
4 Tissue forceps: 1 long with teeth, 1 long smooth, 1 long Russian, 1 Heaney
4 Scissors: 1 Jorgensen, 1 long straight Mayo, 1 long, curved Mayo, 1 Metzenbaum
3 Needle holders: 2 straight, 1 Heaney
1 Long #3 knife handle with #21 blade
6 Retractors: 2 Deavers, 2 Malleables
1 Balfour blade
1 Balfour retractor with 2 or 3 screws
1 Instrument rack with 2 parts

Instruments for a Tubal Ligation

6 Curved hemostats
4 Allis clamps

2 Babcocks
2 Needle holders
3 Scissors: 1 short, curved, 1 short, straight, 1 Metzenbaum
3 Forceps: 1 with teeth, 1 smooth, 1 Russian
4 Retractors: 2 small Richardson-Eastman, 2 Army-Navy
2 #4 knife handles with #10 and #15 blades

Instruments and Supplies for a Cervical Cerclage

2 Ring forceps
1 Large Mayo scissor
1 Large, smooth tissue forcep
1 Vaginal retractor
1 Heaney needle holder
1 Straight needle holder
6 Towels

Newborn Supplies and Equipment

Blankets, thermal caps
Bulb syringe
Stethoscope
Suction catheters
Suction tubing
Suction canister(s)
Endotracheal tubes, stylets, laryngoscope
Oxygen masks: premie, term newborns
Oxygen blender
Oxygen extension tubing
Neonatal resuscitation bag
Newborn pulse oximeter
Predelivery warmer set up
Other:

Newborn Care

Setup for meconium
Setup for intubation
Assisting with neonatal resuscitation
Neonatal Resuscitation Program completion
Participation in neonatal resuscitation
Other:

Operating Room

Review of aseptic technique
Preparation of neonatal warmer
Count before procedure
Count during procedure
Count upon closure of the uterus
Documentation in the operating room
Other:

Recovery Room (PACU)

Operation of bed
Operation of patient warming blanket
Cardiac monitor paper:
    Set speed
    Changing the paper
    Post monitor strip in chart
Vital signs equipment
Medications: location and procedure to obtain
Documentation
Charges for patient care and supplies
Other:

Orientation Log Chart

This is not a skills validation checklist. An orientation log does not validate competency. This type of form may be used to assist the preceptor in confirming the current experiences that the orienting nurse has encountered.

Preceptor's Initials															
Date															
Abruption															
Active labor management															
Admit for cesarean section															
Admit for induction															
Admit high-risk patient															
Admit laboring patient															
Admit low-risk patient															
Admit newborn															
Admit scheduled cesarean section and preparation															
Amnioinfusion															
Assisting with version															

Preceptor's Initials													
Date													
Baby nurse													
Catheterize patient													
Cerclage													
Cervidil													
Cytotec													
Emergency cesarean section													
Epidural													
Fetal death													
Hemabate													
Hespan													
High risk													
IM medication													
Insulin drip													
IV pump													
IV push medication													
IV start													
IVPB medication													
Latent-phase management													
Magnesium sulfate													
Methergine													
Misoprostol													
Monitoring of multiples													
Nonemergency cesarean section													
Outpatient/Triage													
Patient with placenta previa													

Preceptor's Initials																
Date																
Pitocin augmentation																
Pitocin induction																
Preeclampsia																
Prep pt for epidural																
Preterm labor																
Prolapsed cord																
Recovery after cesarean section																
Recovery after vaginal delivery																
Second-stage management																
Terbutaline																
Transfer to postpartum floor																
Uterine rupture																
Vaginal delivery																
Vaginal exam																

Preceptor's Initials _____ Signature _____

Preceptor's Initials _____ Signature _____

Preceptor's Initials _____ Signature _____

Preceptor's Initials _____ Signature _____

Index